What
Your
Doctor
Eats

What Your Doctor Eats

DR CAMILLA STOKHOLM

Vermilion

VERMILION

UK | USA | Canada | Ireland | Australia
India | New Zealand | South Africa

Vermilion is part of the Penguin Random House group of companies
whose addresses can be found at global.penguinrandomhouse.com

Penguin Random House UK
One Embassy Gardens, 8 Viaduct Gardens, London SW11 7BW

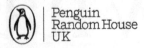

Penguin
Random House
UK

penguin.co.uk
global.penguinrandomhouse.com

First published by Vermilion in 2025

3

The information in this book has been compiled by way of general guidance in
relation to the specific subjects addressed, but is not a substitute and not to be
relied on for medical, healthcare, pharmaceutical or other professional advice on
specific circumstances and in specific locations. Please consult your GP before
changing, stopping or starting any medical treatment. So far as the author is
aware the information given is correct and up to date as at February 2025.
Practice, laws and regulations all change, and the reader should obtain up to date
professional advice on any such issues. The author and publishers disclaim,
as far as the law allows, any liability arising directly or indirectly from the use,
or misuse, of the information contained in this book.

Typeset by seagulls.net
Printed and bound in Great Britain by Clays Ltd, Elcograf S.p.A.

The authorised representative in the EEA is Penguin Random House Ireland,
Morrison Chambers, 32 Nassau Street, Dublin D02 YH68

A CIP catalogue record for this book is available from the British Library

ISBN 9781785045431

Penguin Random House is committed to a sustainable future
for our business, our readers and our planet. This book is
made from Forest Stewardship Council® certified paper.

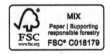

To my patients

CONTENTS

INTRODUCTION

I realise I am not exactly a 'typical' GP. In fact, you might say my practices are highly irregular. For one thing, I know of no colleague who invites patients into their kitchen for cooking tutorials; given I am a doctor and not a cook, this is a very odd thing to do. But we have been calling food a medicine for centuries and some new discoveries have now made this an irrefutable fact. Really, it shouldn't be so odd that a GP is prescribing her own recipes, but perhaps strange that more of us don't do the same.

In truth, I am actually extremely risk averse, and veering even remotely off-piste in medicine doesn't come easily to me. But sharing my personal food diary on Instagram has proven to be one of my most effective treatments. I might look like a 'food content creator' but each dish is carefully considered so that it helps people to apply new medical innovations without even realising it.

I do this, quite simply, because I know it works. Ironically, becoming a doctor is the unhealthiest thing I have ever done. The moment I left medical school I suddenly gained weight, as well as a gaggle of unpleasant symptoms I couldn't explain. Nothing will motivate you to research health like losing your own, but I don't regret my experience; I learned many lessons the hard way so you don't have to. The recipes I share are one part of the approach that allowed me to turn my health around. This book goes 'behind the scenes' of my recipes and is a manual on everything I teach my patients to help them treat, prevent or even reverse disease.

Before qualifying, I used to imagine sitting my doctor down for a few hours and getting them to explain precisely

1

what was happening in my body. Essentially, I wanted their medical degree distilled into a few hours – not the detail, just the CliffsNotes. I needed the practical application of medical science, with just enough context to understand how and why it worked. Of course, this service doesn't exist and doctors have neither the training nor the time to offer condensed tutorials. But now, as a doctor myself, I have learned to make the ten minutes I have with patients equate to hours. How? By giving them homework.

All my regular patients have come to accept that when they leave my office, a prescription isn't all they'll take with them. They will be pointed in the direction of hours' worth of cooking videos on my Instagram and receive a customised list of books, podcasts, documentaries and YouTube tutorials. These will cover the underlying mechanisms of weight gain, chronic disease and poor mental health. As well as addressing current illnesses, I see each appointment as an opportunity to inject health and prevent future diseases. To their surprise, when I follow up with patients I ask how they're getting on with their homework. They might feel like they're back in school but, with some gentle nagging, almost all of my patients become diligent students. The results are astounding. Sustainable weight loss, improved cholesterol and blood pressure, better energy, less pain – the list goes on. Sometimes diseases, like type 2 diabetes, simply disappear.

This approach has made my job infinitely more enjoyable – and, like any dutiful teacher, the more I learn, the more I want to teach. So gradually, the amount of homework has increased, until even I have had to accept that most patients don't have time to read 20 books. Which brings us to *this* book – consider it something of a cheat sheet: it gives you just enough of what you need to know, not just to dodge disease, but also to genuinely achieve good health. A longer and happier life is generally part of this package deal too.

'Slacademic'*

It was only in my sixth year of working as a doctor that I would begin to re-educate myself and it all began on a bit of a whim, when a last-minute research scholarship became available just before I was about to finish my training. Logically, it made zero sense to apply – I had absolutely no plans to work in academia. But like a questionable impulse buy at the checkout, I went for it. Strangely, this whim would change the entire trajectory of my career, my life and, most importantly, my health.

To my amazement I was given funding to research anything I liked. My subject of interest at the time was childhood obesity. As part of my project, I set up free Zoom workshops, ready to teach local parents of obese children what I now realise they probably already knew. I naively assumed general healthy-eating tips could solve everything, but fate intervened in the form of a book my mother gifted me: *The Diet Myth* by Professor Tim Spector. This was several years before the gut microbiome and personalised nutrition had become part of mainstream conversation. Just one book set me off down a rabbit hole of discoveries, propelling me to inhale more and more books, podcasts, conferences and, later, courses. It turns out medicine as we know it is on the cusp of an amazing metamorphosis: what you think you know about health might be completely wrong.

My epiphany arrived just in time, saving me from patronising a group of parents with the same outdated advice they had already been taught. Instead, I provided them with a series of lectures on the new science of obesity. Conveniently, these core principles also underpin the science behind chronic disease, mental health and longevity. As it turns out, we have enormously misunderstood what overweight and obesity are. And, in doing so, we have been completely blinded to meaningful

---

* Within the medical profession, doctors who do research are known affectionately not as 'academics' but 'slacademics'. Medicine is hilarious.

solutions. I now teach *all* my patients the underlying princi-ples of health, no matter their size. What I have realised is that when health is the goal, weight loss can often be a convenient side effect, but the reverse isn't always true. For this reason, I never tell any patient they need to lose weight. I simply show them how to optimise their body and, because they understand the scientific context (assuming they've done their homework), other issues are taken care of too. Of course, no one can exert *complete* control over their health, but you do have much more influence than you might think.

I'm not saying that weight isn't important. But weight gain is only one thread in the complex web of your health. Amazing new revelations about the gut microbiome, hormones, epige-netics, sleep science, the immune system and even just our evolution are unravelling this web. At first sight, they might seem outlandish and very removed from what you have always believed to be true. But, like I said, medicine is in the middle of a metamorphosis – new research is answering all the questions I had when I was struggling with my weight: how does weight gain happen? What makes me hungry and, importantly, what triggers satiety (fullness)? What is the cause of binge eating and why on earth can't I stop? Why do some people never gain any weight and others always do? All these questions and more will be answered in these pages.

Health is like a web, linked and interconnected in ways we previously never realised. We're not just growing bigger, we also have more depression, allergies, dementia, cancer and autoimmune conditions than ever before. Despite amazing medical advancements over the last few decades, we have just been getting sicker. But I can explain that too. And as well as detailing why these diseases are on the rise, I will arm you with the information you need to help avoid them.

You gave me my life back

My methods may be atypical but nothing about what I practise is considered 'alternative' medicine. Many of the concepts covered in the chapters to come are novel – they are too young to have made their way into routine clinical guidelines or medical education. New science can take many years to filter into routine practice so to have *any* clinical experience of applying it is still rare, especially outside of private medicine. I don't have fancy investigations or supplements at my disposal; in fact, all I really have is a patient's mind. My only job is to change it.

I am not in the business of slandering Western medicine and still enthusiastically prescribe medications which improve and even save lives. But I have been humbled by my own experience and know that not everything can be fixed with a prescription. I now see every interaction with a patient as a deal. I'll hold up my end of the bargain, but I also expect that they hold up theirs: in any given scenario there will be things I can do that they can't do for themselves – prescriptions, referrals, x-rays are all my responsibility; conversely, there are many things only the patient can do which I have no real power over. All I can do is teach them what these things are and, with a bit of gentle nagging, encourage them to play their part. Simple changes to when, what and how they eat are just some examples of how my patients have been able to achieve breath-taking results.

Perhaps my most extreme example was a 44-year-old man who was suffering with such severe diarrhoea that he had resorted to wearing adult nappies. Fearful of leaving the house in case of accidents, he had developed agoraphobia, refusing to go out for five years. His symptoms had been thoroughly explored with countless doctors' appointments and several invasive investigations, but no medical cause could be found. After one brief phone call, I suggested a change in his diet – and the diarrhoea disappeared. After five years of not going out, he was finally able to leave his house again. He booked a follow-up appointment with me for no other reason than to thank me and say, 'You gave me my life back.' Amazingly, I came across a very similar scenario in a woman of roughly the same age – the same intervention cured her symptoms too. Teaching them how to boost their gut microbiomes was all it took – not a knife or a pill: instead, all they really needed was new knowledge.

My story

My patients' stories never fail to amaze me, but the one which has surprised me most is my own. To be so unwell was the most humbling experience of my life and I'm sure it made me a better doctor. Believe me, helping others with their problems is infinitely easier when you've had some of your own.

Before I became a doctor, I had always been a very healthy person. Growing up in several countries largely primed me to adopt what I now recognise is a Mediterranean diet. My only long-term health problem in earlier life was a talent for fainting, which I proved to be very good at from the age of six. No cause was ever found, and I was told I would grow out of it. I didn't. With time, I learned how to anticipate and prevent a collapse, but not without experiencing a horrible feeling of dizziness. It was an unpredictable and very frustrating ailment but one I simply grew used to.

When I left medical school, my dizziness got much worse. Around the time I started my first job as a doctor my hormonal acne also suddenly exploded – it made no sense at the time. My weight was next and with it came a very important dose of humility: I had always been a thin person, and in my final years of university nothing I did would make me gain weight. But the moment I started working as a doctor the spell broke and I went on to gain 14kg (10kg of which I gained in just one year). I was the same person, and a medical professional no less

– what could possibly have changed to make something that had always been so easy suddenly become so hard?

In hindsight, it has all become clear. The main thing to change was my *attitude* to food: I'd decided I was too busy to cook. In the blink of an eye, I'd swapped my lifelong Mediterranean diet to a convenient, ultra-processed one. I thought this was okay because I was carefully counting calories and even stopped using extra virgin olive oil because it contained what I considered to be too many. But as the years went by, I became progressively more hungry, and it wasn't long before I entered a binge-restrict cycle: I would ignore my appetite for as long as I could, but eventually snap, gorging extreme volumes of food. And repeat. I forgot there had ever been a time when I ate intuitively to feel full and enjoy my food.

I then spent my years as a junior doctor religiously watching 'fitfluencer' YouTube videos and hanging on to every word they said. 'High-protein' chocolate bars and kale smoothies were my new go-tos. But nothing I did could reverse what had changed. Next, I became crippled by debilitating 'IBS' (irritable bowel syndrome) symptoms – my stomach bloated to pregnant proportions, and I spent my shifts dashing to the toilet every other hour. I also developed fatigue, brain fog, insomnia, more dizziness and, though I was completely unaware of it at the time, all the signs of clinical depression.

Many of my experiences were vague and basic investigations all came back normal. Apparently, there was 'no medical cause' for how I was feeling. I've seen this happen to fellow colleagues and non-medical friends alike; entering adulthood should really come with a considered list of health warnings. But my experience just comes with an added sting of irony: I was a *doctor* – how could I, of all people, not keep myself well?

In a round-about way, however, being unwell and miserable was an amazing education I never knew I needed. And luckily for me, I was born at the right time in history, because in the years leading up to my poor health, scientists were busy unearthing amazing new discoveries; these became readily available for me to learn about at precisely the moment I needed them. In the pages to follow, I will explain everything you need to know to understand what happened to me. When you learn how your lifestyle directly affects your very biology, you will be shocked by the impact you can have on your own health.

In many ways my own case is what gives me the most confidence in my approach. Because it is one thing to be swayed by research, but when you have experienced results first hand, that's a different story. As a sick doctor I learned what it is to be brought down by poor health which simply won't improve – sadly, an increasingly common experience for many of us.

Why this book – and what to expect from it

I need to make it abundantly clear that any advice I am sharing is not a replacement for seeing your own doctor. Sadly, we can't ignore that cancer and other sinister conditions like inflammatory bowel disease are on the rise. If you have new stomach pains, *any* change in your bowels, bloating, unexplained weight loss, blood in your stool, or any symptom that is worrying you, get it checked. Timing matters and denial will not be your friend here. However, we can't ignore the fact that often test results come back normal, and patients are left without answers.

As a population, we are sicker than ever but, despite medical advancements, many doctors are feeling more and more frustrated in their efforts to treat patients. So many of the complaints I see are insidious, non-specific and impossible to diagnose with any test I have access to. GPs have ten minutes to attempt to decipher an array of symptoms often not taught at medical school. There is usually no quick fix or medication, which is as demoralising for the doctor as it is for the patient. Trying to help disgruntled and angry people without the time or resources to do so is a special kind of torture. So while I want to make clear that this book is not a replacement for a doctor's appointment (nor should it serve as fuel for GP-bashing, which has become an increasingly popular pastime), we also need to make medicine less one-sided. Really, healthcare is a team sport – it works best when we get involved too! And this book is the answer. Think of it as your very own tutorial with a doctor. Because when you understand how to practically apply new science to your own body, the potential health benefits are immeasurable.

Having read many health books myself, my hope was to write one unlike any I had seen before. I wanted it to answer the questions I had when I was ill and struggling with my weight and, to do that, I needed it to be a 'two-part series'. So first, I give you the science; believe me, it's only when you understand this that you will be convinced enough to actually use it. That's why Part I is a lesson in how your body really works. In many ways it reads as a story with various characters and plot twists you won't want to miss, so I suggest reading it in order. We will look under the hood and unravel what makes you human (as well as what doesn't). By learning about things like the role of your microbiome, appetite, metabolic flexibility, hormones and genes, you will see your health in a new light. Unpicking our recent history will be the pièce de résistance, helping you to fully understand the predicament we are now in. (It turns out, our ancestors have passed on far more than just genes, much of which you won't be thanking them for!) In Part II, I explain how you can apply the science to your own life in a practical and achievable way. As well as breaking down what and how to eat with a selection of recipes, I look at how the mind and body are intimately connected, and you will learn the surprising impact happiness can have on your physical health.

My hope is that this book will enable you to join the dots to make sense of your health. Like me, I want you to experience a series of empowering epiphanies. If you have ever felt deflated by your current health or anxious about how it might one day change, get ready for some uplifting news. You see we are all here at precisely the right moment in time: medicine is about to get very interesting. Let me show you why.

PART I

WHAT YOU NEED TO KNOW

CHAPTER 1

YOUR MICROBIOME

The organ you didn't know you had

One of the most mind-blowing changes to medicine is the fairly recent discovery that we aren't exactly *just* human. As it turns out, we act as vessels for an amazing ecosystem of microorganisms called the microbiome. It is now impossible to talk about the link between food and health without mentioning these inhabitants – they are one of the biggest plot twists medicine has ever seen! Anything you put into your body, from food to medication, will later be served to them too and what they do with it has changed everything we understand about health. Their ancestry can be traced back to the dawn of our very existence, meaning we actually evolved together, intimately influencing each other. More and more, we have been unravelling just how much the microbiome impacts almost every aspect of our health.

This chapter will unpick these new discoveries, but in preparation, I need to prime you first – because not everything is as it seems. The lines between evidence-based medicine and misinformation, often derived from an ever-glamorous wellness culture, have never been more blurred. Unsurprisingly, the microbiome is providing a new buzzword that many over-the-counter products claim to improve. This science is too new to be part of medical training or formal guidelines – most doctors aren't trained to advise which of these products you should take. Now is the perfect time to make money off anyone who wants to be healthy whether the product is evidence-based or not. Deciphering which is which is harder than you would think and can feel a bit like the film *Inception*: you might be trapped in a dream within a dream, unable to make sense of reality. Allow me to wake you up ...

Do you know what you don't know?

As a rule, most would agree scientific breakthroughs tend to be a good thing. However, the problem with medical innovation is that, at their core, people don't like change. Once we know something to be true, an alternative always seems unthinkable, and this is especially true in healthcare. When the Hungarian obstetrician Ignaz Semmelweis (1818–65) suggested it might be a good idea for doctors to wash their hands in between dissecting dead bodies and delivering babies his colleagues roared with laughter. The assertion almost cost him his career. But then a startling drop in postpartum infection on his ward proved him right. Sometimes the herd can be wrong but letting go of something you have always known to be 'true' is an incredibly difficult thing to do.

People don't like change because it suggests they are wrong – to be offered new knowledge is a double blow most egos can't handle. If you think about it, education tends to be a one-way street: the teacher imparts facts and you memorise them. We almost never question the foundation of their knowledge and ask *why* something is true. (Just like I never questioned my lecturer's statement that in a third of cases, dizziness is actually caused by 'anxiety'*; I now wonder what their evidence was and how we could ever really know that.) Though it feels alien

---

* Non-specific dizziness is one of the most common symptoms we see in GP. There are many complex causes – from inner ear problems, pain-free migraines (yes, that's a thing) to anaemia and low blood pressure. In my case, because my blood tests, heart sounds and blood pressure were fairly normal there was 'no medical cause'. But I now know there were things I could have done to prevent my symptoms, which had nothing to do with anxiety. We often label many symptoms as a direct result of poor mental health because they might be associated with anxiety, but assuming a causal relationship is often an oversimplification of what is going on.

at first, truly learning requires equal *un*learning: you might need to let go of your preconceived beliefs to hear this ...

The truth is we have massively oversimplified health, nutrition and 'wellness': it's been wrapped up in shiny human logic because that's how we like it and, even better, that's what sells. If you can show someone something they can easily understand, they will trust you and buy whatever you like. In fact, buying health is something many of us simply can't resist. A perfect example of this is seen in the placebo effect, which is increased if the 'medicine' costs more. We have known about placebos since the 1700s and yet it still baffles me that symptoms can spontaneously improve with a fake treatment. One example was seen in 2015 when Parkinson's patients received two injections at different times; researchers explained they wanted to prove both were equally effective even though one happened to cost much more. In reality, both injections were just saline, but significant improvements were seen in motor function and, in patients given the 'expensive' one first, there was a 14 per cent increase compared to the 'cheap' placebo. You might have noticed a similar experience with wine – it tends to taste better when you think it's expensive.

Why *do* we prefer expensive things and even mount a measurable healing response when we believe we are taking a pricey pill? Whether we like it or not, money, by definition, is a form of value and so if something costs more, we value it more. In the case of the Parkinson's patients, having an expensive treatment set an expectation which triggered the reward pathway in their brains to release more dopamine – the effect was particularly noticeable because Parkinson's is characterised by low dopamine levels. We also know placebos release our bodies' natural morphine-like chemicals or 'opiates', explaining why they can be such good painkillers. This subconscious belief that expensive things are automatically better is what drives many of us to spend big bucks on an array of supplements, powders and other potions promoted by the influencers we admire. Most consumers don't scrutinise recent meta-analysis of what they're swallowing – but damn, does it feel good going down.

Sadly, the amazing medicinal properties of food are much more enticing to us when we extract a vitamin or specific chemical and put it into a pill because it seems more scientific that way and, of course, is more expensive. But, believe it or not, these isolated chemicals never produce the same health benefits as the actual food itself! No antioxidant, vitamin or food chemical has ever been shown to produce the same result as the food it came from. For example, despite popular belief, it turns out that taking vitamin C only reduces cold symptoms for a few hours at most. In fact, some vitamins are even dangerous, especially in the case of vitamin E, beta-carotene and high-dose vitamin C, which can actually increase mortality. Of course, there are rare medical situations where people do need to take supplements, such as in pregnancy, problems with malabsorption or if there is a known deficiency. However, for the vast majority we are self-medicating needlessly for psychological reward, rather than any true evidence-based benefits. At best, this wastes money; at worst, it could be causing harm.

Something you might not know is that there are at least 25,000 'phytochemicals' (plant chemicals) in food. They have amazing properties and include an array of compounds like polyphenols, resveratrol, flavonoids, isoflavonoids, terpenoids and carotenoids. Just one piece of broccoli has several of these, which genuinely fight cancers and many other diseases. But the key point is that it has *several* types of chemicals, all combined with an array of fibres, delicately and precisely packaged into a structure known as a 'food matrix'. To unravel these and separate them from each other implies that only one component is important, when realistically, they probably all react together in a way we don't fully understand. In fact, of the 8,000 polyphenols we know of, only 150 have been researched – that leaves 7,850 polyphenols we know nothing about, not to mention all the other phytochemicals. The mind boggles. Essentially, we have reduced food down to a small handful of nutrients we can wrap our heads around, and are willing to pay much more money when we see buzzwords like 'protein' or 'added vitamins', not because of any hard evidence they are better than a whole-food source but due to the dopamine hit we get when we swallow them. They say sex sells, but in my view 'the overmedicalisation of our food industry sells'. Sadly, it's an excellent advertising campaign – and it works every time. We are all motivated by what we believe to be true, but we don't know what we don't know. New nutrition and microbiome research is finally helping to bust some myths – supplements have stolen the spotlight from humble ingredients for too long. The curtain is lifting for a new act and there are some surprising performers taking centre stage – simple, cheap and overlooked foods are the new stars.

Bugs: Thugs or drugs?

By now most people have heard of the microbiome, but in 2021, in my last year of training to be a GP, it was completely new to me and frankly, sounded absurd. Until recently, without the right technology, we simply weren't able to examine all the micro-organisms in our body, yet it turns out we are covered in them! Most people talk about the microbiome in the gut, but we also have communities living in our skin, eyes, mouth and vagina (among other places) and they seem able to talk to our human cells, as well as each other. So far bacteria have been the main focus of research, but we also have a mixture of other bugs like viruses, parasites, fungi and archaea which we know less about. Technically, we can't claim to be simply human anymore; instead our bodies are 'holobionts': some sort of part-human, part-ecosystem, hosting a symbiotic community of a staggering 38 trillion micro-organisms. Just under half the chemicals in our blood are produced or manipulated by our microbiome; they also alter our hormones, immune system and the medication we take. In fact, if you were to sequence all the genes carried in the body, 99 per cent are those of our bugs and only half the cells we carry are human. We are one and the same, and understanding our health cannot be done without getting to know the tenants we host.

At first, this sounded like science fiction to me but the more I learned, the more I grew fascinated by a window into health I could never have imagined. I found myself falling down a rabbit hole of new information not covered in my training, starting with *The Diet Myth* by Professor Tim Spector. It is no exaggeration to say this single book would change the course of my life but, more specifically, it was one particular story within it that gave me the most motivating light-bulb moment of my life. Spector describes a young Chinese man called Wu whose weight was completely disproportionate to his diet – yes, he ate a bit more than his friends, but not enough to explain his morbid obesity with a BMI of 59. Professor Liping Zhao, now a household name in Shanghai (a Chinese Spector, if you will), took him under his wing in 2013. Already a specialist in the microbiome, long before most of the world had caught on, he tested Wu's stool and discovered one particularly nasty strain of a bug called *Enterobacter*. He injected this bacteria into the intestines of mice that had been surgically born into an entirely sterile environment. These 'germ-free' mice surprisingly don't develop normal brains and struggle to gain a normal amount of weight – without a microbiome they are destined to be scrawny and weak. But once they received the *Enterobacter* something amazing happened: they rapidly grew obese. Professor Zhao had discovered a superbug capable of fuelling obesity. He went on to create a personalised gruel for Wu to eat, designed to boost health-promoting bacteria in his gut. The results were astounding. After nine weeks he had lost 30kg and the *Enterobacter* shrank so drastically that by six months it was completely undetectable. The growing army of healthy bugs in

Wu's body had ganged up on *Enterobacter*, beating the bully down until it just disappeared.

It is *vanishingly* rare to have one specific strain of bacteria exert such a powerful effect; to learn this is even possible is truly fascinating. But what surprised me most of all was Wu's willingness to eat nothing but unpalatable gruel. Day in, day out, he ate the same uninspiring mush without a complaint, while so many of us struggle adhering to far tastier diets. In fact, he was so happy with the results that he continued living off gruel for another year, helping him to lose even more weight. When Tim Spector asked Zhao how on earth he had managed to foster such amazing compliance, Zhao replied that his patients understood he was feeding their microbiome: they truly believed this would improve their health. Just as we are willing to spend huge sums of money on supplements and health tonics, they simply *valued* the gruel – and when we truly value something, compliance isn't a problem.

It occurred to me that I didn't need to eat bland gruel on repeat to achieve the same effect. I just needed to place value on the foods a healthy microbiome would enjoy. My mind was opened and I couldn't ignore this novel science. Rather than hold on harder to my previous beliefs around food I felt humbled by the fact that I may have been wrong. Perhaps lemon water, macro splits and meticulous calorie counting were never the answer. In fact, I now realise ultra-processed, low-calorie foods were directly harming my microbiome, achieving precisely the opposite effect to Zhao's gruel.

Maybe reading this you will have the same epiphany, especially when we cover how to feed a healthy microbiome (sans gruel) later on. But I didn't feel disappointed or silly for my mistake, and neither should anyone else; if anything, it felt as if someone had finally set me free from tortured rituals I had never enjoyed in the first place. Spector and Zhao had truly 'wu-ed' me and for the first time in my life, committing to change felt effortless because I genuinely valued their evidence-based advice.

Allow me to spend the next few chapters 'wu-ing' you too, so that, by the time you reach my advice in Part II, following it won't feel like a chore – it will simply make sense.

Is obesity an infection?

To be clear, obesity is never 'just' caused by any one thing. Amazing complexity and nuance underpin everything from our behaviour to the diseases we acquire; food is exactly the same and we shouldn't reduce its value to one macro- or micronutrient. An orange contains several vitamins, pectins, carotenoids, fatty acids, hundreds of polyphenols and even some electrolytes. If I were an orange I would be insulted if someone only wanted me for my vitamin C – it's like type-casting a brilliant actor for being beautiful. The same is true of our health conditions. No health complaint has been over-simplified more than obesity; a firework display of incredible research is emerging to demonstrate just how amazingly complex this condition is and yet the stigma lives on. We subconsciously reward thin people in society, affording influencers extreme wealth earned because of the shape of their bodies. This assumes they have complete control over their weight. They don't. There are several malleable and fixed factors which decide your weight, and your lifestyle is just one of them. To summarise this simply as 'willpower' is a dramatic oversimplification of the truth. The microbiome is another factor and, as you will soon come to see, a thin body won't be a reputable currency anymore. I told you medicine was about to get interesting.

Now like I said before the case of Wu is highly, *highly* unusual – for most there won't be just one naughty bacteria driving morbid obesity. But we do know for certain that the microbiome plays an important role in weight gain. The first time this made international news was in 2015 when a 32-year-old lady developed a devastating gut infection called

Clostridioides difficile (*C. diff*).* Historically, this would only happen in hospitalised patients after a long course of antibiotics but worryingly, over the last decade, thousands are now getting it without setting foot in hospital or receiving any antibiotics. This is bad news because, at worst, it can kill you and, at best, it can cause a chronic gut infection which is infuriatingly difficult to treat. Ironically, we have always tried to treat it with the same thing that caused it in the first place: antibiotics. We now understand that *C. diff* behaves like a thug disrupting the party for the rest of your microbiome – similar to Wu's strain of bacteria, which was also calling all the shots. Amazingly, 'donating' a healthy person's microbiome into an infected gut sorts the problem out nicely– the light drowns out the dark. Putting someone else's bowel movement into your own gut is called a faecal transplant and, apparently, this is something the ancient Chinese were doing 1,500 years ago. I won't say how, but fortunately, we have come up with more palatable techniques like freeze drying a sample and putting it into capsules to swallow. It is remarkably effective, curing 90 per cent of infections compared to 25 per cent when we use antibiotics. The procedure is also remarkably safe with only 6 reported infections out of 55,000 cases.

Back to our *C. diff*-infected lady – she was successfully treated with a faecal transplant and went on living her normal life, changing nothing in her diet or exercise regime. However, having never had trouble with her weight, over the course of 16 months she went from 62kg to 77kg, moving her from a healthy BMI to the obese range.† Nothing but her new microbiome had changed: just like Wu, her bugs were triggering obesity.

---

* Previously known as *Clostridium difficile* (medicine likes to keep us on our toes by rebranding names for bugs, drugs and several diseases).
† BMI is not a perfect measure of how healthy someone's weight is because muscle is more dense than fat. As a result, many very muscular rugby players fall into an obese BMI range but actually have a low fat percentage. It still remains our cheapest, crude measure but obviously needs to be interpreted case by case.

She seemed to be the first human mimicking what scientists had already been seeing in mouse studies in which obesity was directly caused through microbiome transplants.

One of the most interesting groups of people to study are identical twins: they are genetic clones of each other, so any differences they do have can help us to tease apart what is caused by genes versus the environment. We will explore this more in Chapter 5 but, for now, I will tell you that the majority of these 'clones' are almost exactly the same weight – so when scientists find one who is obese while the other is not they get very excited. Amazingly, if we take their stool samples and humanely transplant them into those special 'germ-free' mice I mentioned earlier, something remarkable happens. In a controlled lab environment, the mice receive the exact same food, exact same calories and exact same exercise: the mouse with the obese twin's transplant grows obese, while the other mouse stays lean. This sounds ridiculous and the first researchers to perform this experiment thought so too – so it has been repeated over and over again, each time with the same results. Same calories, completely different weights. With one experiment they were able to repeatedly prove that it really isn't 'just' about calories in versus calories out.

Interestingly, when the mice were given roommates with the opposite microbiome a change was seen again. Like many animals, mice eat each other's droppings, taking in a self-imposed faecal transplant. The mouse who received the obese transplant was completely protected from becoming obese when living with a lean friend. So it looks like it was also possible to transfer bacteria which kept them thin; however, this effect no longer happened when they were fed a standard American diet (SAD) high in sugar and fat. On the other hand, the weight-reducing transplant was sped up with a high-fibre and low-fat diet. In other words, the donated microbiome significantly influenced health, but diet clearly sped up the negative and positive outcomes.

Amazingly, we have discovered one bacteria which can keep us thin in spite of an SAD. It's called *Christensenella* and when researchers transplanted it into mice it stopped them from gaining weight even when they lived off junk food! One in 10 lucky humans is infected by this helpful critter, most of whom seem to be completely protected from obesity and a dangerous type of internal fat called 'visceral fat', no matter how unhealthy their diet. But before you start popping it as a probiotic, bear in mind your body's ability to host it is bizarrely genetic. People seem to 'inherit' the bacteria from their mother during a vaginal delivery, as well as the genetic traits to support it. If you know anyone who is disproportionately skinny, despite wolfing down buckets of unhealthy food, they might be one of the 10 per cent. And, if not, they could be helped by another microbiome resident but, in this case, it is a parasite called *Blastocystis*, found in 25 per cent of Brits and 4 per cent of Americans. *Christensenella* and *Blastocystis* have received the most press for their association with being thin, but another study in Boston also found bacteria called *Lactobacillus* and *Bifidus* protected mice from negative consequences of junk food. This isn't an invitation to use our microbiome to shield us from junk food; what we eat can be a potent medicine as well as a poison in a plethora of ways. But it is simply interesting to acknowledge some people host bugs that predispose them to weight gain while others do the opposite.

How does the microbiome affect weight?

One of the most important jobs of the gut microbiome is to help us digest our food: the human component of your body is rather lacking on this front with a measly 17 digestive enzymes, while the microbiome has upward of 60,000. These are vital in helping us release valuable nutrients from the foods we eat but their presence also hints at one mechanism which might drive excess weight gain. Some bacteria are just showing off – like overly keen students, they are working very hard to release as much energy from the food for you to absorb as they possibly can. Others behave like parasites (partly because some of them genuinely are parasites) and like to keep more of that energy for themselves. In essence, no matter how meticulously you calculate the calories you eat, there is no way to calculate which ones your microbiome will give to you or keep for themselves.

It's not that surprising that when scientists try to guess who is more likely to gain weight by sequencing someone's human genes and their microbiome's genes it is the latter which gives better predictions. The same is true when you're trying to predict who will be better at losing weight: research is rapidly unearthing which gut bugs are health-promoting and which aren't. More than that, we also know a 'diverse' microbiome seems to help with weight loss and promote health. In other words, having a big variety of these critters seems to be useful – just like a rainforest has loads of different species which actually support each other to thrive, our microbiome does the same.*
My preferred metaphor is that your gut is like a party: you need a lot of people to turn up, but if they're all the same, something will feel a bit off. If everyone loves to dance the floor will get too crowded; not enough and you're shaking-your-groove-thing all alone. You need a cosmopolitan mixture of people who all like to do different things for everyone to really have fun. The main thing that seems to predict this diversity in our gut is the variety of plants we eat, and 30 or more different ones a week seems to be the sweet spot. Whether this involves eating different vegetables, grains, spices or even drinking coffee, the key is to recognise anything you eat that is a plant won't just be feeding you! Twin studies show that those who had more fibre

---

* There is some emerging nuance here, though. If you compare two people's gut microbiomes the person with more diversity doesn't necessarily have a 'more healthy' microbiome. Quality matters too so if one person has a less diverse mixture which is heavily dominated by health-boosting bugs this might actually be 'healthier' than a very diverse mixture with more unhealthy bacteria present.

in their diets had better microbiome diversity and gained the least weight, but they weren't just eating bran flakes or gloopy fibre replacements – quality counts too. High-quality foods packed with phytochemicals called polyphenols show an independent benefit for weight and the microbiome beyond that of fibre alone. Part II will break down how to feed a healthy microbiome in much more detail, but you might already know brightly coloured foods are full of polyphenols. Far from bland or boring food, your microbiome actually thrives off a diet which is both abundant and vibrant.

So why then does a less diverse microbiome seem to be linked not just to weight gain, but to worse health in general? Because most thoughtful guests bring a gift to the party and in your microbiome these are chemicals called 'postbiotics': the 'good' bugs bring helpful chemicals and the less palatable guests/gatecrashers prefer unhelpful chemicals. Imagine your guests bringing you chocolates or guns – both have the potential to influence the party quite significantly. For example, in 2019, the PREDICT 1 study found that, of the 1,102 British and American participants, those with less microbiome diversity had a worse metabolic response to food: it spiked their blood sugar and fat levels more, largely because of the unhelpful postbiotics being sent into their blood. In other words, our microbiomes influence our metabolism of food through these chemicals – in a way, they change our very biology. This has downstream consequences for our risk of diabetes, dementia, heart disease and stroke, to name but a few. It also dramatically influences the mechanisms through which our bodies store fat, which we will explore in the next chapter.

For the first time in history, we are finally realising that one food can have a completely unique effect in different people's bodies. Some of the factors influencing this, like genes, can't be changed, but the microbiome is incredibly adaptable, which means you can change some aspects of your biology if you know what you're doing. If you create a diverse range of helpful bugs, they will produce a pharmacy of postbiotics which behave like powerful drugs, dramatically shaping your health in a plethora of ways and altering your body's response to food. Invite too many harmful bacteria, though, and they'll generate poisons that trigger disease.

Another vital impact on weight is our microbiomes' ability to manipulate hunger and fullness. The diabetes medication Ozempic has received a lot of press in recent years because of its very convenient side effect: dramatic weight loss. Opinions about its use in weight management vary, but no matter what your attitude is, it has at least brought one fact into the mainstream: finally, we have acknowledged that excess weight is, in part, caused by altered appetite signals. Most people simplify weight gain as a result of consuming too much food when really the question should be *why* are we eating more than we need? The body has fine-tuned mechanisms to precisely trigger hunger and fullness (or 'satiety') according to its needs, ideally maintaining a constant weight. If that mechanism isn't working, there is something wrong with the system, which we will explore much more later. The point is, Ozempic has provided amazing evidence that mimicking a fullness hormone called GLP-1 can reverse obesity. If simply altering appetite can achieve such dramatic results it turns what we believe about this condition on its head: how and why you eat is not entirely in your control! Importantly, Ozempic only works while you are taking it – removing the drug brings back the abnormal appetite signals and with them all the weight that was lost. Would you like some good news? Amazingly, the microbiome can influence the release of GLP-1, as well as other related appetite hormones like ghrelin and leptin. Like I said, believe it or not, you can literally change your own biology and the microbiome is but one of the many powerful tools I will teach you to use. In chapters to come you will learn how to literally mould your own experience of hunger and satiety in ways I never knew possible.

Beyond altering appetite signals, what's even more bizarre is that our bugs can even affect the very way we taste and crave food. We know, for example, that people who admit to chocolate cravings compared to those who are 'chocolate indifferent' have different microbial chemicals in their urine. Some of this is genetic – it might explain why my non-identical twin and I are different: I enjoy chocolate but never experience a craving for it, while my sister craves it every day. Perhaps this was because I inherited a different gene or maybe we happen to host different 'chocophile' bacteria. We now know bugs affect our sense of taste because germ-free mice (who, remember, lack a microbiome) have altered taste receptors in both the tongue and gut – not having a community of bugs means they experience sweet and salty flavours differently. Changes in taste-receptor expression have even been seen after gastric-bypass surgery which, absurd as it sounds, is an operation that reduces weight partly by altering the microbiome. We have always assumed these operations worked by reducing the calories you absorb but strangely, this effect is ultimately minimal. Part of what is actually happening is a change in appetite and food preferences – something we could never have fully understood before discovering the microbiome. Without realising it, patients start to find healthier foods more palatable. It might sound absurd but, if you believe you harbour complete conscious control over what you choose to eat, you're wrong. The wonderful news is that we can capitalise on this fact: if you boost your microbiome your cravings will change too!

Can you see why I initially thought the microbiome sounded like science fiction? I realise it seems crazy that your perception of flavour can be influenced by bacteria but I have actually seen it play out in practice. One of my patients admitted she had previously hated Brussels sprouts and felt indifferent about sauerkraut: a few months after changing her diet, like I suggested, not only did she enjoy their flavours but she genuinely started to crave them. I have had a similar experience with bitter foods like radicchio, which no longer taste bitter to me and I now absolutely love. The reverse is true as well – if you are accustomed to eating SAD food this seems to feed a group of bacteria that hijack your hunger signals, taste receptors and even mood, driving you to eat more of the food they thrive off. Let me repeat that: bacteria can send chemicals to your brain altering your hunger cues and perception of taste, so that you eat more of what they want. Though we have co-evolved with our microbiomes, they need to look out for themselves and sometimes they prioritise their own survival over our health. Individual groups of bacteria each seem to thrive off different types of food: if you consciously start to eat healthier foods, you'll find after a couple of months it becomes something you crave more and more thanks to your helpful bugs.

How does the microbiome influence disease?

Our non-human component is not separate from us: we evolved together so we are one and the same. These bugs intimately affect almost every part of your body, including its potential diseases. If I am going to make you truly *value* this precious commodity – so much so that feeding it becomes an effort-less reflex – first, you need to appreciate all the diseases it can protect you from or bring you closer to.

AUTOIMMUNE AND INFLAMMATORY CONDITIONS

Inflammation has become the buzzword of our time but not without reason. Increasingly, we are able to understand how it drives disease and interlinks so many conditions. For example, if you have psoriasis, an inflammatory skin condition, derma-tologists will automatically check your blood pressure. As a medical student this seemed a bit odd to me: it's like a painter/decorator suddenly going to inspect your plumbing – the two clearly have nothing to do with each other. But, unlike a house, your body and its systems are beautifully interconnected and influence one another dramatically. If your skin is inflamed, so is your body – this increased inflammation can affect your blood vessels, driving the build-up of the clogs which might, one day, give you a heart attack. The clever dermatologist isn't having a career wobble, momentarily wishing they were a cardiologist: they are assessing your other risk factors for heart disease. We see the same consequences from conditions like gout and rheumatoid arthritis – allow them to go unchecked and they also increase your risk of a heart attack.

What does this have to do with your microbiome? Well, you may have heard that most of your immune system actually lives in your gut. One cell beyond the internal lining of your gut is where 70 per cent of your immune cells hang out – and when that close, it would be rude for your microbiome to not at least say hello. But it does more than that; in many ways the microbiome is commander in chief, scheming and treating immune cells like troops going off to battle, even when there's no clear enemy. Remember those gatecrashers and the guns they bring with them? If you have enough unhelpful bacteria they like to shed fragments called LPS, creating 'bullets' known as endotoxin, which behaves like a poison to the body. This opens the door for a phenomenon never taught at medical school; it used to be poo-pooed in academia but is finally being recognised as real: leaky-gut syndrome.

Your gut lining should be like a brick wall with clear doors guarded by some terrifying and impenetrable bouncers. They have a serious job to do because your gut is essentially your body's main contact with the outside world – letting outsiders into your bloodstream is reserved for the most V of the VIPs. When your gut lining becomes 'leaky', the cement between those bricks dissolves and the bouncers fall asleep – not only can thugs then shoot guns between the bricks (our cell walls), but they can even walk straight through the door. In other words, those nasty bugs you didn't invite to the party can sneak endotoxin into your bloodstream.

When a border has been breached like this any army would be on high alert. Your immune system and body in general do just this, entering a state of low-grade but chronic inflammation. If caused by a dangerous threat, like a bacteria known to cause disease, this makes sense and is protective. Short-lived inflammation primes your body to fight off threats and quickly, so when it's temporary, inflammation can save your life. The problem is when it's allowed to bubble away in the background, unchecked for years or even decades. A traditional Western diet is now known for being rich in ultra-processed foods, refined carbohydrates, sugars and various fats, while lacking the fibre our bugs love. It should be no surprise that this way of eating seems to trigger chronic inflammation and part of how this happens is through conversations with our microbiome. For example, one French study found a junk-food diet with very few vegetables promoted inflammation markers in the blood and was associated with reduced microbiome diversity – this effect was present regardless of body-fat levels. All the participants were overweight or obese but it wasn't the level of body fat that predicted inflammation: it was their microbiome. Having said that, we know fat cells themselves play a vital role in inflammation; we used to think they were just inert vessels for fat globules with no other role, but we were wrong.

It turns out your fat tissue is sort of like an 'endocrine' organ, which means it can actually produce hormones. Other examples of these organs are ovaries, testicles, adrenal glands, the thyroid and pancreas. We have long known our body fat influences oestrogen for example, which is why a higher fat percentage increases your risk of oestrogen-sensitive cancers. However, until recently, I did not know fat cells could communicate with the immune system. Each fat cell is surrounded by special white cells called T cells (TREGS) which communicate with the rest of the immune system; however, if we are overweight these TREGS can't do their job properly, which allows chronic inflammation to go unchecked. This is why osteoarthritis pain gets much better when people lose excess weight; patients are often told their pain is exacerbated by the extra pressure the weight exerts on their joints, but this doesn't explain why hand pain improves too. In fact, losing weight helps fat cells communicate normally with the immune system and, just like taking anti-inflammatory painkillers, removing the inflammation reduces the pain. This altered immune system also explains why obesity was an important risk factor for Covid-19 complications.

Through the course of this book, you will see more and more how massively we have oversimplified excess weight, dumbing down its causes and even the very role of the fat cells themselves. Importantly, science is unravelling so much incredible nuance, which completely dismantles any stigma we have had. Unfortunately, opinions are hard to change and new knowledge can be slow to spread. In years to come, I hope we will view fat phobia as something old-fashioned and ignorant! But I also hope offering help to my overweight patients won't cause offence – it would be no different from asking an asthmatic if they would like an inhaler. A complex, multifactorial condition does not define a person – if I give you an inhaler, I'm not trying to insult your lungs or criticise you in any way. The same is true of obesity or overweight – it is impossible to cause offence when we earnestly understand their latest science.

Ultimately, whether from poorly controlled psoriasis or over-filled fat cells, chronic inflammation will increase the risk of developing many diseases. Now that we have discovered the microbiome and its link to our immune system, other things are starting to make sense. Just over a hundred years ago a food allergy had never been seen – in fact, it's only been a recognised medical condition for about 50 years. You can't order anything without being asked about your allergies now. Worryingly, since the 1950s rates of autoimmune conditions like Crohn's disease, multiple sclerosis and type 1 diabetes have increased by

300%! The avalanche of autoimmune and allergic diseases we are seeing is mirrored even in one factor influencing our microbiomes: C-sections. A baby's first injection of healthy bacteria comes from a vaginal delivery; having never been exposed to bacteria before, the birth canal coats them in an army of their mother's bugs. Missing this step means their microbiome can start off on the wrong foot. As C-sections have increased, so have food allergies, coeliac disease and other autoimmune conditions. One meta-analysis even saw a 20 per cent increase in asthma and food allergies in those delivered surgically. That said, if you were born by C-section, please don't worry – you aren't doomed to an unhealthy microbiome (as we will see in Part II, there are many other factors which influence our ecosystem of bugs and it is incredibly good at adapting in a matter of weeks). But it is interesting that we can map rising C-sections so closely to disease.

GUT HEALTH

When I start any conversation about the microbiome with my patients, most reply, 'Oh yeah, it's that gut thing – do you just want me to take some probiotics?' They're not wrong that there is a microbiome in your gut (clearly), but this, like so many aspects of health, is an oversimplification.

As mentioned earlier, you also have separate microbiomes on your skin, in your mouth, in the vagina and a few other places – they amazingly influence each other and, as I hope you are starting to gather, have a previously unfathomable impact on health. But for now, the gut is the star of the show and no discourse on the microbiome can go without acknowledging this. We have previously pinned everything on genes and bad luck when it comes to autoimmune gut conditions like Crohn's, ulcerative colitis and coeliac disease, but we must always have known a puzzle piece was missing. For example, in America, 35 per cent of people have the coeliac gene but only 1 per cent actually get the disease; however, over the last 50 years, rates have increased by 500 per cent. It is now clear that specific changes to the microbiome drive leaky-gut syndrome and ignite these diseases; you could say our genes are like a gun, but the microbiome pulls the trigger.

Coeliac disease is close to my heart because I have tested positive for the gene and also have a family history of it. Luckily, my microbiomes haven't switched it on yet. Even closer to my heart is an umbrella of symptoms collected under the term 'irritable bowel syndrome' or IBS. This isn't a condition that defines a disease – a 'syndrome' just refers to a collection of symptoms. I now joke with my patients that it stands for 'Is Bull Shit' because our old theories and attempts to treat it seem archaic, dismissive and downright belittling. Historically, some doctors have rolled their eyes at this debilitating condition because for many years we have recognised an association with mental health: around a third of sufferers also have anxiety or depression. Patients are labelled as experiencing 'psychosomatic' symptoms generated by their minds and, rather than discussing their real physical symptoms, many clinicians are trained to probe 'deeper'. Gently, they will ask about stress, mood and any history of childhood trauma or sexual assault. We know stress *can* certainly trigger an IBS flare, just like it can directly trigger psoriasis and other visible conditions (but no doctor rolls their eyes at a rash). As we will see in later chapters, psychological stress has an enormous impact on many diseases but for some reason, we place enormous emphasis on its role when that disease is 'functional'*. Of course, stress management can be invaluable, but when used as the primary scapegoat, stress detracts from the complexity not just of the condition, but of the human being experiencing it.

The problem is we haven't been able to understand the mechanisms driving these associations; what's more, many

---

* 'Functional' just means a condition has no worrying pathology. Migraines are a perfect example as are IBS, chronic fatigue and fibromyalgia.

have conveniently ignored the 66 per cent of IBS patients with no mental-health history. Fifty years ago, IBS was incredibly rare and almost unheard of, but now more than 1 in 10 have a diagnosis. Of course, that doesn't capture the countless number who never seek medical attention. In just half a century, IBS has become one of the many conditions on the rise and we are finally starting to understand why. Something has clearly changed and it will probably come as no surprise that people with IBS appear to have very low microbiome diversity. In fact, some researchers are already cautiously trialling faecal transplants as a treatment for IBS, with one study relieving symptoms in 58 per cent of candidates. Fortunately, there are other much less extreme techniques we can all use, which I will cover in Part II.

Importantly, there is one condition which has huge overlap with IBS and, unlike functional diseases, it *can* be proven with a test and is also treated with medication. But in my experience most doctors have never heard of it: SIBO (or small intestinal bacterial overgrowth). I first came across SIBO as a junior doctor working on the gastroenterology ward, where I treated a patient with this 'rare' condition. As the name suggests, it involves the overgrowth of certain bacteria in the small intestine, which should normally have very few bacteria. Food passes through your small intestine first, where the majority of nutrients are absorbed, before reaching the large intestine, where the majority of your gut microbiome sets to work. When our bugs ferment our food they produce gas but this isn't supposed to happen in your small intestine. As a result, one of the main symptoms of SIBO is extreme bloating within one to two hours of eating: patients find they look genuinely pregnant after a meal and this can feel very uncomfortable.

SIBO has many other systemic symptoms, like fatigue and brain fog, showcasing how much leaky gut and a misbehaving microbiome can impact other body systems. SIBO is usually managed with antibiotics but sadly has a notoriously high treatment failure rate and often recurs. Specialists will imply it is a rare condition, but the truth is we don't know; it is now estimated that anywhere between 4 and 78 per cent of IBS patients have SIBO. In the UK, if I refer any patient with IBS-like symptoms to a gastroenterologist, it will often be rejected as 'just IBS'.* If you're lucky, you might be offered a dietician appointment but, to be completely honest, I have yet to meet a patient who is truly happy with the treatment they have received. As GPs, we don't have access to SIBO tests and we receive surprisingly little training in managing IBS. I was taught to offer a basic patient leaflet and try a handful of symptom-relieving medications. Of course, you can always read local guidelines but at the time of writing this, the new research into the microbiome is not included in these. I personally suspect many patients are given a vague diagnosis of IBS without formally excluding alternatives like lactose intolerance, endometriosis, SIBO and coeliac disease with absolute certainty. Though coeliac disease can be screened for with a blood test, it is notoriously inaccurate with several false negatives. If the blood test is negative but you still have a high index of suspicion, an endoscopic biopsy is the gold-standard investigation but this is a referral I have also had rejected, again with the advice that it was probably 'just IBS'.

Sadly, for the time being, it is often only the patients who shout the loudest or who are willing and able to pay privately who receive meaningful help with this condition. However, as a starting point, there are a number of non-invasive changes I will explore in Part II which have significantly helped me and my patients. But of course, it should go without saying that

---

* It is impossible to generalise in healthcare and I've had rare exceptions, as I'm sure other GPs around the country have too. But, as a rule, once dangerous causes have been excluded, it is very difficult to get further investigations or specialist input for IBS. Understandably, most funding and resources need to be focused on sinister health complaints. As a result, many people with debilitating symptoms deemed 'functional' (not dangerous) don't receive much medical input.

anyone experiencing new abdominal symptoms should always see their doctor to exclude sinister causes first.

BRAIN AND NERVE HEALTH

If what we have covered isn't surprising enough now imagine that you actually have two brains in your body: one in your head and one in your gut. An independent nervous system lives in your bowels and is now being referred to as your 'second brain'. Amazingly, our two brains can communicate with each other in what we now refer to as the gut–brain axis. It explains why you experience butterflies in your stomach when you're nervous but, more than that, the gut can also send signals to your brain. In fact, the gut microbiome can 'talk' to the brain via chemical messages, hormones, the immune system and neurotransmitters. Both the gut microbiome and our brain can actually create and respond to nerve hormones like serotonin, dopamine, GABA and norepinephrine. In other words, the brain and microbiome can literally speak and respond to each other.

We now know the gut microbiome produces 90 per cent of our serotonin and 50 per cent of our dopamine – these are the neurotransmitters we try to correct in anxiety and depression, among other things. So having an unhelpful mixture of bacteria or 'dysbiosis' doesn't just cause IBS symptoms but can lead to a depletion of neurotransmitters, also directly causing mental-health symptoms. At last, we can explain why there is an association between conditions like anxiety and IBS: patients aren't imagining their pain because of their anxiety; the microbiome could be causing both IBS *and* anxiety. Interestingly, endometriosis is another condition linked to dysbiosis and has a similar association with anxiety. There may be many other patients whose physical symptoms are labelled partly as a result of anxiety when the two don't have a causal relationship – they are simply both manifestations of the same underlying cause: an unhappy microbiome.

Remember the medicinal postbiotics helpful bugs can produce? Some of these are called short-chain fatty acids (SCFAs) and they can cross another brick wall in the body: the blood–brain barrier. Very few things can cross this tightly sealed barrier but SCFAs are given a free pass, and for good reason. They are vital for repairing the crumbling cement we get in leaky-gut syndrome and seem to have a similar effect on our blood–brain barrier. A whole new area of research called the psychobiome now explores the extensive ways in which our microbiome influences the brain, the breadth of which could fill a whole book. In short, research now suggests the microbiome can affect everything from Parkinson's and Alzheimer's to ADHD, autism, mental health and our general cognitive abilities. Remember, we evolved as hosts to these guests inside us, so it is hardly surprising they impact so many conditions – in reality, it would be easier to list the ones they don't affect, which is difficult to do with any real certainty. Ultimately, if you have anything going on in your mind from severe schizophrenia to low-grade anxiety or forgetfulness, a leaky gut and a misbehaving party of bugs could be a big part of the picture.

CANCER

It is hard to cover the full breadth of conditions influenced by our microbiome and I can't realistically explore each of them in one chapter. But cancer certainly deserves centre stage because there is no person not directly or indirectly affected by it.

The NHS website now tells us one in two people will get cancer in their lifetime – I always remember quoting one in four just a few years ago. Rates are on the rise and we're getting it younger and younger, which is terrifying when you stop to think about it. The number of 20–29-year-olds getting bowel cancer is going up by 7.9 per cent each year. Young surgeons now pine for the days when tumours were only something they removed in patients much older than them. I won't insult the discipline of oncology by attempting to describe cancer's cause and every influence in a couple of paragraphs – you should know (and probably already do) that it is exquisitely complicated. We will never find one cure for cancer because it is an umbrella term for so many conditions, all as unique and complex as we are. But unsurprisingly, the microbiome affects everything from its genesis to its growth and cure.

We realised during the AIDS epidemic of the 1980s how vital our immune system is in protecting us from cancer: when it stopped working from HIV, we saw thousands upon thousands of people develop aggressive types of cancer at every age. Remember the chaos caused by breaching a leaky gut? If you allow chronic inflammation to go unchecked, your white cells are distracted by a ruse: any real threat can sneak in and take over your body and cancer is just one example. It's odd to think, but we actually all have cancerous cells in our bodies at any given moment – it's part of the process of cell production – and every now and again, a mistake is made and the body shoots off a cancerous cell. A healthy immune system notices and deals with it. And so, although it is a dramatic oversimplification of the amazing chain of reactions involved: a good microbiome helps keep your immune system tough enough to clean up the cancer cells we all produce by mistake.

Remember that I mentioned microbiome communities have been found in many places other than your gut? They seem to coalesce with every aspect of our being and cancer is no exception. Amazingly, we now know tumours actually host a separate microbiome themselves. In fact, this is something we knew 100 years ago but at the time, not having discovered the role of the microbiome, we couldn't make sense of this. Why would there be bacteria living in tumours and how on earth did they get there? This is still a topic we don't fully understand, but what is clear is that these micro-organisms are doing something. In a way, this shouldn't surprise us – we now know of 11 pathogens which cause cancer and are finding more. The best known example is the HPV virus which causes cervical cancer –

now that we have a vaccine this might soon become a cancer of the past. Maybe one day the bacteria living in tumours will be sequenced and harnessed to target unique therapies or at least provide some insights into the tumour's cause. What we do know is that our microbiomes seem to play a role in both initiating cancer as well as protecting us from it, largely through those 'gifts' they bring to the party. For example, if the wrong bugs start fermenting your bile acid (a useful digesting tonic stored in the gallbladder), they will produce dangerous secondary bile acids which seem to promote cancers, including bowel, oesophageal, lung and gastric cancers. However, the helpful SCFAs produced by good bugs stop cells from turning cancerous and help to eliminate them.

One of the most famous studies exploring our microbiome's role in cancer asks a good question: why do African Americans have 65 times more colon cancer than rural Africans? Same genes, different environment. Participants in America and Africa provided stool samples and even underwent colonoscopies to take a closer look at their bowels: the American group were found to have many polyps (a precursor for cancer) while the rural Africans had none. They then swapped diets for two weeks; the Americans ate a traditional African diet which was high in fibre and largely focused on plants. Within just two weeks their healthy, cancer-fighting SCFA butyrate levels increased by two and a half times. For the other group, swapping their traditional diet to a SAD cut butyrate levels in half. The African diet dropped secondary bile-acid levels by 70 per cent, while the Western diet increased them by 400 per cent. In other words, in just the space of two weeks, a microbiome-boosting diet dramatically reduced levels of this carcinogenic by-product while a 'traditional' American diet made rates explode. Now imagine what a lifetime of this diet is doing to your risk not just of bowel cancer but all the other ones too.

Hormones

Another area heavily influenced by our microbiomes is the metabolism of our sex hormones (which actually has downstream consequences for cancer risk too). One example of this is our estrobolome: a 'clique' of gut bacteria which metabolise our oestrogen hormone. For tumours, which are sometimes amplified by oestrogen, such as some breast cancers, this means the bacteria can fuel or slow its growth through altering hormones. If you have a harmonious community of bugs adjusting your oestrogen levels to just the right amount (don't forget, men have oestrogen too), this results in strong bones, low cholesterol, clear skin, a better sex drive and even better female fertility. If it releases too much oestrogen, this can be linked to conditions like endometriosis, breast and womb cancer. Finally, if it releases too little this can exacerbate polycystic ovarian syndrome (PCOS) which, alongside endometriosis, is one of the commonest causes of sub-fertility in women.

PCOS isn't just the absence of enough oestrogen, it is also characterised by too many male sex hormones, which your microbiome can also adjust. In other words, if you want well-functioning ovaries, the microbiome needs to carefully release just the right amount of both oestrogen and androgens. Strangely, if a couple are struggling to conceive, many people automatically assume the woman's fertility is the main issue. I regularly have appointments with women who agonise about improving their fertility with a healthy lifestyle, forgetting it takes two to tango here. If a man has leaky-gut syndrome this will send those unhelpful 'endotoxins' through the bloodstream to his testes, reducing both sperm and testosterone.

It turns out anything requiring a careful balance of hormones – whether that's fertility, libido, menopause symptoms or even acne – can be heavily affected by our microbiome. Like I said, this previously unrecognised 'organ' we once knew nothing about coalesces with every aspect of our being and we should cherish it completely.

Are you Wu-ed?

I hope I have convinced you to value the parties you are hosting – you are a mere venue and the clientele you attract will impact your life significantly. Most of all, this chapter should fill you with hope, not just for your health, but for the health of future generations: we have finally discovered a missing puzzle piece in our biology and have so much more to learn.

For the time being, we know a diverse microbiome is associated with all-round better health. Slowly, we are working out which bugs are implicated most in various diseases, and in the future, we might be able to harness this information. Even chemotherapy is influenced by our microbiome, explaining why some respond better than others. Maybe one day, every cancer patient will receive results on their personal microbiome and that of their tumour, allowing for the direct targeting of the cancer, while priming the microbiome to slow its growth and prevent other diseases. Amazing research now also explores the microbiome's role in skin health, diabetes and many other arenas. The intricacies of each disease are interesting but almost not necessary to learn because the answer for each is the same: you just need to place value on your microbiome and feed it what it likes. You can already do that by consciously eating more plants, aiming for at least 30 different types a week. There are many more tricks which will follow in Part II but first there is more new science you need to understand. The microbiome is a vital component but the complex impact of our genes, hormones and metabolism is just as important, for understanding weight gain, and for health in general. Like me you need to be 'wu-ed' to truly value what it is your body is capable of. Next up it's your hormones – when you familiarise yourself with them, you'll see everything you think you know about weight gain could be wrong!

Microbiome: Key points

1) Everything is not as it seems. Research into the microbiome has unleashed an explosion of nutrition research high-lighting food's enormous complexity. Don't be fooled by expensive supplements – whole foods may look simple on the surface, but they are far more potent for your health than you might think.

2) Obesity is an enormously complex condition and the microbiome is but one thing influencing it, as demonstrated repeatedly through research. Some gut bugs protect their host from weight gain, while others can fuel it.

3) Most of our diseases are heavily influenced by the micro-biome. Increased rates of dysbiosis could explain soaring rates of immune-mediated diseases, cancers and mental health/skin/gut/hormonal/metabolic issues.

4) Eating at least 30 different types of plants a week with plenty of polyphenols is a great start to optimising a diverse and healthy microbiome.

CHAPTER 2

HOW DO WE ACTUALLY GAIN WEIGHT?

There are few topics which upset us more than our weight. We don't criticise someone for being short or having dry skin, but for some reason, the shape of our body is perceived as something which is completely our own responsibility. Being thin is a powerful currency, especially in the age of influencers; in fact, it is often the only credential they need to be taken seriously. You might have been enticed to mimic the behaviours of someone based on their appearance – surely if it worked for them it should work for you too, right? But have you mapped that person's microbiome? Perhaps they are one of the lucky 10 per cent who harbour the skinny bug *Christensenella* (see p. 23).

Now I'm not about to absolve or blame anyone, but in chapters to come you will see there are many other influences which make our experience of weight gain completely unique to us – some we can change, others we can't. I want to demystify the amazing nuance so many ignore. Meanwhile, in this chapter, I will break down the mechanisms our bodies use to store fat, which have been massively misunderstood for decades. But mostly, I want to remove the automatic status being thin affords; this misplaced power fuels misinformation and a disordered relationship with one of life's simplest joys: food.

Are you using the wrong currency?

On first inspection, the question of how we store excess fat seems spectacularly straightforward. Apparently, it's just a question of 'energy in versus energy out'. However, if the microbiome has taught us anything, it is that our bodies are not as they seem. We are mere vessels of a semi-human ecosystem that has the power to dramatically influence weight. But there's more: even what we understand about our human biology has been wrong.

It always makes me think of my family trip to Cuba a few years ago; it was an amazing and beautiful place to see but something didn't make sense. *Everything* was eye-wateringly expensive for us in a way I have never seen in other countries. The nation's poverty made this baffling – even adjusting for 'tourist luxuries', there was no logical way the locals could afford the prices we were seeing. How could this make sense? It turns out they had a different currency. Tourists were asked to pay for everything in dollars and only locals were allowed to pay with Cuban pesos – in real terms this meant we were being charged much, much more! They have since removed this dual-currency system, but we haven't done the same in our own bodies. You too might feel cheated by this. Perhaps you have been paying your dues by religiously counting calories but you're seeing no long-lasting results – something doesn't add up here. What you might not know is your body also has a different currency: hormones. If you learn how to pay with these instead, life suddenly becomes so much easier.

Now a quick Google search tells me that 1 gram of fat is equal to around 9 calories. Many will advise the key to sustainable weight loss is to reduce your current calorie intake* by 500 a day. (We will explore where this theory came from in Chapter 6 and it will surprise you!) Now, according to Google, if you maintain a 500-calorie deficit, seven days a week for six weeks, this will look like 3,500 (calories) x 6 (weeks) = 21,000/7,700 kcals in 1kg fat = 2.75kg of pure fat loss in six weeks. This is a conservative measure and many apps inflate it,

---

* This is something an automatic calculator can *apparently* work out based on your age, sex, weight, height and rough level of exercise.

giving you a precise prediction of your weight loss, including a helpful graph mapped over time. It is enchanting and exciting in equal measure to see that graph: *By a certain date, I will weigh Xkg if I just eat what the app tells me to eat ...* I fully understand the logic – it's really idiot proof, which is what I loved so much about it during my yo-yo dieting days. 'You *just* need discipline,' I would tell myself; I was familiar with the concept of hard work and more than confident I could apply this to my own body. But where did these numbers actually come from and do they really have anything to do with our bodies' communication with food?

What are calories?

The French were the first to calculate the energy of food in 1780. They reasoned that food was just fuel, which, in turn, is just energy. Just like wood, gas or oil, you should be able to determine its energy by burning it. They set a sample of food on fire in a sealed container, which they then submerged in water. Next, a thermometer was put into the surrounding water and the researchers waited to see how hot it got – if it went up by one degree C, the food had one 'calorie'. Some 250 years later, believe it or not, we haven't really changed the technique and still use this 'bomb calorimeter' to calculate calories. However, at the end of the 19th century we did start to acknowledge one fact, which you will have encountered most obviously whenever you eat corn or seeds: that some of our food comes out the other end and, evidently, is not absorbed. Around that time, an American scientist named Wilbur Atwater spent 20 years tirelessly and meticulously calculating the energy of people's stools and deducted this from the energy of their food. With a simple maths equation, he worked out the precise absorbed calories of hundreds of different foods, and we still refer to these today.

Of course, back then, Wilbur didn't realise that we all have microbiomes as unique as our fingerprints – a fact which now means forensic investigators can use a person's microbiome as evidence, similar to genetic testing. We've already talked about how our bugs interfere with the absorption of energy from food, but let's ignore that for a moment and pretend calories are still king. Imagine you still wanted to precisely calculate your calories – the problem is that it's so unbearably challenging, even Einstein would admit defeat. Part of the reason for this is that even very subtle changes to food dramatically influence how much energy you can absorb. For example, heating food helps us digest it, meaning a raw stick of celery gives you 6 calories, but cooked, it will actually release 30. That's quintuple (five times) the calories, just from cooking it. Do food labels account for this fairly sizeable difference? No. But it gets worse …

Food is more than a calorie

Food has a vital structure of fibres and particles called a 'food matrix' (we touched on this earlier). Cooking it is one way to change this, but we do much more than cook our food. Take the humble almond, for example: eat it raw and you will theoretically absorb 4.6 calories per gram (although most packets tell you this is 6.1 calories). Roast them and this goes up to 4.9; chop them and this changes to 5; pulverise them into a smooth butter and it's 6.5 calories per gram. That's a 40 per cent increase but, again, the food label won't necessarily reflect this (manufacturers are legally allowed an error rate of 20 per cent). Restaurants now also provide 'helpful' calorie counts, but these can deviate by 200 per cent – so that 300kcal sandwich which fits perfectly into your calculated deficit was actually 600kcal. Whoops. Even if I wanted to count calories again, from a purely mathematical point of view, I realise it is futile. Why bother trying when you know the numbers themselves are unreliable?

Ignoring the genuinely devastating impact of eating disorders, largely fuelled by a belief that food needs to be counted and restricted, one of my biggest bones to pick with calories is their blinkering effect. Calories cause tunnel vision, making us ignore food's other impacts. Coming back to the example of almonds, if you crush their food matrix into a butter, you release their fat globules from teeny tiny 'cages' within the matrix. The body can't access all these globules when the almonds are whole, meaning many end up in your stool; however, if a machine chews them first, you can absorb all the fat and *fast*. This then has a knock-on effect on your blood vessels – a part of the body we don't often think about. We see a similar pattern with sugar molecules: change the structure of the food, doing nothing to its calorie content, and this alters how freely you absorb the sugar and, again, how it hangs out in your blood.

In a way, our blood vessels are like a shop walled with shelves of delicate objects; the shopkeeper definitely wants customers but if a huge group of shoppers rush in and start colliding with the walls, no matter how much they want to spend, it's not good for business. The lining of your blood vessels feel the same way – constant, high impact exposure to sugar and fat molecules damages the inner walls. Damaged blood vessels means a poor blood supply to organs like your heart, kidneys, eyes and brain. This is why certain diseases cluster together: diabetes (with too much sugar in the bloodstream) is linked to kidney failure, heart disease, a long list of eye problems, stroke and even dementia. In other words, we should all care about the health of our blood vessels.

Fortunately, the food we eat can compensate – remember the medicinal plant chemicals called polyphenols? They're like a respectful, understated billionaire walking into the shop calmly and saying, 'Yes, I think I'll just buy all of it, please.' In fact, in the presence of a high-fat meal, if you throw some polyphenols into the mix, they seem to compensate for the damage or 'inflammation' caused to your blood vessels. Does this mean I only eat 100 per cent unprocessed food with its original food matrix intact? No, of course not! As a rule, food doesn't need to be perfect, nor can we define it as 'good' or 'bad'. But it is more than just calories. Importantly, what we eat has been tinkered with in the last 50 years and the impact on health is profound in more ways than one. Food companies have concocted an array of what can only be described as 'food-like substances'* which we have recently started to call ultra-processed foods (UPFs). These foods completely alter the matrix of each ingredient meaning, though the calories may be the same, the downstream impact on our bodies and health are not. Again, it really isn't 'just' about calories, after all, and we need to run away from this damaging idea as quickly as we can. Rather conveniently, the foods which boost our microbiomes also keep our blood vessels happy – humble, whole foods really are an unassuming medicine I wish I could prescribe.

Have we fallen out of love with food?

We will talk more about the astounding benefits of polyphenols in Part II but, suffice it to say, we eat more than just calories. We don't even fully understand most of the medicinal chemicals found in whole foods, but finally, we are starting to acknowledge them. The saddest thing about calories is that they have displaced so much from our plates. Whether it was intentional or not, food giants have dazzled us with 'low-calorie' packaging and conned us into eating food-like substances which harm health. They even fund the research that supports claims that calories and lack of exercise are the causes of obesity, conveniently distracting us from the role of their products. These 'low-calorie' foods replace our traditional recipes using whole ingredients – we value them more because of buzzwords like 'high protein'. Eggs and tinned beans miss out on this marketing campaign though they are the ones who deserve it.

---

* A term I have borrowed from Dr Chris van Tulleken's brilliant book *Ultra-Processed People* (Penguin, 2023).

Beyond impacting health, food carries other significance – a fact many of us are shamed for or try to ignore. What about its ability to stir up nostalgia? Nothing on earth can bring me back to childlike wonderment like the taste of a childhood dish. If alcohol is a social lubricant, I'd argue food is a social glue. Why else is it customary in countries all over the world to cook food for someone who is bereaved? For me, food has become a surrogate culture. Being half Danish, a quarter English and a quarter American is a lot on its own, made more confusing by the fact that I grew up in Denmark, Switzerland, Australia and Italy, before later moving to the UK. 'Where are you from?' is a common question most don't find hard to answer, but I do, especially because I mostly went to international schools where the main thing pupils had in common was that we weren't from the same country, let alone the country we were living in. I wouldn't say I was raised without a culture but, in its jumbled hodgepodge form, it has been hard to align with the single cultural identity most people share. But I *can* align with food: no Dane eats pickled herring or salty liquorice with more gusto than me. I also have no Italian heritage, but I know the Tuscan hand sign for 'good food' and can follow their idiosyncratic eating rules: spaghetti must be eaten with a fork and nothing else; no dairy with seafood; cappuccinos are only allowed before noon, etc. Food is a language in its own right; speaking it integrates you in any culture. Tell someone you like their food and you are saying you like them too. But calories erode this cultural dialogue – when I began calorie counting like my 'fitfluencer' gurus taught me, my childhood food, drenched in extra virgin olive oil filled me with dread. My culture – food – wasn't as important as my discipline, and nostalgic treats that once brought joy were replaced with guilt. Food became a transaction of protein and fuel – any other value it once held was gone. The same is true for so many people: in our attempts to understand food we have stripped away so much of its other value. Social rituals, heritage, nostalgia and joy are no longer reasons to eat if the food doesn't fit our 'macros'.

How does the body store fat?

Back to how the body *actually* knows when and how to store fat. In hindsight, it amazes me that I never stopped to think about this in more depth. I was always vaguely told the body simply manages energy that comes in and energy that goes out. Somewhere, these numbers are crunched and poof – fat either arrives or disappears accordingly. But the mechanisms aren't quite what they seem, and there are some leading characters in this story we seem to ignore. That's because we don't actually have a mysterious 'calorie centre' somewhere in our bodies furiously punching data into a calculator. Instead, our bodies communicate this information in intimate detail using chemical messengers called hormones. Allow me to introduce you to them.

I like to imagine a busy control centre somewhere in the body a bit like the stock exchange: pancreas, muscle and fat cells all in suits, shouting furiously as the numbers fly in and out. They believe a dashboard showing energy in and out is what decides if their 'stock' (or your weight) is up or down that day. In reality, the mechanism is far simpler: it's just a switch. When it's switched on, the body gains fat and when it's off, it burns fat. The two can't happen at the same time, so they take it in turns. Who flicks the switch, you might ask. Well, let me introduce you to the godfather of our hormones: insulin. When he's in your bloodstream sugar is transported into your cells where it is needed, and you are in a state of 'energy storage'. It's only when insulin levels drop that you can effectively use your fat stores.

This might sound like an absurd oversimplification. Ah! But you assume insulin is simple; mafia overlords never are, they can be influenced dramatically but, ultimately, they still have the final say. So much confusion and debate surrounding weight lives on because most people simply don't understand how insulin works. Instead, we have blindly followed an 18th-century belief that our bodies interact with food in the same way that fire does. Reducing food can very obviously cause weight loss but that food is more than a combustible fuel and your body is not an engine. For some it feels unnatural to let go of calorie counting because, of course, attaching a number to a food does allow you to monitor it. But believe me calories are like those dollar bills I paid in Cuba and hormones are the pesos. They're your body's local currency and, *trust me*, life becomes so much easier when you skip the exchange fee.

HOW DO WE KNOW INSULIN CAUSES WEIGHT GAIN?

Do you remember the case of the C. *diff*-infected 32-year-old who had never struggled with weight but rapidly gained more than 10kg? Something out of her control caused this. A similar thing happened in 2005 when a 20-year-old also rapidly gained just over 10kg in the space of a year. The odd thing was that nothing about her diet or lifestyle had changed. And there was something else: her blood sugar kept dropping dangerously low (hypoglycaemia or 'hypo'). She had also been diagnosed with type 2 diabetes a year earlier – some diabetes medications can cause 'hypos' but here's the catch: she wasn't taking any! Instead, she was controlling her diabetes with lifestyle, so there was no logical reason for her blood-sugar dips or weight gain. It just didn't make sense. In the end, doctors diagnosed an incredibly rare pancreatic tumour called an 'insulinoma' – it was misbehaving and producing far too much insulin. When they surgically removed it, the weight melted away and so did the diabetes.

This is a baffling story for many reasons. The fact that it has been published at all is a testament to how incredibly rare it is to have both diabetes and an insulinoma; only a small handful of similar cases have ever been seen. But the most interesting part of this story is that, in our eternally complicated biology, there was one simple cause and effect here: her body was producing too much insulin, which was forcing her to gain weight. If you struggle with your weight, you might also be producing too much insulin, even if you don't have a rare insulin-secreting tumour.

We can mimic the effects of insulinomas artificially by simply prescribing insulin – something doctors do all the time in diabetes. In the case of type 1 diabetics, patients have an autoimmune condition attacking their pancreas meaning they can't produce insulin; this was a fatal condition 100 years ago, leaving young children to waste away and die completely emaciated. Why? Because, without enough insulin, they completely lacked the ability to store fat, and weight loss is still one of the biggest signs of type 1 diabetes. But in 1923, we were able to prescribe a replacement, saving countless lives. It is a tragedy beyond words that a century later, we now have a whole new eating disorder called 'diabulimia': type 1 diabetics purposefully don't take their insulin, so they can lose weight. And, of course, it works. They would rather be thin than take the miracle cure keeping them alive – the consequences to their health are dire and serve as just one example of how pervasive our society's fat phobia is.

Type 2 diabetes, on the other hand, isn't caused by an inability to produce insulin but, instead, the body simply won't respond to it properly. This is usually the result of many years of high insulin levels in the body, largely due to lifestyle* – the cells become used to the high levels and need more and more to achieve the same effect. We call this 'insulin resistance', and not only is it the cause of type 2 diabetes, it is also one of the main drivers of almost all the chronic diseases we are most likely to die from: heart disease, stroke and dementia all walk hand in

---

* To be clear, type 2 diabetes is enormously complex and is influenced by genes, childhood factors, the microbiome and other lifestyle factors. The disease develops when susceptible individuals spend many years eating food in a way that spikes their insulin too much without compensating with techniques that manage it. I will explore this much more later.

hand with a body that is resistant to insulin. Giving diabetics insulin obviously makes them gain weight and several studies show that there is a direct correlation: increasing the dose of insulin also increases the weight gain. Even reducing calories won't compensate for insulin injections; in one study, patients gained 8.7kg over the six months from starting treatment, even though they restricted their food intake. The greatest irony is that, in the most severe cases of type 2 diabetes, we treat patients with the very thing that is driving their disease: more insulin. It exacerbates their insulin resistance so that, in time, we slowly need to make their insulin dose higher and higher. At the same time, they are nagged to lose weight while we are prescribing what's causing the weight gain in a vicious circle.

Importantly, insulin protects patients from other deadly complications of type 2 diabetes, and I am not for one moment inviting people to stop taking their prescriptions. But it is worth acknowledging the uphill struggle that treating insulin resistance with more insulin causes, and I hope we will stop shaming diabetics for not achieving weight loss, as if it were an easy thing to do. Many other medications also cause weight gain by spiking insulin, such as sulfonylureas, olanzapine, quetiapine and gabapentin. When I prescribe these, I warn my patients to expect weight gain; it's not in their control here – their switch is being turned on for them.

Behind the scenes, our hormones are really calling the shots. We now know people who live with obesity simply have higher levels of insulin* – even after fasting, there could still be insulin in their bloodstream (when, really, there shouldn't be). Remember if insulin is in the bloodstream, the switch is turned on, so you are *only* storing fat – the reverse can't happen at the same time. For some people, their hormonal messages obstruct their energy-storing system, meaning they are permanently in a

---

* The underlying causes for this may vary (obesity is a fascinatingly complex condition) but the only way to achieve high fat storing is high insulin.

fat-storing state. The great news is, however, that they *can* flick that switch back, even if it used to be stuck, and we will explore how later. But before we do that, there are some plot twists yet to come in this chapter that you'll want to know about first.

Cortisol – insulin's 'associate'

Remember mafia overlords don't work alone. Allow me to introduce insulin's second in command: cortisol. You don't want to get on his wrong side. In my first year as a fully cooked GP, fresh out of training, I came across an interesting patient. We initially spoke on the phone and his main complaint was a swollen face. When I saw this written in the appointment slot, I immediately assumed it was an allergic reaction, but it turned out, it had been swollen for several weeks. There was no pain or other symptoms, just an unusually round face. I probed more: he had also gained a dramatic amount of weight. My interest plummeted. I couldn't help a knee-jerk thought that weight gain wasn't a medically relevant 'symptom'; I wrongly jumped to the conclusion that his weight was within his control. When he came in to see me I realised his face *really* did look round, which is described quite impolitely as a 'moon face' sign in medicine. He showed me pictures of him from just a few months earlier (I could see the dates), and these were, indeed, evidence that he had always been slim. This was clearly quite a sudden and drastic change from his norm. His weight wasn't spread equally either. It all pooled around his middle, with slim legs and arms. This also has an unflattering term in medicine; we call it a 'lemon-on-stick' appearance: imagine creating a figurine with cocktail sticks as the limbs, an olive as the head and a lemon as the body. It sounds absurd, but serves as a helpful visual when you see the disease it reflects in real life: Cushing's. This man had all the signs of a disease caused by the body producing too much cortisol and, just like the patients with insulinomas, it makes you suddenly gain huge amounts of weight. The opposite is true in a condition called Addison's, caused by too little cortisol: it makes you lose weight, and your skin develops a bronze tinge. (By modern beauty standards this might sound quite appealing, but patients also collapse and can rarely experience life-threatening complications, so it's not a disease I would wish for.) What both Addison's and Cushing's demonstrate quite neatly is that cortisol can affect your weight dramatically.

I can artificially increase cortisol in my patients by prescribing it synthetically as a steroid, which is something I quite often do to treat certain conditions. A short-term course won't cause too many problems, but some patients take these steroids for months and even years. And I can promise one thing: they will absolutely gain weight. But why does this happen if insulin is the big boss deciding when and how we store fat? Because cortisol directly spikes insulin.

Let's go backwards and look at our evolution to make sense of this: as cavemen, if chased by a sabretooth tiger, we needed quick access to energy to get away. Cortisol is our main stress hormone and can quickly give you access to all the blood sugar you require. This is amazing engineering: energy stores are usually only needed gradually and so are locked away in the liver, muscle and fat. Cortisol basically acts like a high-speed getaway vehicle, racing to magically unlock those stores at speed, so you can literally run for your life. The design flaw is that this is only helpful in the short term: you're not supposed to spend months running from said tiger. In our modern lives, we have managed to create chronic stressors which bubble away under the surface and constantly drive higher-than-average cortisol levels. This stream of artificially raised blood sugar, in turn, pushes your insulin levels up, which then increases fat storing, insulin resistance and therefore the production of more insulin: the cycle then starts again. It's a vicious circle and one many of us recognise; if you can remember a time when you quickly gained weight, was there a new stress in your life? For many of us, stress and weight gain happen in unison, even if we don't realise it.

It should therefore come as no surprise that people living with obesity have been found to have high levels of long-term cortisol – something we can test for in hair of all things. There are many studies showing increased cortisol levels are linked to insulin resistance and one which even showed our perceived level of stress correlated beautifully with raised cortisol, blood sugar and insulin levels. That's right – how you rate your own levels of stress scientifically predicts a spike in insulin: the fat storing mafia overlord who also drives all our chronic diseases and even speeds up how fast we age. Stress isn't a wishy-washy, fluffy term for softies but the physical manifestation of your body's chemistry: if you leave this 'mafia' to do their thing there will be [New Jersey accent] *consequences.*

We are finally starting to appreciate that weight gain is not 'just' a sign of your willpower – there are clear outside factors we have ignored but, more than that, we've been asking the wrong questions. Staring at a dashboard trying to make numbers add up has been a decoy from what is really happening – there's a simple switch in your body. Is it turning on and off properly? Or is it becoming stiff and frequently stuck in the 'on' mode, permanently making you store fat? If so, why is this happening so much to so many of us? Yes, for many it is partly related to consuming more energy, but the question is: why does this happen? We have ingenious mechanisms to stop us from eating when we have had enough but for some reason these can stop working. Your local currency answers many of these questions! Now that you have met the big bosses – insulin and cortisol – let me introduce you to their minions. Appetite is heavily influenced by hormones too but here's the shocking thing: you can exert influence over them too! Over the next chapters I will teach you how you feel hungry and full – it's more complicated than you might think.

Weight gain: Key points

1) Being thin is widely perceived as a status symbol in society. Whether this is subconscious or not doesn't matter, but it needs to stop. A thin body on its own is not a valid credential for sharing health advice to others, nor is it a symbol of moral superiority.

2) Calories are an 18th-century notion that cleverly distracts consumers from the quality of their food. What we eat is more than a fuel, and implying otherwise detracts from its other health, social, cultural and emotional value. Unassuming whole foods prepared with nostalgic recipes are worth so much more than a calorie.

3) Being in a fat-storing state is not part of a spectrum: you are either currently storing fat or burning it and can't do both at the same time. The presence – or absence – of insulin in your bloodstream is what decides which state you are in.

4) Insulin can be influenced by many factors. The more insulin resistant you become, the more you produce and the more fat you store. As we will cover in upcoming chapters, how you live your life can directly fuel insulin resistance: poor sleep, high stress and eating lots of sugar are just some ways you might be doing this right now. (But there's much more detail to come ...)

5) Our stress hormone, cortisol, serves a vital function when it is released briefly. However, if it is chronically raised, it directly contributes to insulin resistance and therefore drives more fat storing and disease. Stress is not a wishy-washy notion: managing it is incredibly important for your health.

CHAPTER 3

APPETITE

Where does it come from?

Anyone who has ever experienced unwanted weight gain will know how confusing an experience it can be. Learning about the influence of the microbiome, insulin and cortisol in the previous chapters has, hopefully, made *what* is happening in the body more clear. But we have yet to establish *why* these changes develop in the first place – an angle that is rarely explored.

To completely blame the individual implies they have absolute control over their body. But think about it: do you believe you can override your biology at will? Could the power of thought conjure up a feeling of thirst? Can you spontaneously fall asleep at any moment simply by choice? Of course, we have influence, but we do not have absolute control over our bodies and so, by definition, our weight is not at the mercy of the mind. Our bodies have evolved with an amazing ability to maintain an almost perfect equilibrium in everything from body temperature to fluid levels: weight is no different. The intricate web of systems which monitor and calibrate our weight are nothing short of awe inspiring, but for many of us, they have stopped working. I want to slowly unpick all of the reasons *why* this is happening but to grasp this, you first need to understand where appetite comes from. People might dispute the idea that we only eat due to hunger but we do – there are just several forms of hunger. When your hormones decide you are full it feels impossible to eat. If you are overweight it's not simply because you eat too much – more specifically, it could be because your appetite signals aren't working properly.

An Inca-redible epiphany

A few years ago, I was lucky enough to travel to Peru and hike the Inca Trail to see Machu Picchu. This involved a four-day trek, which, in my memory, was essentially a never-ending staircase. At our highest point, we reached 4,215 metres above sea level which meant the experience was breathtaking in more ways than one. On our final day, we took a train back down to Cusco (just a measly 3,399 metres above sea level). But as we travelled down, I developed a condition called altitude sickness and it was a truly odd experience. I felt slightly nauseous, but didn't vomit nor did anything dramatic happen to me. The nausea cleared within hours, and, over the following days, I felt completely well bar one symptom: I had absolutely zero appetite. I can't stress enough how bizarre this felt. Like anyone else, my appetite can sometimes reduce when I am ill, but it has never just disappeared. For three days I was almost completely unable to swallow anything, which seemed so ludicrous that I tried to ignore it, paying for three meals a day, confident I could overcome this odd phenomenon. Each time I tried to eat I was surprised at how foreign the food felt in my mouth – swallowing it felt unnatural. And after a few bites, I would admit defeat, leaving confused waiters to clear away my almost untouched food. 'You didn't like it?' they'd ask. But that wasn't the problem – the food was delicious. I wanted to want it. But nothing I did would allow me to eat it. I realised that hunger isn't just a desire for food – it is a physiological reflex you can't fake or force.

The altitude sickness had altered my appetite hormones so much that I couldn't face eating anything. But I am not an anomaly – we see this in medicine all the time especially in patients with cancer – one of the reasons they lose weight so quickly, even if they are usually prone to overeating, is they too have no appetite. Patients taking the diabetes/weight-loss drug Ozempic will notice a similar effect: because their GLP-1 receptors (more on these to come) are stimulated they feel too full to eat. A simple desire can't overcome this – it feels almost impossible to ignore a lack of appetite. Many of us eat for enjoyment but I couldn't even stomach my most guilty pleasures in Peru – it was like something switched in my brain and told my stomach, 'Sorry, we're not accepting any new visitors today.' For the first time in my life, I was able to appreciate the amazing control that appetite signals can exert over us. Thinking you *should* be able to override your biology doesn't mean you actually *can*.

The exact same thing is true of eating when we *are* hungry – we can attempt to ignore this sensation but only for so long. This doesn't make us weak, nor is it just a case of 'being human': if we are physically capable of eating far beyond our energy requirements, there is a fault in the system.

Ozempic works because it targets this faulty appetite, thus altering eating patterns long enough to turn off that insulin switch (see p. 50) and allow for fat burning. I need to stress again that I am not in the business of slandering traditional medication and of course, for some, medicine is necessary. Equally, however, for many conditions, there are less invasive lifestyle techniques we can try first. And that is why I am writing this book.

How do we feel full?

As we saw in the last chapter, hormones are the local currency of our bodies and they are the ones who really call the shots. To understand appetite, you need to appreciate the hormones influencing it, but I want to avoid turning this into a textbook. The subject is vast, and for those interested I have put together a full list of hormones in Appendix 1 (see p. 303). However, for simplicity I will focus here on a handful of the most important ones: cholecystokinin (CCK), peptide YY (PYY), ghrelin, GLP-1 and leptin. Don't worry, there is no quiz at the end. The point of Part I is simply to convince you to *value* the science. And I promise everything will make sense in Part II, where I explain how to practically apply everything you have learned to your own life.

Back to my odd experience in Peru – what was going on in my body to ruin my appetite? It turns out the reason I couldn't eat during my altitude sickness was because my body was telling me I was already full.* We know that a hormone called leptin spikes in altitude sickness, explaining my peculiar inability to eat. Unlike other fullness or 'satiety' hormones, leptin doesn't temporarily spike as a result of the food we eat but is instead produced by our fat cells. This is incredibly clever because it creates a communication system between these cells and the brain. Leptin reports back to the brain if we're running too low or, indeed, too high on fat. The more fat we lay down, the higher our leptin levels are, signalling to the brain to feel fuller because 'We've got enough down here.' Even though I had a healthy weight, the altitude sickness made my brain think I had far more fat stores than I needed and so made me feel constantly full. This clearly doesn't make sense in obesity because if the leptin-brain feedback loop were working, obese individuals would be physically unable to eat, but here's the plot twist: we know it doesn't work.

In the majority of people living with obesity, their brains simply don't register the high leptin, meaning they miss out on one of our most powerful appetite regulators. How this happens is complicated; for the majority, it was working to begin with, but after years of climbing leptin levels the brain becomes desensitised and stopped responding to it. Just as our bodies become resistant to chronically high levels of insulin, the brain does the exact same thing with leptin. In fact, insulin and

---

* There is some evidence that altitude sickness also affects our hunger hormones, but I will focus here on its primary impact on satiety.

oestrogen* also have a similar way of feeding back to the brain like this, but leptin is the main focus in research.

Ultimately, our clever bodies have more than one way to double check if we need more or less fat and can stimulate a feeling of background fullness when we've stored enough. This balance or 'homeostasis' sets the stage for something called set-point theory, which was first proposed in 1982. The idea is that the body is designed to keep us at the same weight – it has worked hard for those fat stores and learns what level it wants to aim for. When the system works, many people simply stay the same weight; even a spell of overeating doesn't suddenly cause weight gain the next day. The body simply compensates, like a seesaw finding just the right balance. Kidney specialist Dr Jason Fung uses a useful analogy in his book *The Obesity Code*: he says your set point is like a thermostat. If the temperature goes too high, it triggers the air conditioning; too low and it starts the heating. Should you walk into a room and find it boiling hot, you wouldn't blame the heater for staying on too long because the real problem is that the thermostat isn't working. People are the same: we shouldn't criticise them for eating too much, but instead ask why their 'thermostat' hasn't stopped them from doing this.

Our background thermostats provide a fascinating puzzle piece in the obesity conundrum: why do people eat more energy than they need? If the body learns to ignore important regulators like leptin, it is able to override normal appetite breaks, leading to an abnormal appetite. But these aren't the only stop signs along the way. Again, the body is incredibly clever when it comes to working out how much energy it has and needs. After assessing what is already 'in the tank' it can also monitor

---

* As mentioned, I don't want to turn this into a textbook – appetite signals are incredibly complex and leptin is the most important 'background' hormone to focus on. However, the example of oestrogen is interesting! When it drops in menopause women find they feel less full, and this is one reason why weight gain is a very common symptom: their body is asking them to eat more.

how much is coming in by stimulating hormones in response to food. What, when and how we eat has changed beyond recognition in the last 50 years: for many people their inbuilt system isn't necessarily broken, it's just not being used the way it was designed to be. The food many of us eat doesn't stimulate our fullness hormones properly, and worse than that, sometimes it actually stimulates hunger instead. As I keep saying, food is not merely a fuel source – it is perceived as information by the body. As it travels down your digestive system, hormones and other mechanisms communicate its arrival. And by knowing what has arrived, the body can decide how much more it needs. There is a sequence to this communication, and to understand it, we need to travel down your gut from your food's point of view.

IT STARTS IN THE MOUTH

We begin in the mouth, where chemical messages cascade out to the brain, stomach and pancreas as a heads-up. It's like you have a promoter outside a restaurant with a walkie talkie, letting the barman, waitstaff and cooks know if it looks like customers are about to arrive. This is very helpful – the stomach can get some scalding acid ready, rather than being caught off guard. Meanwhile, your pancreas can anticipate that blood sugar will be arriving soon, so it sends some insulin in anticipation. That way, the sugar molecules won't hang around unnecessarily, bumping into the lining of your delicate blood vessels. Wonderful news! It's almost as if your body actually wants to protect you from disease. The problem? We have created food-like substances with artificial flavourings and sweeteners that have no calories or nutrients, but no one had the courtesy to let your mouth know this. So even if you haven't consumed any actual calories, your body perceives that you have and carries on getting everything ready for them to arrive.

This is what we describe as the 'cephalic phase' of eating and it really answers a lot of questions. If you get people to swirl something sweet in their mouth without swallowing it, whether it has calories or not, we see a significant spike of insulin in the blood. In fact, this happens with any flavour except bitter flavours. (For example, plain black coffee shouldn't cause an insulin spike.) In rats, if you cut the nerve connecting the brain to the tongue, the insulin spike from flavour disappears. This is proof that insulin responds to taste, with or without calories. The really interesting thing is that people who live with obesity see a much bigger spike in their cephalic-phase insulin response (CPIR) than people who are lean. I told you it was complicated. We have been encouraging people to chew gum and sip herbal tea or artificially sweetened drinks, which apparently 'don't count', but they do – they are flipping us into our fat-storing states, and even more so in obesity.

How long it takes you to chew your food is also a way for the body to monitor how much food is coming in. In our evolution the longer we chewed the more calories we were taking in, so our clever bodies have an inbuilt satiety-feedback loop here too: chewing triggers fullness hormones. Many studies show that the longer it takes to chew something, the fuller people feel and the less they eat. But there's a catch: they will enjoy it less. And this is a fact the food industry have really homed in on: food that is soft and easy to chew quickly is irresistibly pleasurable to us. The downside is that this allows it to bypass one of our fullness mechanisms: because we don't spend long chewing it, we don't trigger as many fullness hormones. The customers walked straight into the restaurant while the promoter was having a coffee break; no one gave the restaurant a heads-up to expect guests.

THE STOMACH

The food you have carefully chewed (or perhaps not) makes its way to your stomach next – a glorified balloon with a tiny hole at the bottom. This hole or 'pyloric sphincter' is clamped shut and will only let food into your gut once it is liquidised enough. This allows a perfect trap for our second fullness or 'satiety' checkpoint: our stomach's stretch receptors. As your stomach becomes stretched, it is safe for your body to assume there must be some energy on its way, so it sends messages to your brain to warn that you are starting to feel full. Before walking into a restaurant, you have to ask staff if they have space – if a huge group of people stormed in without asking, staff might struggle to accommodate them. Your stomach is in a similar predicament and is trying to take inventory before letting more food in – the problem is that many modern foods have stopped talking to it. Our evolution assumed more calories would require more time to liquidise, but this is no longer the case. Whether you are eating 'pre-chewed' UPFs, blitzed up smoothies or fruit juices, the energy in the food doesn't reflect how long it will stretch your stomach. I'm not demonising any of these foods but it's worth remembering that food is a language – our body wasn't taught to speak this one. If food doesn't need to sit in your stomach for long it can bypass a vital satiety mechanism.

THE SMALL INTESTINE

Our guests have now barged their way into the top part of your gut called the small intestine, where they can now be absorbed into the bloodstream. But not so fast ... We have another 'stop' sign here – because in the first part of your intestine your gut cells can detect food has arrived and start triggering satiety hormones. This is called the ileal break and the main hormone here is CCK, which is triggered by dietary fat; however, it only lasts for about 30 minutes. This means that the fat you eat plays a big role very early on and tells you, 'Woah, woah, woah! You've had enough.' Later on in the day, it won't send as many fullness alerts, but that's okay, you have other hormones for that. The interesting thing here is that since the 1980s, people in the West have been intentionally eating less fat, not realising they are skipping one of their first appetite breaks.

I have already mentioned our friend GLP-1, whose receptors are stimulated very effectively by Ozempic. Of course, this triggers satiety because GLP-1 is itself another important fullness hormone released in the intestines after a meal. It forms another part of our ileal break because it spikes quickly after you start eating. If it works well, this promptly stops you from eating more than you need. It even sends messages to your stomach telling it to hold tight and delay emptying, thus slowing digestion down and allowing stretch receptors in the stomach to work for longer. We know it is stimulated by proteins and fats but also seems to be triggered by fibre. Of course, as we saw in Chapter 1, fibre is very important for a healthy microbiome, which is also involved in stimulating satiety. One study found 45 different bacterial strains capable of stimulating GLP-1, which is just one example of how gut bugs produce the equivalent of medication for us.

Another vital role of GLP-1 is to stimulate insulin and promote the body's sensitivity to it, which explains part of how the microbiome can be involved in preventing type 2 diabetes. Importantly, people living with obesity get less of a GLP-1 spike from their food, which we now think could be contributing to their abnormal appetites. Boosting your microbiome with at least 30 plants a week is one way we might be able to alter our very biology, all by working with our bodies' hormones. Of course, I need to caveat this by saying again that obesity is an enormously complex condition and I'm not proposing that 'just eat more fibre' should replace advice to 'just eat less'. However, it is one of many powerful tools we can all make use of without a prescription or any side effects.

As my carefully drawn-up table in Appendix 1 will tell the more curious of you, there are a number of other fullness hormones knocking about. The other biggie is one any gym bro will get very excited about: PYY which is stimulated by, you guessed it, protein. Now this hormone is particularly interesting because, unlike CCK, it is mostly stimulated further down the gut. It can take food several hours to reach the lower part of the gut, which is why a protein-rich meal can keep you full for longer. It is also a very important hormone for gastric bypass surgery (a type of weight-loss surgery), which essentially reconnects the gut to a lower segment of bowel. As mentioned in the microbiome chapter, this surgery doesn't primarily work because of reduced calories – it actually alters the microbiome *and* appetite. By skipping part of the bowel, food quickly arrives at the segment where lots of PYY can be stimulated. In fact, we know that after a gastric bypass, patients trigger both more PYY and GLP-1, as well as less of their hunger hormone. Just like my experience in Peru (see p. 59), it simply feels impossible to eat when their bodies are signalling that they are full. Ultimately, it treats the root cause of the problem, not by altering willpower but by correcting appetite mechanisms which have stopped working.

THE LARGE INTESTINE

By the time our guests reach the large intestine, most of the nutrients we need have already been absorbed – now it's time for your microbiome to feast on anything else that is left.

We will talk more about what they eat in Part II, but I just wanted to give your bugs another shout out here because, remember, they produce a lot of your body's chemicals and that includes appetite regulators. One study evaluated the levels of gut hormones in healthy subjects and gave them some prebiotics, which the microbiome love to feed off. The researchers noticed increased fermentation by the microbiome, an improved blood-sugar response to food and – here's the clincher – decreased appetite. Not only did they spike GLP-1, as mentioned above, they also triggered PYY. So just by feeding a healthier microbiome you could alter your appetite hormones to feel full; this is just one example of how you can work *with* your biology, rather than against it. Trying to ignore hunger is a miserable experience and for the vast majority simply doesn't work anyway. Counterintuitive as it may seem, to anyone trying to lose weight my advice is to eat food that genuinely leaves you feeling full.

How do we feel hungry?

Hunger is not merely the absence of fullness – it is very important for our survival that the body can specifically prompt us to want to eat. But what actually makes us experience hunger? Unlike our long list of satiety hormones, we actually only have one hunger hormone – ghrelin. But this does not mean hunger is somehow simple. Like insulin, I warn you not to underestimate this guy because *this* is where things get really interesting. Life is much easier for restaurant staff when customers book in advance – it means they can anticipate the work needed. The body is the same – it actually tries to predict your behaviour and accommodate your needs – but, without realising it, many of us behave like rude guests.

Hormones clearly have a huge effect on us – but can we affect them too? I would like to share with you the findings of my favourite jaw-dropping study, illustrated in Figure 1. In this study, 6 healthy subjects were asked not to eat anything for 24 hours and had a blood test every 20 minutes. They discovered something so flabbergastingly amazing that I still feel baffled by it now: even though participants ate nothing all day, their

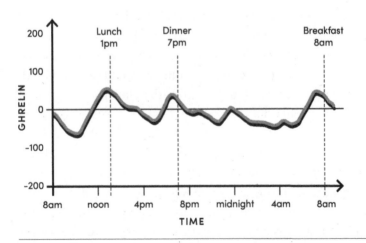

Figure 1: Ghrelin spikes across 24 hours

ghrelin spiked at their usual mealtimes. In other words, your hunger signals aren't random: they are programmed by internal cues to arrive like clockwork. I appreciate this might inspire less dumbfounded excitement for people who aren't me, so let me elaborate: you (or usually the cultural norms you find yourself in) have dictated when it is time to eat and your body has responded. Like a smartphone remembering something you *usually* do, so your body does the same. It knows you *normally* have breakfast at 8am so, doting as it is, that's when it spikes your hunger hormone for you. What is so exciting about this? Well, if your behaviour is the driver of this, then, by definition, you have the power to change your own ghrelin spikes. Eureka!

Let's take a closer look at the graph which, on first inspection, seems to make no sense. The hunger-hormone levels are on the vertical axis and the time of the day is on the horizontal. If I asked most people to suddenly eat nothing all day, they would imagine a day filled with unbearable, climbing hunger, until they eventually reached their limit and collapsed. But that's not what happens in practice or, evidently, in the bloodstream. We have all had busy days when we forgot to eat – maybe we have a whiff of hunger but, engrossed in whatever we are doing, it just disappears. This is mirrored in the blood: at 8am when the subject normally has breakfast their ghrelin spikes right on cue! But, when no food arrives, it doesn't continue to rise endlessly. Instead, it simply drops. (In fact, in my experience it only takes about 20–30 minutes for hunger to disappear when fasting, and this makes sense from an evolutionary point of view. Our ancestors weren't always in a position to eat – they had to go find their food. It would be unhelpful to leave a person famished all day because this, as you might know, is quite a distracting feeling. Instead, ghrelin gives you a gentle nudge to eat but then leaves you alone, so you have time to find food.) The graph also shows a spike at lunch which quickly drops too. Finally, it spikes once more at the subject's usual dinner time, but is actually reduced compared to the breakfast and lunch levels. Rather than feeling progressively more hungry, subjects became *less* hungry.

A biology textbook will tell you ghrelin is produced by the stomach because it is empty but clearly, something else must also be controlling its release. How on earth has it learned to align with our usual routine like some sort of computer? You may have heard of our 'circadian rhythm' – the internal clock which helps to decide when we should be awake or asleep. A cyclical release of hormones is what guides us to wake and sleep but, just like with ghrelin, we can exert some control over this. For example, if you were to fly abroad to a different time zone, your body would eventually align to fall asleep at the same time as the locals. This is largely driven by exposure to light – our clever bodies have worked out that less light coming into our eyes means it is time to sleep.

Amazingly, as it turns out, every organ and individual hormonal pathway we have runs to its own time and, in essence, has a circadian rhythm. But there is one 'master clock' which connects to all of these separate organ clocks. This is called your 'suprachiasmatic nucleus' (SCN) and it lives in your brain, where it is able to communicate with the brain's hunger centre. Long story short, a combination of your SCN's signals and the usual timings of your own meals is what decides when you feel hungry.

What happens when food doesn't ring ahead?

Now, if our hunger hormone has a circadian rhythm influenced by the brain *and* when we choose to eat, imagine how confusing repeated flavour hits on the tongue are to the body.

If you sip on a sugar-free drink, chew gum or generally graze regularly throughout the day, you are warning the body to constantly expect food. This sends a ripple effect through your organs and glands: your stomach might get some acid ready even if no food arrives. Your liver, gut and pancreas all have their own rhythms too and didn't evolve to expect food/flavour persistently throughout the day or late at night. Your pancreas will repeatedly release more insulin each time you are exposed to flavour, turning that fat-storing switch to on mode all day. The body is an incredibly accommodating host and will rev up the appropriate hormones, acids and digestive juices as best it can – but many of us are overworking these systems and not respecting their predictable, rhythmic patterns. It's no wonder our bodies start to grumble at us with indigestion, heartburn, lethargy, poor sleep, constipation and bloating (among other things). Many of us behave like ungracious guests, expecting our bodies to do what we like whenever we like it.

Our food environment has changed beyond recognition, but so have our eating habits, at least in some countries. Over the last 40 years, a new mantra of 'eat little and often' has ingrained itself into wellness culture, as well as formal medical advice; in fact, this is still the advice weight-loss services offer. In 1970, snacks made up one tenth of our calories, but they now make up one quarter. American adults eat between 4.2 and 10.5 times a day and tend to fast for 9 hours or fewer – that means the only time in the day when they have several hours of no eating is when they are asleep. In the 1970s, the vast majority of people only had three eating episodes a day *in total*. This has now gone up to an average of six, not including 'perceived' eating with fake flavours but no calories. Grazing has been normalised in many Western countries and parents are now encouraged to pack separate snacks for their children's school day. Having mostly grown up in European countries this was not my experience – my classmates and I generally only ate at lunchtime. Breaktime was spent playing outside when teachers certainly didn't prompt us to eat.

Etiquette also reflects a society's perceived norm: in Japan, for example, it is considered very rude to eat on the street – food is almost always a seated affair. In fact, only half of Japanese people report regularly eating snacks and they have an average of 4.68 eating episodes a day. This is interesting because just over 3 per cent of Japanese people are obese (one of the lowest rates in the world) and Japan is also home to some of the long-est-living people on earth. There are many complex reasons for this, but I suspect an eating culture which doesn't promote a constant stream of insulin is one of them. It is very interesting to consider food as a language that has changed over the last few decades: in the 1970s it 'rang ahead', politely informing the body's circadian rhythms what to expect so they could accom-modate what was coming. Fake flavours, random timings, late shifts and few breaks mean our digestive system is overworked and confused. If you give your gut (and its co-workers) predict-able hours and enough rest, staff morale will improve and so will your health!

What else impacts our hunger cues?

I hope I have convinced you that, though he is an army of one, our hunger hormone is far from simple. He is intelligent enough to memorise your normal routine and try to mirror your life-style. Like a highly skilled personal assistant anticipating your every need, he predicts what you want before you even know you want it. But believe me, we've only scratched the surface: ghrelin is in cahoots with our bodies' 'mafia' and can work in some very mysterious ways.

POOR SLEEP

Exposure to light and the arrival of food both seem to mediate our SCN signals: when you see light and eat food, this seems to impact the natural tempo our brain sets for the body. Don't forget, each system in the body has a circadian rhythm, includ-ing the microbiome. In fact, if you take a stool sample from someone who is jet lagged and put it into a germ-free mouse, this promotes worse blood-sugar control and obesity. You would be surprised by how little sleep disruption it takes to have an impact – for example, going to bed just three hours later than usual is enough to disrupt your blood sugar. Circadian research expert Satchin Panda refers to this as 'social jetlag' in his book *The Circadian Code*. We know shift work increases the risk of disease because of a disruption to our circadian rhythms but this 'social jetlag' can produce the same effect. The implications are profound for health and appetite – we know just one night of sleep disruption can also reduce leptin and spike ghrelin, giving us less background satiety and more acute hunger. We will talk much more about sleep in Part II, where we navigate how to apply all of this science to your own life – for now, simply know that maintaining a healthy weight without good sleep is a difficult thing to do.

CORTISOL AND GHRELIN ARE FRIENDS

Remember insulin's 'associate' cortisol? In a brief moment of stress he helps you quickly access your energy stores to run away from a threat. If allowed to spike long term, he increases your blood sugar, insulin and fat storing. It turns out cortisol has an associate of his own: our hunger hormone, ghrelin. We know raised cortisol has a dramatic effect on appetite but, interestingly, in two ways: if it shoots up briefly, like nature intended, you will lose your appetite. Most of us have experienced this – you don't tend to feel suddenly hungry during an exam or your driving test. This would make for an inconvenient distraction from the task at hand, which is why our ancestors didn't start wondering what was for dinner while running from a tiger. However, if you have low-level chronic stress with constantly raised cortisol and a subsequent ghrelin spike, not only will you feel hungrier, you will also specifically crave high-fat, energy-dense and hyper-palatable foods. (Rather conveniently, we have a lot of these foods around.) But why does this happen? It turns out, ghrelin has a powerful effect on several areas in the brain which influence self-rated hunger levels, but more than that, it also affects how we *feel* about food. Studies show that when people are given an injection of ghrelin, their thoughts of food become more vivid, meaning they literally fantasise about it.

HEDONIC HUNGER – THE PLEASURE OF FOOD

Importantly, our behaviours, wants and desires aren't entirely under our own conscious control. For example, low testosterone or high cortisol could rob you of your libido, changing your behaviour *for you*. Although it's a different type of 'hunger', our desire for food can also be changed. Amazingly, appetite isn't just experienced in the stomach – you can feel it in your brain too, and cortisol can influence this. Interestingly, research shows that rats lose their appetite as their cortisol rises: the more stressed they are, the less they eat. Humans aren't quite the same – about 30 per cent will lose their appetites, but the rest actually eat more when stressed. However, despite their natural reflex to eat less, we can reproduce this human response in the stressed rats: all you need to do is offer them hyper-palatable foods instead and they actually eat more. Why? Because these foods influence the same reward pathways in our brains that addictive drugs like cocaine do. Here we see how desire and behaviour can converge in spite of our natural instincts. The food we eat is changing our brains and, it seems, our behaviour. But there is actually an evolutionary reason for this: these foods stimulate pleasure chemicals in our brains, which counteract the negative effects of stress. The body is protecting itself – seeking out more of the same pleasure is an inbuilt mechanism, not a conscious choice. If you don't have physical hunger pangs but still eat to seek pleasure this is still due to hunger – but this time it's coming from your brain and is called 'hedonic hunger'. The key thing to remember is that it increases with chronic stress and exposure to hyper-palatable UPFs.

In 2021, the author of *Ultra-Processed People*, Dr Chris van Tulleken, offered himself up as tribute in his own version of 'the hunger games' by taking part in an experiment. He valiantly spent 30 days eating a diet with 80 per cent of his calories coming from UPFs – a diet many teenagers already follow. His blood tests showed lower levels of satiety hormones and a spike in both his ghrelin and markers of inflammation. Remember how psoriasis triggers inflammation that increases risk of heart disease (see p. 28)? Well, evidently, just 30 days of a UPF diet does the same. However, the most daunting results were seen in his MRI scan which showed his brain had literally formed new connections between his appetite centres and his reward pathways. The centre that drives addictive behaviour was whispering sweet nothings to the area regulating appetite – the scan literally demonstrated how his hedonic hunger was being ramped up. After just one month of eating UPFs, Van Tulleken was able to alter his biology to behave like that of someone living with obesity, triggering abnormal appetite signals through both his hormones and even his brain. Just imagine what is happening to the average child in Britain who gets 70 per cent of their calories from UPFs. Again, as I keep saying, obesity is incredibly complex and this isn't the whole story – our genes also play an important role, and we will explore this soon, but the arrival of UPFs over the last 50 years explains part of why obesity is on the rise, despite our genes not changing.

GLUCOSE CONTROL

I hope I have convinced you that, despite appearances, our hunger signals are every bit as complex as our fullness pathways. Clearly, we have evolved to inhabit an infinitely complex vessel along with an army of non-human organisms who work with us to maintain harmony in the body. It's like the story of Goldilocks – it's about reaching a level that is *just* right, whether that's our body temperature, fluid balance or, indeed, our weight. When it works well, this vessel and its inhabitants – let's call it a 'body' for convenience – tinkers beautifully with appetite hormones and mechanisms, until it prompts the host to consume precisely the right amount of energy needed. When things run smoothly, weight is kept stable. Of course, for many of us these systems have been disrupted.

As well as the tightly controlled feedback loops already covered, there is one more measure our bodies rely on to warn us that our energy 'tank' is empty: glucose – or, more specifically, a drop in glucose. In a way, our blood sugar is like the emergency light on a dashboard telling us, 'Quick, eat something. *Now.*' This isn't something your body will let you ignore; if blood sugar drops dangerously low in 'hypoglycaemia', patients lose consciousness, have a seizure, enter a coma and eventually die. Understandably, the body takes this alarm very seriously and wants you to eat something to quickly replace the sugar. The problem is that how and what we eat has changed dramatically over the last few decades, let alone centuries. We simply didn't evolve to eat highly processed foods or refined sugar sources. In nature, sugar and carbohydrates are usually accompanied by fibre, which slows digestion and the speed at which we absorb the sugar into our blood. As far as our body is concerned, we're practically snorting the stuff. When we allow our blood sugar to shoot up rapidly, the body attempts to compensate with a quick explosion of insulin but, in all the excitement, it produces a bit more than we need. This rapidly drives sugar out of the blood and into our cells but this sudden drop in blood sugar panics your body. It's scared we might go into a coma or even die, so it desperately attempts to source more sugar in the best way it knows how: hunger won't quite do it because we're in a bit of a rush; instead, ghrelin spikes rapidly to make us *hangry*.

It's only in the last decade that we've even started to acknowledge that our blood sugar can influence appetite and eating habits. Relatively recent technology has allowed an explosion of research in this field. As mentioned previously, in the 2019 PREDICT 1 study, the use of a continuous glucose monitor (CGM) allowed us to see blood sugar at work in the 'real world'. This amazing bit of kit is like a laboratory condensed into a tiny device sitting on someone's arm, telling us what their blood sugar is 24 hours a day for 14 days. When you measure this against appetite and eating the results are fascinating: how the blood sugar dips two to three hours after a meal predicts hunger. What's more amazing is that blood-sugar control seems to influence our cravings: if you put people wearing CGMs into an MRI scanner and ask them to rate how much pictures of food make them want to eat, the brain lights up like a Christmas tree when blood sugar is dropping. Just a drop of 1.1mmol/L after a blood sugar spike made the craving centres of the brain glow when subjects saw pictures of high-calorie foods; unsurprisingly, a picture of broccoli didn't have the same effect.

The fact that a drop in blood sugar triggers ghrelin explains why certain foods paradoxically stimulate hunger *more* than fullness. Take a packet of crisps, for example: they spend enough time in your mouth to alert the pancreas to stimulate insulin but aren't chewed for long enough to promote fullness cues. They have very little fibre and are mostly made of simple starches, which the acid in your stomach takes no time to liquidise, so they don't stretch your stomach – another fullness stop sign we have skipped. A small amount of fat might trigger fullness for 30 minutes, but there is no protein to allow for long-lasting satiety. Finally, because the stomach liquidised them so quickly, they shoot into the intestines like a fireman's hose, meaning they are then *rapidly* absorbed into the bloodstream. A big blood sugar spike is followed by a rapid fall. Your body then panics and the dashboard starts blinking, warning you to feel *hangry*. Sound familiar at all? Endocrinologist Dr Saira Hameed describes this as eating 'packaged hunger' in her book *The Full Diet* and counsels her patients to consider what they are eating in terms of hormones: will it trigger fullness or are you just eating more hunger?

Ready for another plot twist? Remember our cephalic-phase insulin release? Just the presence of flavour on your tongue can cause an independent insulin spike, even if no calories are involved (p. 63). Well, bizarrely, this means you actually drop your blood sugar and stimulate ghrelin! We see this with artificial sweeteners; not only is a sugar-free diet drink putting you into a fat-storing state, it's also priming you to feel *ravenous*, and specifically for sweet, hyper-palatable foods. In fact, the huge irony is that artificial sweeteners probably increase your risk of diabetes, weight gain and all-cause mortality. So really, much of the food you eat won't make you full but instead you are eating a trigger for more hunger. As I mentioned earlier, food really isn't just a fuel: it is perceived as a language by your body and you might be speaking the wrong one.

Ultimately, if you think what, when and how you eat is entirely under your conscious control, think again. We are the inhabitants of amazing engineering, all geared towards keeping us alive – the systems just aren't working in our current environment. Our body didn't evolve counting calories as they came in – instead it assumes more energy is coming if food takes longer to chew and stretches the stomach for a length of time. Protein, fat and fibre talk to our body and microbiome via hormones to make us feel full. We have long assumed ignoring hunger was the only way to lose weight, but the opposite is true! If you turn to traditional recipes, using wholefood ingredients, they will work *with* your body's inbuilt 'thermostat'. You will stop eating when you have had enough. UPFs and our irregular eating habits confuse our biology and overwork our digestive system. Not only does this increase your risk of well-known diseases like type 2 diabetes, it can also trigger vague symptoms we struggle to diagnose like indigestion. But the good news is we absolutely can change our biology and, better than that: I can show you how. Next, we'll explore how you can alter the way your body processes energy. Importantly, food is not something that needs to be restricted – instead, it actually just needs to be choreographed. Time it well and you can literally realign many of the intricate circadian rhythms of your body; when they're finally synchronised, the downstream consequences on your health are astounding!

Appetite: Key points

1) It feels almost impossible to eat when your body tells you it is full. We see this in cancer patients, Ozempic use, gastric-bypass surgery and, in my odd case, even altitude sickness. The fact that we sometimes eat more than we require is not the issue at hand: we need to understand why.

2) We now bypass many of our satiety cues, but can optimise them by chewing slowly and eating protein, fat and fibre with each meal.

3) Supporting a healthy microbiome by eating at least 30 plants a week helps to stimulate satiety hormones appropriately.

4) Your hunger hormone, ghrelin, has a predictable circadian rhythm which you can exert control over. Ghrelin only lasts in the bloodstream for 20–30 minutes, meaning the sensation of hunger will quickly disappear while fasting.

5) Ghrelin is heavily influenced by poor sleep and chronic stress. This can drive hedonic or 'pleasure' eating, which triggers a drug-like effect in the brain. Hedonic hunger is exacerbated by UPFs, which can rewire your brain's pleasure and appetite centres.

6) Erratic blood sugar spikes can trigger ghrelin, causing extreme hunger or 'hanger'. This allows food to stimulate more hunger, not less, even if it has zero calories.

CHAPTER 4

CAN WE CHANGE OUR BIOLOGY?

A new global Ipsos study has found that, at any given moment, 45 per cent of people around the world are on a diet. In fact, the diet industry has been worth billions for most of my life but something has recently changed: we now have 'fitfluencers'. Over the last few years influencers have shaken up the world of marketing beyond belief – if you add a real-life story to a product or idea, people can't stop buying it! As long as they are thin and toned, they can charge anywhere between $500 (£400) and $20,000 (£16,000) for a single sponsored post. Having a following is now synonymous with power. Children no longer want to be firemen or ballerinas when they grow up: they want to be TikTok stars. And who can blame them? It takes so little to win over an audience who believe weight is entirely under the individual's control: the fitfluencer implies they deserve 100 per cent of the credit for their appearance and offers you 100 per cent of the blame for yours. Like me, you might become transfixed by this apparent expert: they may have no academic credentials, but they are at least an expert on their own body. All you need to do is copy them.

Of course, it's not that simple because they have conveniently ignored the astonishing impact of their completely unique microbiome and genes. Your gut bugs can dramatically influence your weight as can your insulin and cortisol. How you eat is governed by your appetite hormones which, in turn, can also be influenced by your personalised microbiome. Fitfluencers would be worth less money if they pointed out this nuance – luckily for you, I'll do it for them. We will navigate genetics more in the next chapter, but for now, I want to explore the very premise of dieting – a practice rooted in flawed 'science'.

Traditional 'diets' are scientifically flawed

As we saw in previous chapters, the human body clearly has magnificent engineering with ingenious software, wired to drive behaviours we've always assumed were conscious decisions. Your 'choice' of what, when and how to eat is being manipulated by your microbiome, hormones, brain pleasure pathways and even social cues. If someone offers you food as a polite and friendly gesture, refusing it inherently feels rude. As a child, you might not even be allowed to refuse food because caregivers will demand that you finish your plate, even if you are full. And so you learn to ignore satiety signals. Traditional diets ignore the body's amazing complexity and ask you to override your biology through sheer force. Evolution simply fights back. In fact, strict dieting is such an aggressive insult to our biology that our body will compensate over time. Scared of losing its fat stores, it learns to hang on even tighter meaning people who diet regularly end up weighing more than those who don't!

Twins provide perfect human experiments to test this on. In 2012, a Finnish study looked at 4,129 individual twins where one had been a lifelong dieter and the other had not. You would assume the twin conscientiously trying to lose weight would be thinner than their sibling, but after 25 years, they actually weighed more. The identical twins who dieted were on average 0.4kg heavier than their non-dieting twin, while in non-identical twins the difference was 2.2kg (BMI 1.7). So, let's say you have spent several decades dieting on and off. Now imagine you had long-lost siblings who shared either half or all your DNA – having never been on a diet, they would both weigh less than you. This wasn't a fluke; other studies have demonstrated the same results: people who intentionally restrict food are more likely to gain weight in the long run than those who don't. But to announce 'diets don't work' tends to ruffle people's feathers because we all know someone who *did* lose weight. And of course, an army of fitfluencers appear to be living proof, and they will show you precisely how they restrict food to create a 'calorie deficit' – evidence enough that willpower is all it takes, right? But each person's body is incredibly unique: to compare your biology to someone else's is futile and meaningless. If you look at a systematic review of the diet studies we have, fewer than 1 in 6 people maintain a 10 per cent weight loss for more than 12 months. For everyone else, evolution fights back.

How does our biology protect fat stores?

It's important to remember when our bodies were 'designed': 300,000 years have fine-tuned our genes to keep us alive in spite of adversity. Our ancestors were faced with famines and extreme starvation but managed to survive because the human body is amazingly resilient and knows how to compensate. If you starve yourself, the body doesn't recognise or, frankly, care whether this is intentional on your part: all it cares about is keeping you alive in what it perceives as a famine. The first thing it will do is ramp up your appetite and alter your emotions around food. If you start to lose fat, the fat cells will produce less leptin, which means you have less background fullness. It turns out, this is actually leptin's main job: its evolutionary value wasn't to stop us eating, it was to warn us when fat stores were dropping and send us an explosive firework of a message to eat. That's not all diets do to appetite hormones. If this were a war in the fight to protect energy stores, I like to think of ghrelin as a ferocious warrior who shows no mercy. Both a drop in leptin and a rise in ghrelin will produce changes in MRI brain scans which directly demonstrate how weight loss makes the sight and thought of food highly emotional for us. Our hormones literally prompt us to pine for food like a lovesick teenager cruelly separated from their dreamboat.

Before long, persistent restriction will trigger you to binge, gorging food with animalistic fury: this is precisely what ghrelin and leptin are asking you to do! We can even see it in MRI scans and yet you might feel shame for this evolutionary reflex. Embarrassed by what you believe was a conscious choice, you respond by restricting food even more. But this aggression is met with a counterattack - the body, exhausted and crippled by fear of starvation or even death, has no choice: if you continue to restrict energy, it will simply be forced to reduce its energy losses. Fertility? Hair growth? Muscle mass? Bone strength? These are unnecessary luxuries the body is willing to forgo in the name of survival. This is why anorexic patients become emaciated, stop having periods, lose their hair and develop bone thinning. These bodily functions are considered a waste of energy. This is an aspect of our metabolism most people are unaware of; in fact, though we all talk about it, most people feel confused about what metabolism actually is. Put very simply, metabolism is just your body's overall energy use. Fitfluencers will tell you it is a constant number you can use to calculate your calorie deficit, but in reality, it is under your body's control. Remember how your hunger and fullness hormones unite to maintain a stable weight? Well, your metabolism is an important part of that equilibrium: it does everything it can to keep you at the same weight. If you restrict energy in, it will restrict energy out.

This is infuriating news for our fitfluencers who might smugly declare your body's energy is 'just the law of physics'. Apparently, you 'just' need to consume less than you burn. They don't understand that our body is more intelligent than a physics equation – in the war to win back energy stores, it has undercover tactics! Focusing just on the calories you are taking in is an excellent decoy to distract you while it reduces the total calories you burn. The most famous study to demonstrate this looked at contestants from a well-known American TV show called *The Biggest Loser*, in which obese participants provide so-called entertainment as viewers watch them being tormented by shouting coaches. (They are trained furiously in the gym with strict calorie restriction. Knowing what I know now, I'd describe this as nothing short of televised abuse and am embarrassed I ever watched it.) In the study, those who achieved their weight-loss goal were followed up by researchers for six years: almost all of them gained all the weight back and some gained more than they began with. You would instinctively assume they 'fell off the wagon' and returned to their old ways but they didn't. When researchers measured their metabolisms, they were burning 500 calories less than would be expected for their size; even six years after the extreme restriction, their frightened bodies were still reducing metabolism, terrified their fat stores might be stolen again.

The Biggest Loser study wasn't the only one to show long-lasting biological changes: in 2011, researchers put 50 overweight or obese participants on a highly restrictive diet for ten weeks to examine the effect on hormones. A whole year later, participants still had a change from baseline in their levels of leptin, PYY, CCK, insulin and ghrelin. That means one year later, their self-reported score for perceived hunger remained higher than it was before. One year! Dieting makes you feel hungrier for a *long time*. We also know it doesn't take long for cortisol levels to rise and thyroid levels to fall when you start a diet: your body is a highly intelligent army and has a lot of tricks up its sleeve, doing everything it can to keep the status quo. The question is: is there another way? Can we train the body to reroute and start using fat stores without fighting back? Can you lose weight without feeling like you are starving but actually feeling comfortably full? Is it possible to change your own biology? Of course it is.

What is metabolic flexibility?

On reflection, it's a bit strange that we feel hungry when our bodies have more than enough energy stored away. In a roundabout way, I've realised our energy system is a bit like my family's relationship with butter. We always have a butter dish on the counter so it's soft and spreadable, ready to use *now*. But, due to the butter-loving Danish side of my family, we keep a back-up bar in both the fridge and the freezer.* Now imagine every time the butter dish is empty, instead of using our extra stash, we just bought more – some for the counter and some for the fridge-freezer. It would be a strange and inefficient thing to do but that's precisely what many of us do in our own bodies! The issue is that we can't access what is stored because the door to the 'fridge-freezer' is stuck, so we rely on sourcing new energy. If you are 'metabolically flexible' you can effortlessly open that door and use your saved energy stores. Importantly, having this will reduce your appetite, boost your energy and protect you from disease. The good news is that I can teach you how to switch on this flexibility and it's easier than you might think.

So, what is it that's keeping the door to our energy stores stuck? Insulin. If the body has too much insulin around, the fat-storing switch is turned on. As you might recall, we can't burn and store fat at the same time – leaving the switch on means you are storing fat and can't access your energy stores. We know insulin spikes in the bloodstream after eating, which makes sense – you need a chance to absorb that energy into your cells. This can be stored as 'glycogen' in the muscle and liver, which is our body's 'fridge', and, just like cooled butter, you can use this relatively quickly. Once the fridge is full it has to go into the 'freezer', which is your fat tissue – just like frozen butter, this is harder to use. Being metabolically flexible means you can effortlessly access your glycogen and fat for energy when you need to. When you're not eating, insulin should fall in your bloodstream so you can open this door. However, for people living with obesity, even when they aren't eating and are in a 'fasted state', their insulin levels actually remain high. That switch is truly jammed, far too stiff for anyone to budge, no matter how hard they try. The trick is to 'flip the metabolic

___
* Danes really like butter.

switch' – an expression coined by Anton, et al. in their knock-out paper 'Flipping the metabolic switch: understanding and applying the health benefits of fasting'. They unpick the nitty-gritty science of how to finally loosen up the switch so you can enter fat burning again. If you learn to flip your switch, this can lead to not only weight loss but also reduced appetite and better energy as well as a reduced risk of cancer, heart disease, type 2 diabetes and brain diseases. It can even slow down how fast you age! Metabolic flexibility is something we should all want.

It turns out the key to retraining your body is the same as in comedy: it all comes down to timing. Because it's not just *what* you eat that counts but *when* you eat – or more precisely, when you *don't* eat. This employs a technique broadly described as intermittent fasting (IF). I will discuss how to apply this to your life in Part II, but first, as always, I want you to *value* the science. The key thing to know is that at some point between 12 and 36 hours of not eating, the body simply flips into its fat-burning mode. That's because, for most people, it takes about 12 hours to deplete their glycogen stores. For example, if it takes *you* 12 hours and you finish eating at 7pm, that means by 7am your glycogen 'fridge' is empty and you're now using fat from your 'freezer'. However, of course, this depends how many stores you have: more glycogen stores initially take longer to clear. When people first start IF, they might not enter fat burning for the first few days or even weeks if they are very overweight. This can be disheartening and they might think IF doesn't work, but it is working – they just can't see their glycogen stores reducing. The longer you persist, the smaller this initial 'fridge' storage becomes and eventually a 12 hour fast will 'flip your switch'. You will finally be able to efficiently open your freezer and use your fat stores.

There are many studies that demonstrate the amazing impact of IF, but one of the first was in 2012 and it completely baffled scientists at the time. Researchers took mice and let them essentially eat junk food, which was high in fat: one group was left to eat whenever they felt like it, while the other only had access to the food for an eight-hour stretch. They ate the same food, consuming the exact same number of calories. Amazingly, those that only had an eight-hour eating window were protected not just from obesity, but also avoided high insulin, fatty-liver disease and inflammation; they also had better motor coordination and activated chemical pathways associated with longevity.* The scientific community was in uproar by this preposterous and clearly 'fake' outcome which defied everything we knew to be true. In response, the experiment was repeated over and over again: each time with the same result. Why does this strange phenomenon happen? Because, remember, every part of the body has its own circadian rhythm – from our sleep hormones to our stomach acid, they follow their own rhythm, guided by the master clock in your brain. Each hormone and digestive enzyme tries to play a symphony in time to the life you live. If you simply close your eating window appropriately, you give the body time to rehearse properly. For example, insulin works best earlier in the day for most of us – that's why late-night eating is an inefficient use of your body. It asks your pancreas to pump out *extra* insulin it hadn't planned to give you, bringing more fat storing and insulin-resistance with it. The mice were allowing their bodies to capitalise on each system's circadian rhythm – rather than overworking them. That's why the health benefits go so far beyond weight loss!

Training your cells: The role of mitochondria

Metabolic flexibility also helps improve the chemical sequence involved in turning fuel into energy in your cells. If you studied biology at school, you might recall learning about

---

* By longevity pathways I mean they triggered signals in their bodies associated with living longer. Fasting prolonged their lives.

mitochondria, which act as the powerhouse of the cell. We eat energy the body can't use yet, so the cells run it through their mitochondria to produce other chemicals they *can* use. Memorising each chemical pathway was the bane of my life as a medical student and I won't put you (or myself) through the details. It is enough to understand that your cells receive sugar, protein or fat from food and, when you're not eating, the body generates them itself. For example, your liver can actually make its own sugar, which is why you don't crash into a coma from hypoglycaemia when you're asleep and not eating. Bizarrely enough, mitochondria *technically* aren't human, which feels less outlandish now that we understand the microbiome. In fact, they are ancient 'organelles' who somehow became stowaways in our cells. You don't even have DNA for your mitochondria as such – your mother's egg has its own set of stowaways waiting to jump into your cells next. This is why mitochondrial diseases can only be 'inherited' from your mother. Anyway, I digress. The point is, your mitochondria are sort of like pets in your home – not the same species, but still family. It is your responsibility to look after them – and many of us don't.

Imagine you bombard these mitochondria with more energy than they can reasonably exchange – they will feel overworked and stressed. Our modern way of eating often doesn't reflect the environment they evolved to deal with and it's taking its toll on them. It's a shame because these little non-human 'pets' we employ to exchange energy for us, humble as they seem, are actually directly responsible for our energy levels, risk of disease and, most importantly, how fast we age. They are a secret fountain of youth, and though they don't command the spotlight, they are secretly the stars of the show. Ladies and gentlemen, no one is talking about them, but the most exciting thing is that mitochondria are where your body and mind meet. And I know I've said it before, but this time I really mean it: *this* is where things start to get *really* interesting.

What happens when we overwhelm our mitochondria?

Each cell in the body contains thousands of mitochondria and, because they aren't human, these mitochondria contain their own DNA (called mtDNA).* As we have seen, one of their main jobs is to convert sugar into energy for us. Honestly, this is a *dramatic* oversimplification! Whole textbooks have been written on how we metabolise several other energy sources but, for simplicity, I will focus on the idea of sugar. Just know that there are many types of sugar and anything you eat that isn't pure fat or protein arrives in your bloodstream as a sugar. So by the time energy from foods like pasta, rice or bread have reached your mitochondria, it will all be in the form of sugar. For several reasons, many of us send our mitochondria far more sugar than they evolved to deal with and they're feeling the pressure. This burden of work and its downstream consequences are explored in a fascinating theory called allostatic load: 'allostasis' is a body Goldilocks would approve of, in which everything is harmonious, balanced and *just right*. Put that system under stress and it will cumulatively increase your risk of disease – this state is called 'allostatic load'. If you inject too much sugar, too quickly, too frequently and for too long into your bloodstream this will overwhelm your mitochondria – and what you eat is part of this. But there's something else, other than eating, which makes your body shoot sugar into the bloodstream: cortisol – insulin's second in command.†

As we saw in Chapter 2, brief stress is fine: your body is giving you the sugar you need *now* to run away from the tiger.

------

* It's thought at some stage during our evolution mitochondria were probably a type of bacteria which bumped into another cell – the two got on so well they decided to stay together, intimately evolving to rub each other's backs.

† Cortisol: this is another oversimplification. There are other stress signals (catecholamines and glucocorticoids) involved but for ease I will use 'cortisol' as my main 'character' and umbrella term for stress chemicals.

But if it is chronic, it consistently spikes higher blood-sugar levels. In other words, chronically raised cortisol will constantly send your mitochondria too much work and, with time, they will burn out. Cortisol can also bind to receptors on the mitochondria and bully them directly, stressing them even more. The first thing our stressed mitochondria do is send off too many reactive oxygen species (ROS) or 'free radicals'. These are dangerous little 'bullets' we all produce; a small number are manageable and our bodies can 'neutralise' them; however, left to roam free, they cause a lot of damage through what we call oxidative stress. Fiddling with our own DNA and bumping aggressively into our cells, they slowly damage the body, trigger inflammation and switch on disease. This process speeds up ageing and promotes dementia, heart failure, cancer and type 2 diabetes. And as this stress accumulates, we see changes in mitochondria's mtDNA, which is one predictor of how fast we age! We know mtDNA damage builds with years, but this can happen at different rates. That's why we now distinguish 'biological age' from 'chronological age': many of us simply have cells and mtDNA that look much older than our years. Put bluntly: we don't all age at the same rate. Amazingly, oxidative stress like this can alter our mtDNA and speed ageing up in both diabetes *and* chronic psychological stress – that's because high blood sugar and cortisol both upset our mitochondria. The second predictor of how fast we age is the length of our telomeres – these are sections of our DNA. If they shorten faster that means you are ageing faster. Cumulative mtDNA damage, ROS and oxidative stress all speed up this process. In other words, constantly spiking blood sugar whether through food or stress literally shortens your life.

As I said before these 'pets' in your cells are the body and mind's meeting point: they are where psychological and physical stress collide. If you are under chronic psychological stress this pushes up your blood sugar and also directly upsets your mitochondria: both will shorten your life. Strangely, mitochondria weren't a big topic of conversation at medical school. I vaguely remember needing to memorise (and then promptly forget) a list of vanishingly rare mitochondrial diseases; to date, I have only met one patient with inherited mitochondrial dysfunction. But, in reality, mitochondrial dysfunction is something I see every day: it is seen in diabetes, heart disease, cancer, dementia, Parkinson's and autism. What's even more interesting is that mitochondrial dysfunction appears to be implicated in poorly understood conditions like fibromyalgia, long Covid and other post-infectious fatigue syndromes like myalgic encephalomyelitis (ME) or chronic-fatigue syndrome (CFS). We now know viruses like Epstein-Barr and Covid-19 can upset mitochondria. Fibromyalgia, a condition which causes fatigue and widespread muscular pains, is classically triggered by psychological trauma. Sadly, when a condition is linked to a life stress, the medical community can sometimes be dismissive, rolling their eyes at yet another condition that's apparently just 'in your head'. But given the direct impact cortisol has on mitochondria, have we simply been looking in the wrong place? The pain isn't imagined in someone's mind; a traumatic life event primes their subconscious to assume it is constantly in danger and drives chronically raised cortisol. Subsequent mitochondrial damage triggers their very real symptoms. We know psychological stress also increases risk of heart disease for the same reason, but no one has ever rolled their eyes at a heart attack.

Though they were skimmed over in medical school, mitochondria are taking centre stage in what we now understand, not just about disease, but about health. If they aren't happy, they can drive oxidative stress and chronic inflammation with many downstream complications. If you live a chronically stressful life and overwhelm your mitochondria with too much sugar you will simply age faster. I've said it before and I'll say it again: you do not want to get on cortisol's bad side.

Time-restricted eating (TRE)

Intermittent fasting (IF) is something we all do every day: for six to ten hours or so a night we all voluntarily lose consciousness and don't eat anything. Patients are often asked to fast before a blood test or even an operation and no one bats an eye. In Spain, France and Italy over a third of the population skip breakfast thus extending their fast even longer. However, many people feel very anxious about fasting – it has been drilled into us that breakfast is 'the most important meal of the day'. I was taught it was the main thing 'revving' up my metabolism and skipping it would make me eat more later and gain weight. Cultural 'wisdom' like this seeps so deeply into our 'knowledge' that no one questions it. But where did it come from?

Some of these ideas came from poor-quality, small-scale studies of people living with obesity, which point out an association between not eating breakfast and gaining weight. However, there are plenty of associations which don't reflect a cause-and-effect relationship. For example, we might notice that people who eat at Michelin-star restaurants have better health outcomes than people who don't. An influencer could start to promote a 'Michelin diet', encouraging people to eat elaborate seven-course meals with a wine flight pairing as a way to live longer. But does the health improvement come from the Michelin-star food or, just maybe, could it be that people who can afford Michelin-star restaurants can also afford better healthcare, gym memberships, good-quality food and cortisol-dropping activities? I'm not knocking Michelin-star cuisine – this is just an example of the flawed logic we can take from bad science. Not every association we see in science has a cause and effect – sometimes they coincide for other reasons.

Luckily, we have lots of statistically meaningful research out there and many studies show no effect on total calories consumed if skipping breakfast; in fact, they show a slight drop in calories, as well as weight loss. Increasingly, knowing what we do about our 'metabolic switch', narrowing our eating window fits with so much of the body's evolutionary engineering. Studies suggest hunter-gatherers regularly had long periods without food and wild mammals have biology geared up to do the same. Wolves might eat once or twice a week; the only way they can survive is to be metabolically flexible. Importantly, in a fasted state they need sharp brains to be able to coordinate a hunt with their pack. Fasting doesn't hinder brain function, it fuels it; and humans see similar benefits too. I am not proposing that we should eat like wolves – they simply serve as an amazing example of metabolic flexibility at work and reflect the evolutionary advantage it once gave us when we were either hunting or hunted. By letting the body use its 'fridge-freezer stores' appropriately, it wastes less time searching for excess energy. When you stop wasting time inefficiently sourcing fuel you don't need, it enables pathways that will improve brain function, prolong your life and prevent disease. Time restricted eating (TRE) is a form of intermittent fasting and is the only type I personally use. As we saw with the mouse study earlier, it simply narrows down the window of time when we eat. The mice had an 8-hour window, but many people also use a 10- or 12-hour window depending on their situation. It can be a powerful tool for weight loss but even where people don't lose weight, studies show they still boost their microbiome and reduce their risk of metabolic syndrome, type 2 diabetes, cancer and cognitive decline while also slowing down ageing. Let's take a closer look at some of these amazing benefits.

REDUCED HUNGER

You might recall from the circadian release of ghrelin study (see p. 68) that our hunger hormone does not spike persistently when we aren't eating. Think of those wolves: if they felt ravenous all the time they wouldn't have the brain space to focus on their next hunt. It makes no sense to constantly feel hungry. You might have memories of feeling unbearably famished and recall that the longer it went on, the worse you felt. I have had these experiences countless times but, after trialling a continuous glucose monitor (CGM), I realised they always coincided with erratic and even slightly low blood sugar after something I ate. Blood sugar generally doesn't behave like this during a prolonged fast because it is being steadily produced by your own body. If you are 'hangry', in my experience, this is almost always triggered by 'packaged hunger': you ate something that caused an uncontrolled blood sugar spike, insulin then over-reacted, making the blood sugar plummet, followed by a spike in ghrelin. You will feel dizzy, shaky and unwell until you eat something.* If you feel like this you *should* eat – the trick is to avoid it happening in the first place, which we will cover in Part II. I have rarely experienced this feeling in the morning, but only when my dinner triggered erratic blood sugar – again, it was what I ate that caused it. My point is that fasting is not the cause of these symptoms: it's not what you didn't eat but what you did eat that has made you feel uncontrollably hungry.

I know for a fact – not just through science, but through my lived experience – that time-restricted eating progressively dampens down your appetite signals. As someone who used to experience constant 'hanger', I now just get a calm, peckish feeling around 12pm and 7pm because that is when I usually eat. I remember once I didn't have access to food for 24 hours while travelling; in the past, this would have been an unbearable torture. But my peckish wave passed after 20–30 minutes, my energy was stable and my mind sharp. Why? Because after just a few months of time-restricted eating, I'd trained my body and mitochondria to become metabolically flexible. As we saw in the circadian ghrelin study (see p. 68), my own ghrelin has

---

* A drop in blood sugar (hypoglycaemia) can be dangerous, and more severe forms are experienced in rare conditions like insulinomas (insulin-secreting tumours). People with diabetes who are on medication that affect insulin can also experience dangerous hypos. For the rest of us, mini-hypos are triggered by the food we eat and being metabolically inflexible.

simply realigned to spike according to my new behaviour. It takes about 12 weeks for this to happen because that's how long a change in behaviour takes to alter gene expression – we call this 'epigenetics'.

Amazingly, the genes you are born with are simply an instrument, but you are the musician – it might take a while to learn a new song but, with practice, you can easily play it. That's why our environment dramatically affects our risk of diseases coded for in our genes and why identical twins, who are genetic clones of each other, can get different diseases. One of them turned the gene on while the other didn't. But I digress. Your genes code for things other than disease and the timed release of ghrelin is just one of those things. The key, again, is that it takes time for a new behaviour to alter your biology, so if you are changing your eating, sleep or exercise, be mindful that it takes three months of discipline – afterwards, it should become easy.

Why does appetite gradually reduce when you get into the habit of fasting? It's one thing to synchronise *when* your ghrelin spikes over a few months but, within a few days, you will find even the amount of ghrelin produced will reduce! When you start TRE it downregulates your brain's appetite centre in the hypothalamus. In fact, it can take as little as four days for TRE to tell your hypothalamus to reduce ghrelin and increase leptin. Remember how I felt in Peru? By decreasing your hunger hormone and increasing your background satiety, without thinking about it, you will simply want to eat less. *Four days!* In no time you are literally manipulating the appetite hormones which affect your inbuilt reflex to eat – this achieves the *opposite* effect of dieting. But that's not all TRE does to your brain ...

IMPROVED BRAIN HEALTH

So once you have flipped your switch and start burning fat as fuel, what happens? Whole textbooks have been written on the subject but the only thing you need to know is that our mitochondria can exchange more than one energy source; when they run out of sugar they simply convert fat to 'ketones', which your brain happens to love. It's the equivalent of serving wine all night and then swapping to champagne; rather than feeling short-changed when fasting, the brain just got an upgrade. This is why people will describe amazing concentration and clarity during a fast; it's also why I recommend patients see me in my morning clinic before I break my fast at lunch. My mind feels much sharper. These ketones also reduce brain inflammation and improve nerve repair, which is why ketogenic diets are still prescribed for patients with poorly controlled epilepsy – feed the brain its version of champagne, and you prevent seizures.

TRE also promotes new nerve growth and connections which increase something called neuroplasticity. Until recently, we believed the brain stopped developing in early adulthood, but we were wrong. It continues to be a little bit malleable for life, and by increasing a protein called BDNF*, fasting promotes this. For this reason, fasting results in less depression, better memory and reduces your risk of neurodegenerative diseases like Alzheimer's and Parkinson's. In fact, low BDNF is linked to depression and, like fasting, some antidepressants work by increasing it. Bizarrely, our fullness hormone CCK can get into the brain and, in high numbers, can drive anxiety. Time-restricted eating helps by containing CCK to manageable levels, thus reducing one mechanism for anxiety. So not only does fasting help you concentrate in the moment – in the long term, it is also thought to boost memory, prevent neurodegenerative diseases like dementia and even make you happier and less anxious. Sounds pretty good so far, doesn't it?

GUT HEALTH

The gut is one part of the body in desperate need of rest that we just don't give it with our modern way of eating. If mice are left

---

* Brain-derived neurotropic factor (BDNF) plays an important role in the development and function of a healthy brain and nervous system.

to eat all day, they develop features of IBS but if you narrow their eating window, this spontaneously resolves. This might surprise us, but it shouldn't – the constant, repetitive stream of food most people expose their digestive systems to leaves very little time for rest and recovery. The staff are being overworked and kept late against their will – so don't expect good service.

Every part of your digestive system has a circadian rhythm – even your saliva prefers production during the day and for a reason: it helps to neutralise acid in your stomach (which, incidentally, also favours daytime production). So if you eat late at night, you ask your stomach to produce more acid but get less saliva. Food then sits in your stomach for two to five hours. Ideally, the body prefers you to be vertical for this part of digestion (for fairly obvious reasons). However, if you eat shortly before going to bed and lie flat with increased acid levels, it's no wonder you might get heartburn. Any laxity in the door between your gullet and stomach invites that acid backwards up the gullet, and voilà. There is limited research in the area, but plenty of anecdotal evidence that TRE is a powerful tool to reverse the cause of heartburn, but instead, we pump people with acid-reducing medication. This doesn't fix the cause or even stop stomach contents going into the gullet – they're just less acidic, so you don't feel the burning. But if you stay on these tablets for a long time you *do* damage your microbiome and, therefore, increase your risk of gut infections like C. *diff* (see p. 21). I am not suggesting we should stop prescribing acid blockers; there are many examples where they can even be life-saving. But I do think lifestyle tricks like TRE should be tried at the same time; why blindly treat a symptom when you can remove the cause?

Speaking of your microbiome, it needs rest too, and fasting seems to promote its diversity. The main bug that loves fasting is called *Akkermansia* – it feeds off the mucous lining of your gut and releases by-products to support the gut wall and other friendly bacteria. In essence, it cheers up your good bugs and also protects you from leaky-gut syndrome which, you might recall from Chapter 1, is not a good thing. Your gut wall hosts most of your immune system, so allowing it to essentially leak is an excellent way to trigger all kinds of diseases, including poorly understood ones like IBS. Fasting can use *Akkermansia* as an ally to reverse this. This might be why people notice an improvement in rheumatoid-arthritis pain during Ramadan and why their markers of inflammatory chemicals improve too. These chemicals are involved in promoting asthma, allergies, autoimmune disease and inflammatory bowel disease – all conditions which also improve with fasting. If you give your bugs time to rest and repair a leaky gut, the number of symptoms and diseases you can potentially prevent are hard to count.

Have you ever wondered what decides how efficiently your bowel pushes food through? It is achieved through a rhythmic squeezing, generated by an electrical current called the migratory motor complex (MMC). This too has a circadian rhythm. Essentially, electricity courses through the bowel like a Mexican wave of football fans. Like much of the digestive system, this also calms down at night because the gut assumes its 'shift' should be ending. However, if you do some late-night snacking, the food will move slowly through a sluggish bowel or might even move backwards, in the wrong direction. As a result, the bowel wall cramps, causing stomach pains.

It takes our MMC about three to four hours to complete one full cycle; if you eat mid-cycle, it stops the wave, resets and starts again from the top. This means, for people who like to regularly snack in between meals, they are repeatedly interrupting their MMC: the partly digested food cannot transit efficiently, leaving longer for fermentation and more gas production. People are then surprised when they have constipation, bloating and painful cramping. Again, we might give medication to mask the symptoms, but doctors can't treat the cause – only the patient can do that. Time-restricted eating with predictable mealtimes lets your MMC, microbiome and every other choreographed digesting event do their thing in a rhythm that suits them best.

ATHLETIC PROWESS

I don't mean to keep poking fun at the fitness industry – I'm sure most fitfluencers believe they are helping people with their lifestyle advice. But in medicine there's a saying which haunts every clinician: 'you don't know what you don't know'. We all have blind spots in our knowledge – not only is that okay, it's human! If you don't know something it's not a problem – I won't prescribe a medication I'm not familiar with, for example. However, when you are completely unaware of a fact (as opposed to just unsure), that's when you can make a *big* mistake. Many fitfluencers simply don't know what they don't know, and their mistakes aren't completely harmless: we are seeing a wave of devastating eating disorders sweep the world and I feel our fitfluencer culture fuels some of this. Ironically, contrary to what many fitfluencers suggest, persistent calorie restriction can actually hinder athletic performance.

This might come as a surprise but TRE could directly help you to gain muscle. Hugh Jackman famously used an eight-hour eating window in preparation for his role as the Wolverine – why? Because TRE does two things: firstly, it makes you metabolically flexible and therefore brilliant at endurance sports by allowing you to efficiently access your energy stores. But, amazingly, it also specifically activates muscle building. This is partly because of metabolic flexibility: in obesity, where insulin keeps the 'freezer door' closed, the liver is forced to use protein parts to produce new glucose (a process called gluconeogenesis). This is fine if it only happens for a few hours a day but, if you're metabolically inflexible, it happens 24/7. Tragically, this means you lose your muscle mass – your body is essentially eating itself, breaking down the protein in muscle to make glucose because it's not metabolically flexible enough to access its fat stores. Think about that carefully: rather than using the energy you have specifically stored away, your body is unable to access it so uses your muscle instead – this is something evolution only planned to do in cases of severe starvation! But we simply didn't evolve with the constant insulin spikes modern eating now brings – it's causing a huge glitch in our design.

Most people assume obesity is simply the presence of too much fat but, importantly, it is also the absence of enough muscle. We have massively underestimated the role of muscle in the body, and I will explore it more in Part II – but for now, just know that losing it is devastating for your health. With TRE, you flip the switch and reduce your need for gluconeogenesis – instead, protein can be used to build muscle. In other words, you no longer break down your own muscle as fuel. In traditional diets, calorie restriction might seem to produce excellent weight loss at the beginning, but this is because, as well as losing fat, you are losing muscle. That's why a number on the scale isn't necessarily a helpful reflection of health being gained: if maintaining muscle mass is your goal, your waist circumference can reduce while your weight stays static or even goes up. Instead of weighing myself I simply use a tape measure for this reason. Interestingly, TRE even has another clever way of building muscle: it stimulates the release of growth hormone. In a way this is your body's own perfectly legal steroid which builds muscle, bone strength and promotes wound healing. Body builders in the know are using TRE instead of doping – if you could sell all its benefits, it would make you millions. Luckily fasting is free.

PROTECTS AGAINST CANCER

In 2007, the World Health Organization declared shift work a 'probable' carcinogen, likely due to a disruption of our circadian rhythm. We will explore how sleep disruption affects health in Part II – but remember: when we eat also affects our circadian rhythm. One amazing study looked back at women's diet habits and found those who had a regular eating schedule and finished eating within an 11-hour window were significantly protected from breast cancer. That means if breakfast was at 7.30am they simply ate nothing after 6.30pm – this way of eating is hardly extreme and actually reflects how most families ate before the 1980s.

Why is fasting protective? A whole book could be written on the subject but, at the crux of it, aligning meals with the rhythm of your body allows for allostasis: the wonderful state of harmony in your body. When not under stress, mitochondria won't fire off free radicals driving inflammation and disrupting genes; the microbiome will be on board too – less inflammation from both parties means your immune system can actually detect and remove tumour cells appropriately. Even after developing cancer, fasting appears to reduce the speed of tumour growth and improves response to chemotherapy – all because you are letting your body protect you the way it was designed to do.

CHOLESTEROL AND HEART DISEASE

To any younger readers who might think this is a topic only relevant later in life, think again. Heart disease takes decades to progress and the artery plaque that might one day kill you starts to develop when you're a teenager. By reining in your insulin, TRE protects your body from becoming resistant to it. It feels almost impossible to convey how valuable this is in a sentence, but simply put: being resistant to insulin* is an excellent way to shorten your life and promote disease. We see just one example in heart disease – a study found controlling insulin resistance between the ages of 20 and 30 reduced men's risk of

---

* Remember 'insulin resistance' simply means your cells aren't responding well to insulin anymore, which means your body needs to produce *more* insulin. Eventually, this makes your 'freezer door' to fat stores stiff and hard to open. Type 2 diabetes is one example of a condition driven by insulin resistance, but it has a genetic component meaning you can be insulin resistant and not have type 2 diabetes. Obesity and polycystic ovary syndrome (PCOS) are other conditions linked to insulin resistance.

a heart attack by 42 per cent. In fact, the researchers concluded that of all risk factors, insulin resistance was the most important cause of coronary artery disease. Imagine if people in their 20s knew this and how much future disease we could avoid.

Part of the reason for this is because of our precious blood vessels – remember we want them to work properly to deliver oxygen and nutrients to all our organs. Insulin resistance can inflame these blood vessels and potentially narrow them but it does something else too: for a number of reasons it can influence the health of your cholesterol and blood fat, which affect your risk of heart disease. Cholesterol is a beast I will tackle fully in Part II – it has been entirely misunderstood and nothing confuses my patients more! TRE, believe it or not, is an excellent trick for optimising it. This is partly because it boosts your microbiome, which is able to improve cholesterol, but it also helps you to remove excess cholesterol in your stool. As it turns out, bile acid (a digesting tonic made in the liver) is partly made of cholesterol, and TRE makes our liver and gut more efficient at excreting it into our bowel movements. We also see a significant improvement in blood pressure because, for several elaborate reasons, insulin resistance pushes it up. In fact, one study showed an eating window of six hours was just as effective as blood-pressure medication. Not only does this avoid side effects, drug interactions and regular blood tests to make sure the tablets aren't upsetting your kidneys, this free intervention comes with many added health benefits. It's further evidence that if the pharmaceutical industry could bottle TRE, it would be priceless.

LONGEVITY

The idea that there are pathways in the body that predict how fast we will age is relatively new – the fact that we have any control over this is completely profound. Not to sound like a broken record, but I was not taught anything about this at medical school – traditional medical degrees primarily teach you about disease. Optimising health, preventing disease and prolonging life are not a big part of the curriculum but maybe they should be.

In 2016, a Japanese scientist called Dr Yoshinori Ohsumi won the Nobel Prize in Medicine for demonstrating a life-prolonging mechanism triggered by fasting: 'autophagy'. This term translates into 'self-eating', which is what our cells do in the absence of food; they simply reuse what they already have. Let's say you don't have money for a takeaway, so you eat left-overs from last night instead – you save money and time. It also helps to clean out your fridge. Well, autophagy does the same: any build-up of damaged organelles, proteins or oxidised parti-cles can be spring cleaned out of the cell, leaving it revitalised and better able to function. In other words, autophagy slows ageing and, if it becomes disrupted, this is linked to diseases like Parkinson's, type 2 diabetes and cancer, to name but a few. By activating autophagy, fasting protects you from disease and prolongs your life.

AND SO ON ...

It's surprisingly difficult to concisely summarise the health benefits of time-restricted eating because there are so many. It almost goes without saying that TRE is a powerful tool, not just for managing but reversing type 2 diabetes – you are simply retraining your body not to resist its own insulin anymore. The fact that type 2 diabetes is reversible is a relatively new concept which, just under a decade ago, no one was even talking about. And yet Dr Jason Fung has been reversing type 2 diabetes in his clinic for many years, simply by using intermittent fasting. Like so many who dare to do something different, he initially faced huge criticism for his techniques.

People don't like change, and if it's not printed in your local guidelines, you feel rogue, as a doctor, if you suggest a novel approach. Dr Unwin, a GP in Southport, England, has also tired of only treating diabetes with medication and prefers to reverse it with lifestyle. He put 51 per cent of all his diabetic patients into remission and, if they started his programme in the first year of diagnosis, this number went up to 77 per cent. His main focus is a low-carbohydrate diet, rather than fasting, but how it is achieved isn't the point: the fact that a busy, underfunded, NHS GP clinic can reverse disease with lifestyle is amazing. When I diagnose new type 2 diabetes, I tell patients I am not interested in treating the condition: my sole ambition is to get rid of it altogether.

All that said, I haven't really mentioned much about what most people are interested in: weight loss. That's because I consider it the least interesting benefit – a thinner body doesn't really compete with the cancer-fighting, immune-boosting and life-lengthening results TRE can achieve. But yes, for the vast majority, committing to long-term TRE will result in less fat and more muscle – what's more, it will eventually feel easy. But this isn't a diet book and weight loss isn't my goal: this is a book about health; losing weight is just a convenient side effect.

Now think back to the 45 per cent of people in the world currently on diets and imagine what they are going through. Unaware of their microbiome and the local currency of their hormones, instead they are paying with forced calorie restriction. It might work for a little while according to their scales, but the body will fight back for its energy stores by slowing metabolism and spiking hunger. Rather than wage war against their hunger hormones, metabolism and muscle mass, they could work *with* their bodies, not against them. More than that, promoting metabolic flexibility and respecting the circadian rhythm of the body lets it function as it should.

Ultimately, to know you can personally alter how fast your body will age and accumulate disease is so much more exciting than weight loss. I hope I am convincing you to *value* how truly powerful your lifestyle can be. As promised, I will introduce you to factors which are in your control (and those which are not). We all inherit some of our health in ways that might surprise you. Read on to find out how.

Change your biology: Key points

1) Traditional diets ignore our evolution and are based on flawed science. Strict calorie restriction forces your metabolism to slow down and, on average, people who diet regularly weigh more than those who don't.

2) Just like it is almost impossible to eat when your body tells you it is full, it is almost impossible not to eat when it is screaming for food. Binge eating is not a personal choice: it is an evolutionary reflex designed to protect your survival.

3) Insulin resistance blocks your ability to burn fat: time-restricted eating can reverse this by optimising metabolic flexibility and lubricating your fat burning on–off switch.

4) Mitochondria are valuable creatures living in your cells: exposing them to chronic stress and excessive sugar damages them, speeding up ageing and the accumulation of diseases.

5) Time-restricted eating reduces your appetite signals, optimises brain function/mental health, boosts athletic performance, reduces risk of cancer/heart disease/inflammatory conditions, boosts the microbiome and gut health, can reverse type 2 diabetes and also slows ageing. It would be worth trillions if drug companies could bottle it, but luckily for us it's completely free.

CHAPTER 5

OUR HERITAGE

Can we inherit obesity?

In the early 1950s, a British lady named Phoebe Kingsbury began a trend which would ripple through her family for generations to come: she acquired a taste for salad. In postwar England, vegetables were not a big part of anyone's menu; National Food Surveys (NFS) at the time suggest less than one fifth of respondents ate them regularly. Salad was more popular with some 40 per cent enjoying it in the summer months. But Phoebe liked salads so much that they became a permanent fixture with every evening meal, all year round. Soon enough, a dinner table without a salad was like a cat without a tail: not impossible, but definitely odd.

Phoebe was my great-grandmother, and though I'm not aware of a specific salad-ophile gene, I have certainly inherited her view on the subject. Her daughter unthinkingly served salad with every dinner too, and later so did *her* daughter – my mother. In my family, even Christmas dinner is incomplete without a large bowl of fresh, crunchy leaves. Growing up, 'Would you like some salad?' was always a rhetorical question because it was already on my plate before I had time to answer. It became so ingrained into my food culture that I still eat it almost every day, not out of obligation, but because I genuinely enjoy it. I don't think I inherited this through my genes, but it is definitely part of my heritage. And, as it turns out, our ancestors have passed on many other things we never even realised. From weight to our risk of disease, there are many risk factors decided for us long before we have any influence ourselves.

For centuries, a thin body has been an unwritten status symbol: whether we like it or not, being thin is rewarded in society. But this is based on a fundamental subconscious belief that we 'earn' the body we are in. Think about the automatic assumptions you make when you see someone who is thin. Now think of the knee-jerk impression you have of someone who is overweight. Either way, you might assume they 'deserve' it. But is this really absolute? You've seen the profound control our microbiome and hormones exert on us – have we been fooled? I am not proposing anything about health is black or white, and this book neither aims to blame nor console: I just want to open your mind so you can question the foundation of what you believe to be true. Part II will show you we absolutely *can* control many aspects of our health, but this shouldn't detract from those which we can't. Over the next two chapters, you will see just how much of who you are is decided for you. In this chapter we will look at how the genes you inherit from your parents can inform your weight. They act like a set of instructions for the body but we don't actually follow all of them! Importantly, genes can explain a lot, but not everything – your environment can alter how your body interprets and uses those instructions.

Squeezing into genes: Is weight genetic?

In 2023, an acclaimed obesity expert appeared on a *60 Minutes* interview and caused quite the stir by declaring obesity a 'genetic disease of the brain' which could not be treated by lifestyle. In the interview, Dr Fatima Cody Stanford explored metabolic compensation* and why so many now struggle to lose weight. 'But what about willpower?' asked the slender interviewer, taken aback by this notion, to which Dr Stanford promptly replied, 'Throw it out the window!'

---

* Remember this is where your body reduces metabolism to compensate for long-term calorie restriction.

Is there any truth in the premise that we can inherit our weight and, if so, why do people get so upset about this? The answer to this question is all about one thing: nuance. To imply that anything in human health is simple or 'just' caused by one thing completely undermines our brilliant biology. The body is awe inspiring – whole careers and books can be spent exploring just one of its many facets. So absolutely nothing about how your body came to be the size it is will be simple. Rates of obesity have sky-rocketed since the early 1980s, but our genes haven't changed; therefore, by definition, they cannot be the entire answer. But as we have already seen, not all our genes 'turn on'. Identical twins can develop different genetic diseases, like coeliac, for example; something in their life can switch the coeliac gene to 'on' mode in one twin, while it stays 'off' in the other. So while many other factors contribute to excess weight gain, yes, we do have genes that make us more vulnerable, and many of us lead lives which now switch them on.

My favourite study on genetic weight came out of Denmark in 1986. The fact that I am half Danish is only part of why I love it so much; the main reason is that the results were the opposite to what you might predict. Let's be honest, science can be dull at the best of times – who doesn't like a good plot twist? The study simply wanted to compare adopted children's weight to that of their adopted and biological parents. Which parents' weight predicted the child's weight more? The researchers discovered a baffling answer: there was virtually no correlation between a child's weight and that of their adoptive parents, but there was a very strong link to their biological parents: in other words, nature won.

Why does it surprise us so much that weight is decided by birth parents and hardly affected by adoptive parents? Because again, we have always thought body size is in our control; in fact, three out of four Americans still believe obesity is caused by a lack of willpower to control appetite and exercise. The limitation of the Danish study is that, though families all have their unique lifestyles, the overall environment in this small country is pretty similar and Danes have a strong, fairly coherent food culture. Although obesity rates in Denmark are now on the rise, it is less of a problem than in other countries, and data from the 1980s certainly won't reflect current trends. What we really need is an identical-twin study where each twin grew up in a different environment. Luckily, such an example does exist: in 2003, Chinese identical girls were accidentally separated at birth to Norwegian and American parents. Ten years later, they managed to reunite and were, well, identical – they had the same body shape and roughly weighed the same. The only difference was that the Norwegian twin was a few centimetres taller than her American sister, which is now a recognised phenomenon: a diet rich in ultra-processed foods (UPFs) stunts growth. It turns out that if you feed children artificially concocted food-like substances, depleted of natural nutrients, they don't grow as tall. For example, children in the UK are, on average, 7cm shorter than other European children who eat far fewer UPFs. Although our height is strongly affected by genes, environment influences it too. Sorry to point out the obvious here but we don't criticise someone for being short – just like weight, our height is decided by things in and out of our control. In fact, if you were to pluck any pair of identical twins off the street, do you know what the average difference in their weight is? Just 1kg. This is astounding! I fluctuate by 1kg in a day, yet these genetic clones live independent lives and their weight is almost identical. This makes it impossible to ignore the fact that genes absolutely *do* affect our weight.

It is estimated that, on average, 60–70 per cent of our weight is decided by genes, which can influence everything from appetite and food preferences to eating speed and how much we enjoy exercise. If you have a sweet tooth, 50 per cent of this seems to come down to genes; the rest is affected by your culture. Either way, a propensity for obesity is strongly linked to sugar-loving genes; and there's a dose response too: the more sugar-loving genes you have, the more you will weigh.

But it's not just our volume of body fat that genes can influence – even *where* you store it is highly genetic. In 1990, researchers decided to purposely overfeed a group of identical twins and found their weight distribution was mirrored perfectly. They seemed to put on muscle in the same places but also had a propensity for collecting fat in the same spots. This is part of why it is unhelpful to compare your body to that of a fitfluencer – you have different genes! Part of their six-pack could be from exercise but they might also genetically store less abdominal fat. I, on the other hand, store fat on my middle very easily but less so on my legs. It would be strange to praise me for achieving thin legs because, if you stand me next to my father, you'll see where they came from! In my case, I didn't 'earn' them at all. Of course, we do have some influence over our bodies but, unless you're looking at your identical twin, it's really not helpful to compare yourself with another individual.

Obesity genes

Are there specific genes that programme for full-blown morbid obesity? Well, yes. But the chance of you having one is pretty slim. I happened to meet a six-year-old boy in my clinic who was likely one of these rare cases. His mother was at her wits' end because her son was literally eating her out of house and home: it seemed he was incapable of feeling full. He frequently stole his much older siblings' food off their plates and would raid the fridge at all hours of the day. Even locking the doors couldn't stop him; anything vaguely edible was inhaled, whether it was dog food or even fished out of the bin. His mother was struggling to afford these demands and was doing a big food shop every other day. No amount of discipline could stop her child's odd behaviour and so, in desperation, she brought him to see me.

Having recently completed a research scholarship in childhood obesity, my ears pricked up. He looked slightly 'chubby', but his growth chart actually showed he was technically morbidly obese. If you think about it, we base our idea of obesity on adult bodies, but it presents differently in a child: they often don't look obese. For this reason, parents don't recognise it and neither do doctors. In my research I even came across a GP colleague who was baffled to hear his own children were technically obese, having always thought they simply had 'puppy fat'. But remember that unlike adults, children are losing a lot of energy to grow vertically – we therefore can't interpret their weight like ours. Instead, you need to anticipate what their adult weight will be like once the vertical growth stops. As part of my research, I sat in on a tertiary paediatric clinic reserved only for the most 'severe' cases of child obesity: these children were starting to get complications we normally only see in adults. Their blood tests showed evidence of fatty-liver disease and type 2 diabetes, which was unheard of a few decades ago. Amazingly, most of them didn't look 'obese' to me. They had simply been picked up by paediatricians, who were often seeing them for something unrelated to weight. In truth, most obese children are not flagged as such or given any formal health input. This is partly because there are limited services to support them but also because parents, teachers and doctors don't always notice if a child is morbidly obese.

As with adults, broaching the subject of weight is incredibly challenging when it comes to children. In fact, it is much harder because parents can take enormous offence. Sadly, I think this is only because of the misplaced stigma obesity still has. For so long it has simply been misunderstood, and my sincere hope in writing this book is that I can replace that stigma with knowledge. As a GP, if I notice a child is underweight on their growth chart, I can easily refer them for assessment without causing offence. I hope one day the same will be true at the other end of the growth chart: if recognised as a complex, multifaceted condition, childhood obesity could be identified and addressed in early life, preventing future complications. For now, I worry many clinicians don't refer these children because they don't want to offend the parents.

I referred the six-year-old boy to paediatrics to test his genes, but I never learned the outcome – I have my theories, though. My first is that his chromosome 15* wasn't working, causing a rare genetic condition called Prader-Willi syndrome. These children develop cognitive impairment and extreme hyperphagia (medical speak for overeating). But we're not talking about a cheeky splurge; the compulsion to eat is so extreme that there are many stories of individuals dying from severe bingeing. Their intestines are stretched enough to burst open (perforation) or they simply choke or inhale food into their lungs due to their rapid pace of eating. This genetic disease essentially interferes with hormones, lowering thyroid levels, increasing ghrelin (hunger hormone), lowering PYY (fullness hormone) and disrupting the brain's response to leptin, so they can't register background satiety signals. They don't feel hungry – they feel *famished*, and the feeling is there all the time.

My second theory is that the little boy may have had a very rare genetic leptin deficiency. Remember our fat cells produce leptin like a stock boy letting you know the inventory of energy already in storage? We already know the brain is less sensitive to leptin in obesity, but now imagine never receiving any at all. In 1997, scientists discovered a rare leptin-deficiency gene in two morbidly obese cousins. At just three years old, the younger cousin weighed 42kg. Amazingly, when the scientists injected him with leptin, his unrelenting appetite subsided and he gradually grew into a healthy weight. By the age of seven he was a slim 32kg and a normal height. This was a eureka moment at the time – scientists believed they had found the golden ticket to weight loss: leptin. Soon they started injecting it into everyone, whether they were obese or lean, but none of

---

* Each cell has 46 chromosomes that house our DNA. Essentially, one of these DNA 'packages' might have been abnormal, thus causing his extreme hunger.

them lost weight. Why? Because their leptin was working just fine – if anything, those struggling with weight had too much of it because, remember, it is produced by fat cells. If you have greater fat stores, you produce higher levels of leptin, but the longer your brain is exposed to high levels, the less it responds to them; just like we become resistant to insulin, we also become resistant to leptin. Injecting more insulin doesn't reverse insulin resistance and the same is true for leptin. Replacing leptin only works if you have this incredibly rare genetic deficiency.

My final theory actually ties into one of my favourite breeds of dog. Labradors technically have a genetic mutation which drives obesity, and a similar one is found in humans too. Anyone who has ever lived with a Labrador knows not to leave anything vaguely edible out unsupervised! The moment you leave the room they will eat it. No matter how much you've fed them, they are always game for more. Are they inherently weak-willed for having this extreme appetite? No, they simply have a deletion in their POMC gene, which means they are born with a brain that is less sensitive to leptin. It's just a genetic glitch.

In 1998, researchers in Berlin discovered a similar POMC mutation in a morbidly obese child – just like Labradors, his appetite was out of his control. A similar pattern is seen in a mutation of the MC_4R gene, which also blunts the brain's response to leptin, and up to 6 per cent of severely obese children have been found to have a change in this gene. In fact, we estimate 1 per cent of people with a BMI greater than 30 – that is, people living with obesity – have an MC_4R gene mutation. Importantly, that means 99 per cent of obese people do not have this gene. Having one mutated gene driving obesity is actually very rare. This means most people living with obesity do not have a specific disease for it such as Prader-Willi syndrome. But, even without a disease, the combined effect of all your genes can still be very powerful.

Interestingly, these 'obesity genes' were discovered several decades ago and yet many of us are taught nothing about them.

Most people, fortunately, don't have the rare conditions I've described – but that doesn't mean genes aren't important: how they influence weight is simply more nuanced. In reality, there are around 100 genes that code for weight; some help you stay slim and others help you gain weight – in truth, you have a mixture of *both*. Some people will have more genes that tend to promote weight gain with fewer that prevent it. Others have far more 'thin' genes and fewer obesity genes. Researchers have attempted to calculate your precise risk of obesity by averaging out all these genes, but it's futile. It would be impossible to precisely calculate risk because, as I've said before, genes are just a list of instructions: your environment decides how your body interprets them. Some genes are switched on; others aren't. To truly understand why some people gain weight more easily, we need to acknowledge their genes but, as well as that, we need to know what switches them on.

Even our individual response to specific foods can also partly be explained by genetics. Take amylase, for example. This is the enzyme we all use to break down carbohydrates into sugars – but did you know we each have between 2 and 30 different amylase coding genes? And the more you have, the better you are at stripping out every last calorie from starchy foods like pasta and bread. In essence, being 'more evolved', though it protected your ancestors from famines, now puts you at a disadvantage in our current food environment. Because if you have more of these genes, you will store more energy from starch than someone who has fewer. Here's the catch: this is only true if that individual is eating a high-carb diet. If you put everyone on a low-carb diet people with *more* genes have a lower BMI than people with less genes. Is one scenario better than the other? Well, if you take people with low and high levels of these genes and try both low- and high-carb diets, the question is which combination is most protective against weight? The lowest BMI is actually seen in a high-carb diet eaten by people with fewer genes! Diet culture has never implied increasing carbs will help you lose weight, but it only provides a one-size-fits all solution – in reality, we each have a unique response to food. We simply can't say everyone should be on a low-carb diet because clearly, with certain genes, some people respond best to a high-carb diet. Ultimately, there is no perfect diet for everyone and our genes explain part of this – the trick is to find the one that works best for you. This is a philosophy described as 'personalised nutrition' and everything from your genes, hormones, blood sugar and blood fat control to your microbiome will influence what is your body's ideal diet.

Epigenetics

As mentioned earlier, our environment interacts with our genes to decide which of them gets turned on. This is a concept referred to as epigenetics, and it is completely changing our understanding of health. For example, if a Chinese woman moves to America, she will double her risk of getting breast cancer, not because her genes changed, but because her new environment is changing their expression. Similarly, a Ghanaian man is 11–15 times more likely to become obese after migrating to Europe than a Ghanaian who didn't move; his change in environment wakes up obesogenic genes, which would otherwise have stayed asleep in Ghana. Bizarrely, how heritable obesity is seems to depend on which country you live in. On average, across the world, genes seem to explain around 70 per cent of our weight. But clearly, as the Ghanaian man demonstrates, some countries turn on obesogenic genes more than others. One study suggests that, in low-obesity countries, genes only explain 31 per cent of your weight but, in high-obesity countries, genes can control 90 per cent! Generally, living in higher-income countries with a greater BMI average seems to turn obese genes on much more. If we home in on a single country and map how heritable obesity has been over the last 30 years, we see that number gradually increase – over time, our waists have gone up, but so has the power of our obese genes. Finally, we even see a change in heritability in different households within the same country. Research shows a child living in an obesogenic home has an 86 per cent heritability of obese genes compared to just 39 per cent in a home that isn't obesity-promoting. Many things influence how obesogenic your childhood home is, but one of them is socioeconomic status – if your family can only afford cheap, ultra-processed foods, you are twice as likely to switch on your obese genes.

Do we inherit our microbiomes?

Talk about a plot twist: remember how you're technically only 50 per cent human?* We know your army of coexisting organisms are highly influenced by your environment – just a change in your diet can dramatically alter your microbiome in as little as two weeks. But can you actually inherit these bugs? If they technically have their own genes, surely this can't be possible. But, believe it or not, it is.

The first way you can 'inherit' them is through birth, as we discussed in Chapter 1. A vaginal delivery is a baby's first inoculation of intrepid bugs cautiously setting sail to colonise the gut. Your parents also affect your microbiome, just by being around you – in fact, we seem to share a lot of microbiome similarities with anyone we live with, including dogs. Although this technically isn't something you have inherited, it is an example of how your family in early life seem to influence your microbiome which, in turn, can help to decide which diseases you do or don't get. This might be why growing up with pets reduces your risk of eczema; in fact, I now take huge pleasure in telling my young eczema patients it might be worth

---

* Remember from Chapter 1 when it comes to how many cells you have in your body, only 50 per cent of them are human.

investing in a dog – the look of despair on their parents' faces is priceless.*

One study found that some microbes are specifically influenced by your genes, such as the skinny *Christensenella* bacteria covered in Chapter 1. As I mentioned then, your mother donates it to you through a vaginal birth and also passes on the genes needed to keep it happy. The most fascinating and worrying thing we have noticed about microbiome inheritance is that, over time, we could be inheriting progressively less diverse (and therefore less healthy) gut bacteria. One mouse study looked at how changing diets in each generation can influence the microbiome diversity seen in offspring. A grandmother mouse might be born with 1,200 species in her gut, but her offspring would then only have 900; her grandchild would then only have 600. In other words, your diet or, more specifically, the diet of your microbiome doesn't just affect your own health but, through progressively dwindling diversity with every generation, it actually affects your child. It's not genetic, but it is still a type of inheritance because we personally affect our child's initial microbiome: you can give them a head start in life if it is diverse, but you can also do the opposite. In a way, history hasn't been on our side – as our food environment has changed our children have 'inherited' less healthy microbiomes with each generation.

Epigenetics starts in the womb

As I keep saying, your genes aren't set in stone – they are merely a list of instructions, and your environment decides if and how they are followed. The womb counts as part of this

---

* Your skin has its own microbiome which, believe it or not, can 'talk' to your gut microbiome. Dermatology research is being dramatically shaped by new discoveries linking the microbiome to skin diseases. There is some suggestion that living with pets like dogs alters the bacteria on your own skin, therefore affecting skin diseases like eczema.

environment. In other words, even as an unborn foetus, the environment your mother exposes you to is already starting to influence your future risk of disease. It also starts to affect how good you'll be at putting on weight. Now this isn't new knowledge – I even remember being taught this at medical school. A lecturer pointed out that if your mother was obese while you were in her womb, this would prime you to develop metabolic syndrome as an adult. I jotted this down in my notes, in case it came up in my exams, but put no real thought into it, even though it is jaw-dropping information. Let me explain …

Metabolic syndrome basically influences your risk of heart disease and is defined as someone having at least three of the following conditions: abdominal obesity, high blood pressure, high blood sugar, high triglycerides (blood fat) and low HDL (good cholesterol). In other words, your destiny isn't written in the stars, it starts out being written in your mother's womb. Like I said: jaw-dropping. Does this mean we should shame expectant mothers for their weight? Absolutely not! Their own weight was clearly influenced by hugely complex factors – perhaps even starting when they were in *their* mother's womb! Blame is not the point – I am only interested in understanding obesity's incredible complexity. To remove stigma, it is paramount that we recognise how and why it can be easier for some people to gain weight than others. There are many factors we can exert control over, but our individual genes and womb environment are decided for us. Far from a source of criticism, this information should further help to inject compassion into a condition we have always oversimplified.

Many studies demonstrate this effect and it is partly what explains the Danish adoption study: if the mother was overweight, the baby was exposed to an environment in the womb which would go on to increase their own weight as adults, independent of sociodemographic and lifestyle-related factors. Tragically, they might have been teased or even bullied by classmates for being overweight, but these children weren't running the same race: their weight gain actually began in the womb through no fault of their own. Just like our microbiomes, each generation is progressively passing on more and more congenital obesity. (The term 'congenital' simply means it was caused by the womb environment.) For example, cerebral palsy is a congenital disease and can't be genetically inherited – something went wrong in the womb. But we don't chastise these children with disabilities for their limitations.

But how does the womb environment have such a powerful effect on the child's risk of metabolic syndrome and obesity, you might ask. Well, insulin levels in the mother's blood get fed to the baby through the placenta. We know that persistently high levels of insulin will make us become resistant to it – I realise I keep repeating myself here but *this* deserves repeating: the more insulin you are exposed to, the more resistant you become and, therefore, the more insulin your body progressively produces. With time, you become less and less metabolically flexible and more adept at storing fat; eventually, with enough practice, you might reach fasting insulin levels that never drop low enough to enter fat burning. Cue: obesity. Now what if I told you insulin resistance is a time-dependent phenomenon: the more cumulative time you have to build it up, the worse it gets. It's not just about your mother's weight; if your mother had gestational diabetes, you are three times more likely to develop obesity. Why? Because your mother exposed you to high insulin in the womb: she gave you a head start.

Historically, it was impossible to have an obese baby. Infants simply fed on demand and even now, we know you can't really overfeed a breastfed baby. But a study looking at child obesity between 1980 and 2001 saw some worrying weight-gain trends, not just in pre-school children, but in babies under the age of six months. This is partly due to the congenital insulin resistance the babies were born with – they were metabolically primed to store more fat. However, we now know that ultra-processed infant formula may also play a role. A study in

Cambridge revealed that parents were feeding babies hundreds more calories than recommended by the World Health Organization, with some being overfed by as much as a litre of formula a day. In 2008, babies drank 5.5kg of formula a year but are now drinking 8kg – a whopping 40 per cent increase. This should be inherently impossible because babies naturally stop feeding when they have met their dietary requirements – their hormonal regulators of appetite are so finely tuned that over-feeding them *should* be impossible. But whether intentionally or not, food industries have tweaked formulas to make them hyper-palatable; like many ultra-processed foods, they bypass satiety cues, allowing babies to drink more. Combine this with any degree of congenital insulin resistance and it is no surprise we are now seeing obese babies.

Again, I need to stress that weight gain and obesity is enormously complex – I am not for a moment suggesting it is directly caused by formula milk alone. However, over recent decades changes to formula milk might explain one mechanism nudging infants to develop insulin resistance. Many mothers are unable to breastfeed for complicated and often distressing reasons. I am sharing this information not to upset parents or suggest any guilt on their part, but rather to enlighten us all. If we understand the many, many root causes of adult weight gain, it means we can start to come up with meaningful solutions.

Why does any of this matter? Obese children are 17 times more likely to be obese adults. More than that, childhood obesity is directly linked to an increased risk of heart disease and overall mortality in adulthood. As Dr Jason Fung says in his book *The Obesity Code*, we are 'marinating our children in insulin' – and it starts in the womb. But there is hope – because all these risks are reversible. If an overweight child develops a normal BMI by adulthood, their risk of mortality normalises, as if they had never been overweight at all! Catch children while they're young and you can halt the domino sequence of epigenetic and metabolic changes that will go on to program disease. But because so much stigma and misinformation still exist this doesn't happen. From my own research, I know doctors are often too frightened of offending parents and, in truth, there is limited support available anyway. You might recall I set up a Zoom workshop for parents of obese children to teach them everything I am telling you in this book but, to be honest, recruitment was tough! I invited countless parents to the course, but most said no. Some parents broke down in tears and others shouted abuse before storming out of my office – even though I broached the subject delicately and with huge compassion, no one wants to be told their child is technically obese. All they hear you saying is, 'You're a bad parent,' when of course, that's not the case.

Epigenetics in early life

As a GP I know breastfeeding is an incredibly emotive subject and I never impose my opinion on any of my patients. I fully empathise with the plethora of reasons why many women simply cannot breastfeed. A poor milk supply, difficult latch, nipple pain or bleeding, recurrent breast infections, work commitments, time restraints or the mother's need for medication which isn't safe in breastfeeding. The list goes on. At the end of the day, I fully recognise that how someone chooses to parent is ultimately their own choice. But there is an uncomfortable truth most shy away from discussing: the UK has the lowest rate of breastfeeding in the world, alongside one of the highest rates of childhood obesity. To point this out does not mean I lack any level of understanding or compassion for parents but, just because it is upsetting to hear, doesn't mean it isn't true. After everything I have just explained, it is hard not to see how these trends are linked. The World Health Organization have been enormously clear in their message that breastfeeding is the best option for babies. This might be partly because it dramatically boosts the child's microbiome, but I think insulin is another part of the reason: an ultra-processed alternative conspires with our bodies' insulin, increasing future risk of weight gain and chronic disease.

But there is good news. Public-health campaigns have dramatically improved rates of breastfeeding in countries like Sweden (62 per cent), Sri Lanka (82 per cent) and Rwanda (87 per cent). By contrast, in the UK only 1 per cent of babies are exclusively breastfed to 6 months.* There is huge room for improvement here. A dedicated army of breastfeeding counsellors could descend on maternity wards with regular follow-up in place. Compared to other countries, women in the UK get very little support in learning this difficult skill. A campaign could sweep through workplaces where employers could protect and facilitate the ability to pump. If staff are entitled to sick leave and toilet breaks, why not give them the time and privacy to breast pump, perhaps even with access to cooled storage?

In her brilliant book *Every Body Should Know This*, medical scientist and nutritionist Dr Federica Amati even suggests donor breast milk should be the first-line alternative in place of formula – a trend which is already becoming a reality in America. Of course, formula should still remain an affordable option, but not without educating parents fully on the risks and benefits. Polite British culture can make frank conversations difficult for doctors – we are too frightened of causing offence and too burnt out to risk receiving a complaint. For a true health revolution to take place sometimes *culture* is what needs to change first. At the six-week baby check I am expected to ask parents if they are breastfeeding but, in truth, the question is pointless. All I do is write their answer down. I'm too nervous to advise on evidence because I don't want to upset anyone, and for some infants it may even be too

---

* The World Health Organization recommends exclusive breastfeeding up to six months and continued breastfeeding with food until at least two years of age.

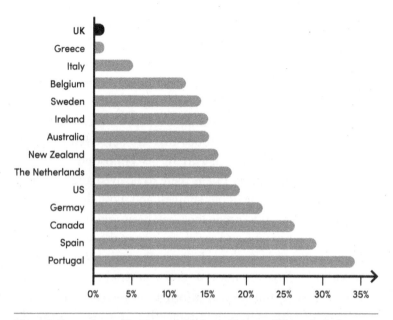

Figure 2: Percentage of babies aged 0-5 months breastfed exclusively

late to establish breastfeeding. From a public health point of view this is a missed opportunity. If culture changed, perhaps doctors and other health professionals could intervene earlier and, if there are difficulties, refer for intensive breastfeeding support. Breastfeeding is also enormously healthy for women: it reduces their risk of ovarian and breast cancer, while also helping them to lose weight gained from pregnancy and, thus, prevent future insulin resistance. If we lived in a society that championed this amazing and free health initiative with policies in place to make it the most convenient and comfortable option, the downstream benefits could be incredible! Sadly, in many countries this hasn't happened yet and individual parents should not be blamed for this.

I hope you have come to appreciate that our microbiomes and hormones have an amazing impact on health, long before we are old enough to influence this ourselves. As individuals, we can't control the microbiome, insulin resistance or epigenetics we enter adulthood with, but we can use this information with our own children. Being mindful of how you spike your own insulin during pregnancy is a good starting point. Of course, I am not proposing tortured restriction or becoming obsessive about food while pregnant – or at any other stage of life. (Orthorexia is an emerging eating disorder characterised by an obsession with only eating foods that are perceived as highly healthy.) As you will see in Part II, my philosophy is one of balance and pragmatism. Life is there to be lived and, as I have said before, food is one of our simplest and most cherished joys. However, historically, pregnancy has been jokingly seen as a window of time in which to throw caution to the wind. If you're going to gain weight anyway, I can see the logic behind 'making it count' with large volumes of food you would normally only consider a treat. But food is information interpreted by your body through hormones: just remember you are sending the foetus that same information.

Childhood sets the stage for future health

After birth, parents also have a valuable window of time to help shape the trajectory of their child's life. Again, to assume you have complete control is absurd – you clearly don't. The culture and environment you live in shapes this enormously. After all, if an entire class of students fail an exam, we need to look at the teacher: if rates of obesity are high in a country, we need to look at the country. Governments and public policies need to do this for us. But beyond policy, I think we need to humbly rethink culture. We know it is easier to switch on our obesity genes in rich countries with high rates of obesity – that is not the individual's fault. It is impossible to shield your child from the impact of UPF advertising, and helicopter parenting isn't the solution. Absolutely banning all UPFs could ostracise children from their peers and is not necessarily the answer. I would always suggest a balanced approach.

However, having grown up abroad in countries with low rates of child obesity, I can't help but notice different cultural norms in the UK. The first is that I have seen parents use food as a reward or punishment: 'You can't have pudding if ...' 'If you're good, I will give you some chocolate.' Teaching children to attach food to emotion like this seems strange to me. For me, growing up, food was just food. I didn't have to earn it. The second thing is that high-sugar foods (often in the form of UPFs) are sometimes culturally acceptable things to give young toddlers and even babies in the UK. In many European countries, this would be considered strange because whole foods are the norm. Finally, the biggest difference I have noticed is that children are served 'child-friendly' food. This simply doesn't exist in many other countries. Children eat precisely what their parents eat – it might be mashed or chopped up for them, but the food is the same. Even as a toddler, I ate dinner with my parents and was served the same food as them, priming me to mirror their behaviour. Perhaps this meant a slightly later bedtime than would be culturally accepted in the UK, but all my childhood friends did the same. Importantly too, when I was full, I was allowed to stop eating and this was a non-negotiable because my parents trusted my satiety cues, teaching me to do the same. These family rituals were not dictated by public policy in any of the four countries I grew up in: they were decided by culture.

New science has unearthed so many truths we were simply unaware of before. Understanding that you can exert control over many aspects of your biology is the point of this book. However, instilling compassion is my second goal: for so long we have judged others and ourselves for body shape. Height doesn't attract this same scrutiny, even though it is also heavily controlled by epigenetics – a conversation happening between our genes and environment. When it comes to weight, we simply aren't running the same race – unless you are looking at your identical twin, comparing yourself to another body is meaningless. That person's genes, womb environment, childhood and microbiome are completely personal to them.

I am not absolving all responsibility nor am I assigning blame with this book – it simply offers answers to valid questions. However, one remains unanswered: how exactly did we find ourselves where we are now? In the 1970s, the majority of the British population had a healthy weight; obesity was incredibly rare and childhood obesity was almost unheard of. In the years since, rates of autoimmune conditions have increased by 300 per cent and our risk of cancer, food allergy and mental-health conditions have all increased too. If you live in the UK, you are now in the minority if you have a healthy weight, and the same is true in the States. What is it about the way we live that has changed us so much when our genes have remained constant? I believe we need a cultural revolution to reverse this trajectory, but to achieve this we need to retrace our steps: history has not been on our side and in the next chapter I will show you why.

Our heritage: Key points

1) Our genes and womb environment dramatically influence weight. If a child is adopted, the weight of their biological parents predicts their own weight much more than that of their adoptive parents.
2) There are a number of very rare genetic conditions that directly cause obesity by interfering with our hunger and satiety hormones. This doesn't reflect the individual's will-power: an abnormal appetite is what pushes them to eat.
3) Most people have a mixture of both obese-promoting and thin-promoting genes: our environment can dramatically influence which genes get switched on.
4) We are all exposed to factors shaping our risk of weight gain and disease long before we have any control over our own lifestyle risks; these include the microbiome, womb environment, whether we were breastfed and food in childhood.
5) Recognising the factors which were out of our control should empower us to change them for our own children. This does not mean fostering a culture of blame but should encourage productive discussions about meaningful solutions.
6) Governments and public policies need to change, but so does culture. As a starting point, it is worth examining countries with lower rates of obesity and the cultural norms which may be influencing this. But understanding the history of a culture which does not might provide even more insights.

CHAPTER 6

A HISTORY LESSON

Where did we go wrong?

You have now been introduced to all the main characters in this previously untold story of your health: your microbiome, hormones, genes and their epigenetic influences. There is much more to come in Part II on what and how to eat – but before then, a final nugget of theory is needed if I am to truly convince you to value the science. Now is the time for me to clinch the deal.

For anyone to make a change in their life they need to believe it is both necessary and achievable. However, it is very difficult to be convinced that change is necessary when the thing in question is perceived as normal or as something 'we have always done'. If something has always worked before, why change it? But herein lies the problem: so much of what, how and when we eat has changed in our recent history. Few people questioned why these changes were happening or considered who might be profiting. In truth, you will see I simply teach my patients to mirror our lifestyles *before* these changes took place but, to fully embrace them, we need to retrace our steps. What is the sequence of events which led us to where we are? More than that, where have so many of our strong views on obesity and diet culture come from? Have we inherited stigma and cultural rituals passed on by our misinformed ancestors? Our lives have long been shaped by advice and 'knowledge' we have always accepted without question. But what if I told you much of this was never based on fact and the 'experts' proposing these ideas lived to regret them. More and more, we can see that people are the product of epigenetics – an intimate mingling between environment and genes. Next, let's examine what else our ancestors passed on: diet culture, stigma and a misunderstanding of the science.

The history of obesity

It might surprise you to learn that people have been desperately worried about obesity for the last 700 years. Even in the middle of deadly plagues, in the 16th century, a politician named John Hales famously declared more men died from overeating than from 'sword or plague'. Two hundred years later, a doctor named Thomas Short despaired that 'no Age did ever afford more instances of Corpulency than our own'. And a couple of hundred years after that, in 1920, an 'obesity expert' named W.F. Christy proclaimed that 'more people floated into their coffins on a flood of beef tea and milk than ever arrive there by the ravages of disease'. These are extremely strong statements, especially given obesity was incredibly rare, at least by today's standards. In fact, I have always vaguely assumed this was an entirely modern issue, but was I wrong?

Have you ever wondered when human obesity became a thing? In fact, I needn't include the word 'human' there because, aside from domesticated pets and some hibernating animals, we are the only species really capable of obesity. The topic is debatable, but some say its first depiction was 35,000 years ago in a German figurine and we've also discovered rotund shapes in the art of *Homo erectus*. Academics will bicker among themselves, some arguing that images like these were merely symbols of fertility but, as far back as 1939, a historian named R. Hautin wrote: 'the women immortalised in stone age sculpture were fat; there is no other word for it. Obesity was already a fact of life for Palaeolithic man – or at least for Palaeolithic women.' Even ancient Egypt lends some insight; at the time, a queen named Hatshepsut was similarly depicted as overweight in images and, what's more, appeared to have rather 'pendulous breasts' in her mummified remains. How modern an issue can this be if we have mummified remains of an obese Egyptian queen?

Sadly, the cruel mockery of a large body is as old as time; we see frequent examples where people living with obesity became the butt of a joke whether in Victorian 'freak shows' or as jesters to amuse royalty. The most extreme example I found was from 2,200 years ago when a Chinese emperor named Qin was buried with an enormous terracotta army. These were handcrafted so they could guide him into the after-life; his tomb was filled with 8,000 life-sized figurines, most of which were depicted as soldiers or accountants (yes, of course you need accountants in heaven). But there was one unique figure, different from the rest: a single obese man so, as well as paying his taxes, Qin still had someone to laugh at in the afterlife. More recently, even our most cherished Christmas film *Love Actually* has at least eight fat jokes in it. Over the course of our history, if we weren't worrying about obesity, we were laughing at it. Knowing what I know now I feel mortified by this and am taken aback by how deeply rooted it is in our history. Finally, we are at a turning point in science, replacing stigma with compassion and facts. I now suspect the people being ogled in Victorian freak shows probably had one of the very rare genetic conditions which drive morbid obesity. Perhaps they were very unlucky like the Chinese man Wu (p. 18), harbouring an abnormally aggressive strain of bacteria which could fuel dramatic weight gain. Or was it an undiagnosed Cushing's syndrome like my patient with the swollen face (p. 54)? We will never know but, no matter the root cause, to mock someone for their body is clearly barbaric.

The history of diet culture

To navigate our current diet culture objectively, I propose you learn where it came from. This is a sticking point so many of us will struggle with for many reasons. For one, the principles of dieting are so pervasive in society: governments, clinicians, teachers and influencers share similar advice with absolute confidence. The origin of that advice feels impossible to track down – whose idea was it in the first place? I hope understanding the involvement of your microbiome and hormones has helped dismantle some of your previous beliefs. However, I propose we get into the detail because it is one thing to accept new logic, but it is another to win over your subconscious mind. Meticulous restriction has become so ingrained in our attitudes and behaviours around food – and they can be so difficult to let go of. I want to show you how food can be treasured instead of analysed. I strongly believe it should provide joy, nostalgia and cultural celebration, while also nourishing us and fuelling our health. But even I struggled to completely let go of my restrictive mentality – until I learned about the history of dieting itself. Like catching someone's affair long after suspecting their infidelity, I finally fell out of love with my romanticised view of dieting. This chapter is the final nail in the coffin within which lie all my old beliefs around weight – and I want to help you bury yours for good.

It seems as long as we have been worrying about obesity we have been trying to combat it. The ancient Greek doctor Galen (c. 130–200AD) wrote about treating his obese patients by 'rubbing them hard' (whatever that means), making them sweat profusely on a long run and then soaking them in a hot bath. Interestingly, he believed in the power of good food and, like me, regularly shared recipes with his patients. Hippocrates was another Greek doctor now famously remembered as 'the father of medicine'. He too treated obesity with lifestyle changes, including vomiting and regular enemas – a method I wouldn't try at home. Yes, diets were already a thing and we see many examples through the ages. By the 1800s, some of our 'modern ideas' start to emerge: Brillat-Savarin, a French lawyer, announced carbohydrates were the problem and his low-carb-diet advice went on to make him a very rich man. More than 200 years later we have rebranded this in famous diets like Atkins, Dukan and now Keto as apparently new trends, never realising our grandparents and *their* grandparents tried the same things. With what we know about personalised nutrition and the genetic differences we have in our amylase genes (see p. 114), I can't help giggling when fitfluencers imply low-carb diets are 'the only way'. Like I said before, they simply don't know what they don't know and their blind confidence in giving health advice worries me.

It might surprise you to learn that the famous poet Lord Byron was a bit of a fitfluencer himself and the results were devastating. He hated nothing more than a fat body, especially when it was his own. Byron was well known to restrict food and chain-smoke to suppress his appetite. He measured himself obsessively and wore uncomfortable layers of clothes in the hope that sweating would shed more pounds. However, there was only so much restriction he could take: eventually, he would break down, gorge on a huge feast and start all over again. Was he the first to trigger a restrict–binge culture? His influence was extreme and impressionable youths flocked to copy his regimes. Doctors of the time worried he was eliciting 'melancholia and emotional volatility' in starving young girls. Little did they know how much worse it was going to get.

Most books will say the first diet was written by an undertaker named William Banting in 1863 (they have forgotten about Galen's 'rubbing hard' and Hippocrates' enemas). His was one of the most important diet books in history – so much so that in Swedish to 'banter' does not mean tongue-in-cheek jest but 'to diet'. In fact, 'banting' was how many described dieting up until the 1920s. Banting sought advice from a surgeon named Dr William Harvey who had just returned from Paris where the low-carb diet had been popular for many decades. He decided to test the idea on Banting whose weight plummeted simply by removing carbohydrates. Interestingly, he didn't feel starved or restricted and was still allowed to eat the equivalent of 2,800 calories (including up to five glasses of sherry). Like the French lawyer earlier, Banting published his own experience and became a very rich man. One thing in history remains constant: if you can teach people how to lose weight, you can make a lot of money.

Through the decades, diet culture grew increasingly absurd, in line with society's growing stigma against weight gain. A spa in Baden-Baden, Germany, famously charged large sums of money to essentially torture their clients; they believed beating, squeezing and 'pummelling' fat tissue would make it recede, especially if you then soaked the victim in a boiling hot bath for uncomfortable durations of time. I can't help but feel today's liposuction operations aren't dissimilar – a plastic surgery which risks rare post-operative complications, including death. The lengths we go to for thinness are baffling. Arsenic diet pills and cigarettes laced with amphetamines are some other bizarre examples I've come across. Perhaps the strangest trend of all was thought up by an artist named Fletcher, who earned the nickname 'the Great Masticator' (read that carefully). He believed food didn't need to be swallowed because you could extract all the nutrients you needed simply by chewing each mouthful 100–700 times before spitting it out. To convince others of his techniques, he even carried around a sample of his stool to show them! Fletcher believed passing firm, clay-like pellets once every fortnight was synonymous with health. You might imagine people recoiling at this strange man, but he was a sensation – everyone from John D. Rockefeller to Franz Kafka was lapping up 'Fletcherism', and 'munching parties' became highly fashionable in England. The most glamorous accessory to buy for your dinner parties was an expensive 'spitting bucket'.

By the 1920s, a new idea had arrived: calories. People deduced that food was just fuel – if you could mathematically monitor how much an engine required, why couldn't you do the same for the human body? Apparently, it was simply the law of physics and so had to be true. Anyone who questioned this notion was labelled 'not academic enough' to grasp the science and, based on this, no real human evidence was required. For the first time in history, rather than eat food to feel full, people were asked to count it instead. The first book on the subject came out in 1918 and was written by a doctor named Dr Lulu Hunt Peters – she had successfully lost 70 pounds using calorie counting and wanted to share this with the world. She argued 'three out of four' American adults were 'disgracefully overweight' at the time and, as a very religious woman, also believed this was a sin. Not only was restricting calories your salvation, it was your duty as a moral person, and she advised 1,200 a day was more than enough for everyone.

A few years later, another doctor, struggling with his own weight, echoed the same sentiment. However, this time, with more mathematical prowess. In 1937, Dr Fishbein acknowledged total calories couldn't be a one-size-fits-all, given the fact that we aren't all ... well, the same size. Instead, he suggested calculating your calorie requirements based on weight and height, then simply reducing this number by 500. According to his calculations, this should equal half a kilo of weight loss each week because, again, it is 'just' physics. He didn't conduct human trials to prove the efficacy of his methods. Read that again: his advice was based on theory, not fact. But here's the kicker: years later, he conceded the results were only temporary when he wrote:

One saw women haggard and sallow, wandering about in a weakened condition, but still proud of the fact that they have taken off in a short period of time anywhere from 10 to 15 pounds. One sees the same women a month later with 10 to 15 pounds restored ... and nothing to show for their experiment but a disappointment and some loss of health.

In his lifetime, he regretted proposing advice that clearly didn't work. But it was too late; his book had been published and the idea released – to this day, personal trainers and fitfluencers still declare with confidence that a deficit of 500 calories is the only way to lose weight. They've heard a 90-year-old idea but none of them questioned where it originally came from. Reading this, you might still be roughly deducting 500 calories from your apparent predicted calorie expenditure. I did this for many years myself, and letting go of this notion felt like abandoning a faith. But it collapsed the moment I learned it was only ever an idea, and even the man suggesting it realised it was wrong.

Like I said, history has not been on our side. Our ancestors pioneered both the stigma-fuelling fat phobia and the diet myths to ignite disordered eating tactics that actually drive more weight gain. Yet behind the smoke and mirrors, we do see several historical acknowledgments that weight gain does not affect people equally. Despite centuries of stigma, a handful of humble, forward-thinking individuals recognised obesity's amazing complexity. As far back as 1780, author James Boswell wrote, 'You will see one man fat who eats moderately, and another lean who eats a great deal'. The latest science suggests this could be because of an especially parasitic microbiome or just winning the genetic lottery, but we still automatically celebrate these people who can eat a lot without gaining weight. They are essentially congratulated for having a 'fast' metabolism and go on to reap the societal rewards of inhabiting a body that is assumed morally superior. But if the reverse were true, like an overweight person who seems to gain weight even when they eat very little, people wouldn't sympathise – they would assume that person is lying and subconsciously shun them for being weak willed.

In 1935, the *British Medical Journal* published an article highlighting the complexity of obesity – even the scientific community was starting to acknowledge nuance in what was, at the time, a rare condition. By 1950 physician-biochemist Professor Sir Charles Dodds wanted to study the bragging people who never gained weight: he tripled their calorie intake and found they didn't put on weight – it was because their metabolism simply shot up to compensate. He repeated the experiment on people with the opposite problem: their metabolism stayed the same, but their weight certainly didn't. Does this change your perception of obesity and the assumptions you might make? It is absolutely easier for some people to gain weight than it is for others. Ironically, this is a fact we have known for decades, but perhaps society has always had selective hearing – because it's much harder to make money from overweight people when you concede it's not entirely in their control.

A cultural revolution:
The one-way street to obesity

As you can see, for many centuries, our ancestors have been very interested in the subject of weight loss even though obesity was incredibly rare. As we saw in the Finnish twin study, a lifetime of dieting causes overall weight gain! Ironically, the emergence of a diet culture is part of the reason for where we are now. But many other things about the way we live our lives have changed too: examining these will, hopefully, dispel the flawed assumption that we don't need to change something 'we have always done'. As it turns out, we haven't always done many of the things we now do – acknowledging this might help you to let go of them.

In the years following the 1950s a cultural revolution would unfold; you couldn't design a better sequence of events to drive obesity if you tried. The kitchen is arguably the main scene of the crime – put simply, its use has changed unrecognisably. In the 1950s, a 'marriage bar' meant women could legally be fired after their wedding day and, in a way, it made sense. Without modern conveniences, the average domestic work of a housewife took 74 hours a week – not including weekends! They quite frankly didn't have time for a career; meals were very time-consuming and highly labour-intensive. Eating was generally a seated affair, often enjoyed with family at the dinner table. Most people only ate three times a day – no one had time to prepare more food than this and, culturally, to eat more often just wasn't the done thing. With post-war rations, food was very expensive and used up 33 per cent of a family's income. Compare that to 8 per cent in the UK and 14 per cent in Europe today.* After the war, people simply couldn't afford excess food. Meals out would remain a lavish luxury for many decades and any form of prepared take-away simply didn't exist – food was a family ritual within a confined window of time. It was precious and not something to be wasted, meaning children were taught to clear their plates, even if they were already full. Seventy years later, some children are taught the same thing now but, in our completely new food environment, this simply trains them to unlearn their evolutionary satiety cues. What we now eat is comparatively cheap and requires very little effort: we eat frequently throughout the day simply because we can. This ability is *very* new in our evolution and not something our bodies have adapted to deal with.

In 1970, the arrival of the Equal Pay Act meant women couldn't be fired for being married or pregnant; they could now

---

* Figures referenced from Avison, Z. (3 February 2020). 'Why UK consumers spend 8% of their money on food'. Retrieved from: https://ahdb.org.uk/news/consumer-insight-why-uk-consumers-spend-8-of-their-money-on-food

work for as long as they liked. Kitchen technology boomed in tandem, making meals far more time efficient; by 1976, 80 per cent of families owned a fridge, and a lucky 30 per cent even had freezers. In the 1950s, most men came home for lunch, but by the 1970s, they were working farther away and ate on the go. Our food landscape needed to accommodate this, becoming something quick and convenient. Some countries never quite caught up with this modern transformation; France and Italy are still well known for making food a slow, leisurely experience. Why rush one of life's simplest pleasures? But for many, life became busy and time needed to be won back somewhere. Many mothers were now employed, meaning they weren't necessarily home when children finished school. For the first time in history, husbands and children alike had to fend for themselves until dinner – cue the arrival of something called a snack.

Most people don't realise the ritual of eating outside of sit-down meals is relatively new – and the food industry couldn't have been happier. However, they soon saw that food needed a longer shelf life and that achieving this made it tasteless and almost inedible. Enter the British Society of Flavourists in 1970 – a body representing new food scientists who could create fake food flavours. Finally, we could artificially inject flavour into anything making the unpalatable not just edible, but exquisitely delicious. In just ten years, they had developed 6,000 chemicals apparently 'safe' for human consumption. If drugs need years of research before they're made available to the public, you might assume these food chemicals should be rigorously tested too. But why? It's 'just' food after all. Instead, as long as they didn't show obvious signs of harm, these additives were 'generally regarded as safe' (GRAS) – a standard food companies often follow today. Who knows what we have been eating?

Far from our three sit-down and labour-intensive meals a day, food was now readily available and all you needed to do was open a packet. Over the course of the 1970s, England would launch 20 new crisp brands, available in small packets you could eat on the go. If you wanted to, you could eat them every day; some still do in Britain, which has one of the biggest crisp-consuming populations on earth. This decade also saw the appearance of freezers in the home, bringing with them ready-made meals. But an even greater technology would grow in popularity during the next decade: the microwave. Now reheating ready meals was something every family member could do individually. For many families, the dinner table became obsolete: not only could they eat separately and in front of the TV, but everyone could have a different dish. The 1980s would serve as the precise tipping point at which obesity rates suddenly soared. With everything we now understand about the microbiome, metabolic flexibility and the hormonal theory of weight gain this is hardly surprising. Our food environment was doing everything it could to dismantle our way of eating. But here comes the plot twist: one last event in the 1980s was instrumental in pushing us over the edge. A new epiphany emerged which changed a generation's way of eating to the extreme. Populations all around the world were taught to fear cholesterol and were given strict instructions to eat less fat. Again, the origin of this advice might surprise you, and its story is rarely told. In fact, it is a sad tale of misinformation and irony. The man behind it would live to regret this.

A new enemy: Dietary fat

When US president Eisenhower had a heart attack in 1955, the media had a new story to home in on: heart disease. Rates had long been increasing and scientists were conscious of this, but without a leading character, it's hard to gain much traction in the press. The masses don't want facts; what they really want is a story, and Eisenhower gave them just that. It's worth bearing in mind that in the time that heart-disease rates were increasing, antibiotics and other medical innovations were prolonging life. People weren't dying more – they were dying less. In 1900 the average male life expectancy was only 44 but by 1950 it had increased to 66. To be blunt, they had to die from something. Without realising this context, scientists grew worried there was something specifically driving more heart disease.

Around this time the American physiologist Ancel Keys published a landmark paper named the 'Seven Countries Study' – a strange name, given he had investigated populations in 22 countries. The problem was that 15 of the countries he investigated produced results which didn't fit his theory: 'dietary fat is bad'. Regardless, the evidence he chose to share implied dietary fat increased blood cholesterol, which was something we already knew increased heart disease if too high. For the first time in history, this information prompted governments to produce specific dietary guidelines and the message was clear: eat less fat and more carbohydrates. The fact that Keys received funding from the sugar industry was never mentioned, and food companies were delighted: he had handed people over to them on a silver platter. Highly processed food began selling like never before; as long as the label read 'low fat' or 'heart healthy', the products would fly off the shelves.

Amazingly, people listened. In America, dietary fat went from making up 45 per cent to 35 per cent of total calories consumed. Refined-grain consumption went up by almost 45 per cent, while egg consumption dropped by 18 per cent. And yet, obesity soared like never before. In years to come, his sources would be re-analysed and, though Keys appeared to cherry pick his data, when examined carefully, even what he *did* share didn't support his hypothesis. As mentioned earlier, he lived to regret the profound consequences of his research; in 1987, the *New York Times* quoted him saying, 'I've come to believe that cholesterol is not as important [as a risk for heart disease] as we used to think'. Given that more than 30 years later most of my patients are still on a self-imposed low-fat diet, I can confirm this acknowledgment was too little, too late. The horse had already bolted and an idea had been released. However, I will let Ancel Keys redeem himself because he was also responsible for running the world's most famous study on human starvation. Sadly, its results have been ignored for over 80 years, but they will amaze you now. If only governments had publicised his Minnesota Starvation experiment (1944–5) instead, we might be in a very different position now.

Starving for science

Towards the end of the Second World War, Keys grew genuinely worried about the millions of European civilians who were dying from starvation. In the Siege of Leningrad, it is estimated that a thousand civilians starved to death a day. One thousand. This unthinkable human tragedy motivated him to understand what happens to the body when you starve it: he put out a call to conscientious objectors of the Vietnam War to do their bit for the country in another way, asking them to starve themselves for science to compensate for not fighting. Years later, the men were interviewed and their reasons for not fighting had nothing to do with cowardice; they were peace-loving men who fundamentally disagreed with the principle of warfare. But to suffer for science – that they could do. A group of 36 volunteers spent a whole year being studied under strict conditions to mimic the lives of the European civilians they wanted to help. No matter how much they ate, each week they were expected to walk 22 miles and do 15 hours of physical work, like chopping firewood. Over time, their calories were reduced and the impact of this on both body and mind is fascinating. As well as losing weight and feeling constantly ravenous, they also became exhausted, irritable and depressed with many reporting horrific nightmares.

Several had to withdraw from university because they just couldn't concentrate; their thoughts were entirely consumed by one thing: food. One participant recalled:

> Food became the one central and only thing really in one's life. And life is pretty dull if that's the only thing. I mean, if you went to a movie, you weren't particularly interested in the love scenes, but you noticed every time they ate and what they ate.

These young men lost their sex drives and, amazingly, even their sperm counts fell. That's because in the face of starvation, the body prioritises 'essential' organs like the brain, while it cuts back on anything else it can. This explains why the men lost 40 per cent of their muscle mass – in a state of famine, the body starts to eat itself, using muscle for fuel. Even body temperature dropped, making them feel permanently cold, and their heart rates slowed down too – the body will do anything it can to conserve energy. And how many daily calories do you think they were 'starving' themselves on – 1,800. How many fitfluencers now encourage us to eat far fewer?

Eighty years ago, the Minnesota Starvation experiment demonstrated clearly what happens when you enforce a strict calorie deficit. After 24 weeks of being starved the subjects lost 25 per cent of their body weight, but here is the shocking thing: their basal metabolic rates dropped by 40 per cent to compensate. Just as we saw in the *Biggest Loser* study (see p. 83), the human body does not conform to the laws of physics and can't behave like a mathematical equation – our clever bodies compensate for lost energy by down-regulating non-essential functions. Their experience might sound familiar to you – while dieting have you struggled to concentrate? Were your mood low and libido non-existent, replaced instead by constant thoughts of food? Willingly starving your body is not the way to make it healthy – Ancel

Keys recognised this *eighty* years ago, but we have ignored his fascinating discoveries.

History has taught us to hate and mock excess fat, while also tricking us into tackling it using 'logical' techniques which only serve to exacerbate it. When the Minnesota men were finally allowed to increase their calories, eating felt like something they simply couldn't stop; as if in a trance state, they inhaled huge quantities in a way that was previously completely out of character for them. One participant needed his stomach pumped after a binge and another had to leave a restaurant to vomit after devouring more than he could physically contain. Maybe this behaviour sounds familiar too. Have you ever devoured an extreme volume of food in a way that felt out of your control? That's because it was: we don't have absolute control over our appetites or behaviours. Bingeing is an automatic evolutionary reflex built into our bodies to protect us from famine. Unaware of this, most simply feel consumed by shame and, just like Lord Byron, return to the very restriction which caused the binge in the first place. Now is the time to break this cycle and unlearn the fake science from our past.

As we have seen, history has been against us and our ancestors have passed on much more than their genes. Obesity is not merely a modern concern: we have been worrying about it for centuries. In that time Ancient Greek doctors, a famous British poet and even an undertaker have informed cultural rituals we now can't escape. Dieting has become so pervasive in society, we no longer remember how to enjoy food. But we can't help ourselves because previous generations taught us subconsciously to reward being thin. Our grandparents and those before them were ridiculing people for the shape of their bodies for thousands of years. Perhaps we can forgive their ignorance, but can we forgive our own?

In the next chapter we will start Part II, where I will show you how to apply all of this science to your own life. Far from offering outlandish or novel advice, my approach to food is actually very traditional. When you mirror the eating habits society took for granted before the 1980s, the problems which followed will naturally ease.

History: Key points

1) Human obesity has existed for up to 35,000 years but was not common before the 1980s. We now understand these sparse cases may have been related to rare genetic conditions, diseases or even problems with the microbiome.

2) Society has been mocking obesity and overweight for thousands of years. On the surface this might seem to be changing but, in truth, many people hang on to stigma. With new science we should consider this as outdated as racism and homophobia.

3) Dieting has existed since 130AD and has long been an industry worth a lot of money. The techniques we use today are rooted in 18th-century concepts, which were 'modernised' 90 years ago. These concepts were never based on human evidence because they didn't need to be – an accepted 'logic' often requires no proof.

4) The landscapes of the workplace and our homes have both changed beyond recognition. Food needed to become convenient, so was replaced with 'food-like substances'* we were encouraged to graze on. Ancient cultural rituals surrounding food drifted away in some countries but still remain strong in others.

5) The flawed epiphany that eating fat was the apparent cause for increased rates of heart disease scared a generation into eating carbohydrates and sugar in its place. This normalised UPFs and obesity rates soared.

6) Our 'new' understanding of metabolic compensation isn't new at all. We have known about it since the 1940s, but science can bring about selective hearing. Many of us willingly impose the same calorie restriction as the Minnesota Starvation experiment and endure the same consequences.

---

* 'Food-like substances' is a term I have borrowed from Chris van Tulleken's amazing book *Ultra-Processed People*.

PART II

WHAT YOU NEED TO DO

CHAPTER 7

HOW TO EAT FOOD WITHOUT WORRYING ABOUT IT

Over the last chapters we have covered an enormous breadth of theory which might feel like a lot to take in. I often find myself taken aback by the end of a book or podcast and don't quite know where to begin applying what I have learned to my life. It reminds me of someone reading instructions to a new board game – I usually still don't understand the game until I start playing it. That's why I wanted to treat this book like a driving test; now that you have finished the theory we can put it into practice. If nothing fully makes sense yet, don't worry – in the second half of this book I promise it will all start to click.

Let's start with the most controversial topic of all: food. However, before covering *what* to eat, I want you to grasp *how* to eat it – a concept which should be simple but, instead, has become enormously confusing, with an ever-expanding stream of 'experts', each telling us to do different things. Can food return to the cherished ritual it once was without the need to count, analyse or restrict it? Surprisingly, this is completely achievable, and I will show you, step by step, precisely how.

Intuitive eating

In a way, it is completely absurd that people should need to learn how to eat. Wild animals get no formal training; even those that spend no time with their parents instinctively know what they're doing. In fact, they're just responding to their inbuilt hormonal cues. Just like us, their bodies are fine-tuned to drive eating behaviours for balance and the correct weight. Even nutrients can be tightly controlled through clever internal systems and external cues, driving the animal to crave foods it specifically needs. We will talk more about this shortly but, for now, I would describe an animal's eating habits as truly 'intuitive'. Breastfed babies have the exact same cues – remember, it is impossible to overfeed a breastfed baby. When they have had enough, no matter how hard you try, they will absolutely refuse any more milk. People assume we grow out of this as we age, but we don't; most people just unlearn their cues through dysregulating, you guessed it – hormones.

Ever since diet culture really gained momentum in the 1920s, eating has turned into a meticulously orchestrated event for many of us. When you stop to think about it, our approach to eating is very strange: we have decided that what and how much we eat is an academic endeavour. Many people still weigh out precise portions to quantify their personal needs – this is again based on the assumption that food is a fuel and that, just like an engine, we should be able to calculate how much we need. But, as we have seen, our energy requirements can adjust. In fact, they often change in ways the individual can't anticipate nor calculate. Whether it's a fluctuation in hormones, an infection, cancer or you simply moved more, the body might need more food to compensate. But through leptin, insulin and all your satiety hormones, your body can communicate this to you. So assuming you haven't dysregulated these hormones or your brain pleasure pathways, if a meal that would normally fill you up doesn't do so today, that's because today is a different day; your body is asking for more food – and it might ask for less tomorrow. Just like breastfed babies and wild animals, we can absolutely be guided by our appetites. But as you have seen, many of us now respond to abnormal appetites. Over the next few chapters, I will show you how to change this and trust your body to tell you when it needs more or less food.

Change your food mindset

Remember my Machu Picchu altitude sickness in Chapter 3? Nothing I did could entice me to eat. Worried my body needed energy, I even resorted to simply buying dessert, but even that didn't work. My hormones were telling my brain I was already full. As I keep mentioning, drugs like Ozempic have taken the world by storm because they allow people to finally feel full. What if I told you that is something you can absolutely achieve yourself? I am not on a diet and I never ask my patients to go on one, but I have comfortably returned to my pre-doctor size.* I now can't count how many of my patients have achieved even more dramatic results, but the weight never goes alone; on its way out, it takes other things with it: indigestion, sleep problems, brain fog, fatigue, low mood, joint pains – and that's not even mentioning the high blood pressure and a plethora of abnormal blood test results. When health is the goal, weight loss seems to follow, and I strongly think part of the reason is psychological. Many people believe aesthetic goals will provide them with the motivation they need to make changes, but I disagree. If I have done my job and convinced a patient of the profound health benefits they can achieve, this is a much greater source of motivation.

Just like Wu (see Chapter 1) agreed to eat unpalatable gruel because he valued and understood the impact this was having on his microbiome, my patients now make changes for the same reason. But I show them that food is allowed to taste delicious and still optimise their microbiomes, metabolic flexibility and the behaviour of their hormones. From Part I, you should be able to understand the awe-inspiring impact this can have on your health. The greatest motivator of all is that my patients tell me they simply *feel* better. And I do too. I no longer feel exhausted and bloated all the time, my debilitating

---

* Note the term 'size', not weight.

stomach aches have disappeared, I can truly concentrate and my mood has never been better. I can genuinely say I feel well and, having experienced the opposite for so long, there is no price you can put on that. How I eat isn't motivated by a desire to be thin anymore – how can it be, now that I know I am actively combatting unpleasant symptoms while simultaneously preventing dreaded diseases like cancer, dementia, heart disease and stroke?

One of the most important changes for me was that these discoveries allowed me to actually enjoy my job. Rather than seeing my patients as disgruntled clients waiting for me to fix problems with a magic bullet that didn't exist, I've begun to view them as teammates. An unwritten agreement between us acknowledges that modern drugs are incredible but can't cure everything. Instead, we need to unite and each do our part to address the underlying cause of their health problems. As I said earlier, the old doctor-patient model no longer serves us. Ten-minute appointments are simply not enough – they lead to burnout and compassion fatigue in the doctor, and frustration and finger-pointing in the patient. Patients need to be able to participate directly in their health *with* their doctor, not against them. In essence, I think what is needed is humility on both sides: the doctor needs to be humbled by the fact that they can't cure every problem. But at the same time, the patient needs to acknowledge how much they can influence their own health. Ten minutes isn't enough time to achieve this, which is why I send my patients home with many hours of guided self-study. When they do as I ask, the results are genuinely remarkable.

Weight: Stop thinking about it

Remember weight loss is just one pleasant side effect you can achieve here. I suggest the exact same techniques to my lean patients because they are so powerful in preventing disease and improving all kinds of symptoms. But for those who do carry excess fat, they absolutely will find this reduced without thinking about it. If any of them want to lose weight I specifically tell them not to think about it – watching a kettle won't make it boil faster but you know it will finish boiling at some point. I have shown you that rapid weight loss will trigger evolutionary reflexes to regain the weight – such as extreme hunger and a reduced metabolism. In truth, sustainable weight loss can take many months or even a couple of years. On the flip side, it takes very little time for these changes to start impacting your health and risk of disease and, in a way, that is the thing I would prefer to achieve quickly. I know it sounds counterintuitive but, if you want to lose weight, you need to stop thinking about it.

After reading Tim Spector's *The Diet Myth*, I got rid of my bathroom scales because they no longer seemed important: a number couldn't tell me all the amazing changes I was creating in my cells and microbiome but it *could* deflate me. Instead, I decided I wouldn't monitor my weight at all and simply trust that the evidence-based science was doing its job. I didn't even notice I had been losing weight, until a bridesmaid dress I couldn't fit into zipped up comfortably – I tried it on 'just in case', even though I was sure it couldn't possibly fit. It was a very pleasant surprise when it did – not a scrutinised event, obsessively monitored for months on end. In a way, when weight loss is a surprise, it feels even better. If you focus on health you won't struggle to feel motivated and you also won't feel deflated; remember that even in the absence of weight loss measurable changes are happening in the body which will improve how you feel and will also prolong your life. I vote for a mass burning of bathroom scales – they cause more problems than they're worth. If I ever want to measure anything, I use a tape measure, which gives me all the information I need and doesn't penalise me for gaining muscle. It is entirely possible to drop a dress size, but stay the same weight if you did this partly by building muscle; the scales will tell you nothing about the value of what you have achieved.*

Choreograph your eating – don't scrutinise it

Since calories became a thing in the 1920s, we have been asking people to consciously starve themselves, implying an ability to ignore hunger is linked to morality when it clearly isn't. From now on, when you look at your food and the pattern with which you eat it, I'd like you to imagine it translated into the hormones it will trigger in your body. Feeling hungry all the time is not a solution for your health or happiness, nor is it an efficient way to achieve meaningful weight loss. Appetite is a cue from the body we have been taught to ignore. I want to teach you how to mould it so that you can confidently listen to your hunger and fullness cues.

To recap, remember that food starts its journey in your mouth. Every time you expose your tongue to flavours (with the exception of bitter ones, like black coffee, black/green tea without milk or sweeteners), it will flip that fat-storing switch (see p. 63) to 'on', asking your pancreas to pump out some insulin. This puts you into a fat-storing state.

Many of us spike insulin repeatedly throughout the day, causing insulin resistance. This sets off a vicious cycle which can, eventually, lead to chronic diseases like type 2 diabetes, dementia, heart disease and stroke. Weight gain is only one of the consequences – clamping the 'freezer door' shut to your fat stores, you become metabolically inflexible and will struggle

---

* For women, it is also worth understanding you will develop water retention around your period and for some, even around ovulation. I often gain up to 4cm around my waist at this time. I also get impressive swelling in my legs. It can look like I have gained weight, but I never panic because it quickly disappears after a few days and is another example of why scales are very unhelpful. I used to think I had randomly gained 1–1.5kg out of the blue, worrying I was doing something wrong. When you focus on the health impact of your lifestyle, rather than the appearance of your body, the process is so much more enjoyable.

to lose weight. But insulin resistance is the root problem, not obesity – weight gain is a mere side effect even though, for many centuries, it has been deemed *the* thing we should worry about. Importantly, thin people can be insulin resistant too – they might have a fatty liver, excess visceral fat* and type 2 diabetes but, for genetic reasons, look thin on the outside. This is because we each have a unique subcutaneous fat capacity – if it's high you are more able to gain external fat but, if it's low, you can't compensate like this and actually develop diseases like type 2 diabetes faster instead. Rather than 'obesity rates higher than ever', news reports should read 'insulin resistance on the rise!' Whether you are overweight or not, insulin resistance is the problem we should *all* be paying attention to.

If you look at how people used to live in the 1950s and '60s, they were spiking their insulin far less frequently than we do now. They didn't snack in between meals or graze on artificial sweeteners (e.g. sugar-free drinks) and they also routinely allowed 12 hours or more overnight with no food/flavour. We now talk about using this as something called 'time-restricted eating' but in the past it didn't need a name: it was just the done thing. Being metabolically flexible was a given and, as such, people didn't feel they were starving because they could effortlessly tap into their energy stores. Having lost this flexibility, many of us have less athletic endurance, find it easier to gain weight and feel both sluggish and hungrier. If we respect the circadian rhythm of our pancreas (and other organs) and return to our old ways of eating, many of these problems improve.

I am not suggesting that everyone needs to eat in the same way – we are all unique and need to adjust our precise eating styles to our own lives and genes. However, when it comes to how the 'restaurant promoter' in our mouth behaves (see

---

* Visceral fat is the type of fat which surrounds your organs – you can't necessarily see this which means thin people can actually still have a lot of it. The problem is that this type of fat massively increases chronic inflammation, thus driving your risk of many chronic diseases.

p. 63), we can definitely all ask him to calm down. If you are not delivering real food don't trick your body into thinking that's what it is about to receive. In between meals don't chew gum or sip 'calorie-free' flavoured drinks; ideally just drink plain water, plain black/green tea or black coffee and give your pancreas the break it deserves. If you are metabolically flexible, you simply won't *need* to snack – a habit which makes this flexibility harder to achieve. More than that, by treating food as a timed and predictable meal you let your bowel self-clean. By leaving three to four hours between meals, you let the migratory motor complex (MMC – see p. 98) do its thing: a Mexican wave of electricity courses through the gut moving everything in the right direction. So many of my patients can't get rid of their indigestion and uncomfortable bloating, leaving them increasingly frustrated that the drugs I prescribe aren't working. But if you eat following the patterns our bowels evolved to deal with, many of these problems go away by themselves.

Now think back to the pancreas flipping that on/off switch; he takes his job seriously but, just like all of us, he wants to leave work on time. Asking him to work overtime comes with some real consequences. For most of us, the pancreas is programmed to work best earlier in the day – late-night snacking will need an extra release of last-minute insulin. It can still push blood sugar into your cells (and fat stores) but less efficiently than it should. As a result, blood sugar lingers longer and you actually produce more insulin, which means more fat-storing and insulin resistance. So what can you do with this information? Like people did in the 1950s, try to finish all your eating at least two to three hours before you go to bed. This optimises how your pancreas works alongside your sleep hormone, melatonin.* Less heartburn, bloating, indigestion, fat storing and

---

* Your sleep hormone, melatonin, rises 2–4 hours before you sleep and can alter your blood sugar control. This is part of why eating a lot (especially lots of sugar) is not good right before sleeping. It can drive worse insulin resistance and all the consequences that brings with it.

better sleep are just some of the benefits you will enjoy. But importantly, this doesn't mean restriction.

In the 1950s, food happened at the table and that was it – once you stood up from your meal, the show was over. Dessert could still feature, but it was at the table. I suggest mimicking our ancestors: see eating – and not eating – as choreographed events with start and finish times. My 'window' of eating (and insulin spiking) opens at 12pm and closes at 8pm with filling and enjoyable meals. Importantly, within those eight hours I have episodes of insulin spiking during my set meals but, when each meal is over, I let my pancreas rest. Excuse the repetition but this is important: in between meals I only expose my tongue to water or bitter flavours like black coffee. If I ever want a sweet treat, it closely follows the meal but isn't something I indulge in randomly throughout the day. This specific timing works for me around my clinics, but you can, of course, pick windows that suit your life. All I ask is that you do actually create them – because most of us don't.

The next thing to remember is that how you eat directly impacts your hunger and fullness hormones. Maybe it's nerve wracking to let go of the frequent eating you have always considered normal because you might worry you will be hungry all the time. But you won't be. The science says otherwise and I am living proof. I used to constantly keep 'emergency food' in my bag because uncontrollable hunger hit me throughout the day. I now can't recognise myself – hunger is a gentle and predictable event which normally only arrives at my usual mealtimes. I have streamlined my hormones and metabolic flexibility to achieve this and my day-to-day life is much more comfortable. Constant hunger pangs are very distracting and inconvenient, but you can change this too.

Firstly, remember the second satiety cue we get from our mouths comes from chewing our food. This stimulates fullness hormones before you have even swallowed anything. Generally, food that takes longer to chew will also sit in your stomach for longer, especially if it is packed with lots of fibre. This is a fullness mechanism many tend to bypass, especially if we are dieting. Protein shakes and aesthetically pleasing smoothies are now synonymous with the bodies society approves of: chiselled and sculpted muscles on beautiful fitfluencers. But these drinks bypass two important satiety cues: you don't chew them and they have already been liquidised enough to leave your stomach quickly. Smoothies can be useful for people who have nausea or a low appetite *because* they skip these fullness mechanisms. For example, I would suggest them to cancer patients or expectant mothers struggling with morning sickness. However, if your goal is to feel full, I suggest avoiding liquidised food.

Many highly enjoyable foods also sneak past our first two satiety cues. Remember, the catch with food that needs more chewing is that we enjoy it less – food companies have taken note of this. Do you remember what happened to food after the 1970s in the last chapter? It was altered into chemically engineered food-like substances because we needed it to have a very long shelf life. To achieve this, we had to strip it of components which might spoil, thus completely altering the original 'food matrix' (this is the structure of food which, as you might recall from the almond-butter example – see p. 46 – can dramatically influence our bodies' response to it). In his book *Ultra-Processed People* (a must-read) Dr Chris van Tulleken describes these UPFs as 'pre-chewed'. Now think about that: chewing directly triggers our satiety mechanisms – why are we choosing to eat food which doesn't? Part of the reason is that food we can eat quickly easily floods our brains with the feelgood chemical dopamine. When it comes to making a substance addictive, speed of delivery matters; for example, nicotine is absorbed rapidly when you smoke it, but when delivered through the skin in a patch it is absorbed *very* slowly. That's why people don't become addicted to the patches but *do* become addicted to cigarettes. Food that is easy to chew or, better yet, requires no chewing at all can give you a quick hit of rapidly absorbed sugar. The effect you see in the brain is similar to that of addictive drugs like cocaine. The rush of intense pleasure is irresistible. Wherever possible, my advice is to pick meals you can slowly enjoy chewing – after all, food is a simple pleasure like no other, why rush it? We will explore examples of these meals that fit this profile in the next few chapters but there are some more things you need to know about the act of eating first.

How to train ghrelin and insulin with eating windows

Just like we can retrain our sleep hormone, melatonin, to adjust to a new sleeping pattern in jet lag, we can retrain our hunger hormone, ghrelin, to spike at new times. It just takes longer. As we have already seen, because of the epigenetic expression of genes, it often takes about 12 weeks for a new habit to change our biology. That means after about three months of eating in a new rhythm, your hunger hormone will learn to spike in tandem. This might sound like a long time but, when you are eating *genuinely* filling food, it's not a difficult process to endure.

How you choose to arrange your eating window is ultimately up to you and dependent on your lifestyle. We are all exceptionally unique and not everyone feels comfortable fasting for long periods of time. Because of the structure of my clinics, I currently find it easiest to start eating at 12pm and finish by 8pm, an 8-hour eating window. More recently, scientists have suggested a 10-hour eating window is ideal. But if this isn't feasible for you, try to keep your eating window to 12 hours or less; for example, 8am to 8pm. Whichever pattern you choose, make sure it fits into an enjoyable life for you and remember that perfection is not the goal here – life is there to be lived, and food is an enormous part of a good life. If my eating window runs later than my 8pm cut-off while I'm out socialising, I don't worry about it and neither should you. And on days when I'm not working and have more flexibility, I often extend my window to 10 hours.

Ghrelin will learn to spike at your usual mealtimes, so my advice is to try to eat at roughly the same time of day and with the intention of feeling full. Of course, this might not always be practical. For example, when I was a junior doctor I had much less control over when (or even if) I could take a break to eat. Choreographing my ghrelin spikes was impossible, especially with my changing shift patterns. However, if your work and lifestyle *do* allow food to be something you can time, make the most of it. Sipping black coffee or tea can help if you feel peckish while you wait for your eating window to open – it helps you ride the wave of a ghrelin spike, which should only last 20 minutes or so. Unlike with dieting, you aren't starving yourself – the goal is actually to feel full. But you are rearranging your hunger signals so that you can choreograph well-timed insulin spikes. In the first three months this will involve riding out a 'hunger wave' while you wait to eat but, with time, you will synchronise your hunger with meals. When the time for food arrives, rather than restricting anything, you should fully enjoy eating a filling meal. But outside of these planned insulin spikes be mindful of whether an *extra* insulin spike is worth it. For example, if a colleague offers you a biscuit, first ask yourself if you genuinely want to eat it or if you are just doing so to be polite. If it is something you truly fancy, then accept it but wait for your mealtime so it can be part of a well-timed insulin spike. If you stick with this approach, you will directly alter your own biology and your entire experience of hunger. This epiphany is one of the most miraculous of my life and has completely changed how, when and why I eat.

It is important to note that strict time restricted eating (TRE) isn't appropriate for some people. As a general rule, there are some groups who should not attempt to prolong their fast beyond 12 hours: breastfeeding or pregnant women, type 1 diabetics and people recovering from an eating disorder. I also tend not to ask children to fast beyond 12 hours because, as far as I can tell, TRE hasn't been thoroughly researched in children. In fact, broadly speaking, what we understand about how children should eat is still very much up for debate. If they have a healthy microbiome and are offered food which prompts appropriate satiety mechanisms, I would argue their eating should be truly intuitive. If they feel hungrier one day, it might simply be because they have greater energy requirements. But the same is true if they are less hungry – something which often happens with toddlers. During this stage, their rate of growth and development can alter, meaning they might simply need less fuel. Many parents agonise about this and worry their child isn't eating enough. They might feel UPFs are the only way to convince their child to eat more, but this isn't necessary. Unless a child is unwell, losing weight or dropping a centile on their growth chart, they are fine. We need to start trusting their appetites – they are inbuilt to precisely tune how much the child should be eating. (This is based on the assumption that we aren't artificially stimulating an excessive appetite through UPFs and uncontrolled blood sugar spikes.) Returning to how they ate in the 1950s is the easiest thing to do – focus on mostly whole foods and no late-night snacking. It really doesn't need to be more complicated than that.

Of course, I don't want to imply changing how a child eats is easy. As much as possible, I suggest allowing them the opportunity to mirror their parents' healthy eating behav- iours,* which many parents do already. However, in the UK, many people are under the impression that they need to provide 'child-friendly' food, which doesn't exist as a concept in other places. Ideally, I think we can learn from countries

---

* This is why a key theme in treating childhood obesity is that you can't just change what the child is eating: you need the *entire* family to change their behaviour too. Eating is a social experience for children and evolution has primed them to copy their parents.

where there is less childhood obesity, like Japan and Italy. Children are essentially served the exact same food as their parents and eat it at the same time. Of course, this can be chopped up or mashed for infants and toddlers, but the basic premise is the same. Eating becomes a social ritual: they want to copy what you're doing while you're doing it. For some, this is realistically difficult to facilitate around work shifts but, whenever possible, it should be prioritised. I also strongly suggest taking a gentle approach; change is allowed to happen gradually. By working small changes into how we feed children – and ourselves – we allow time to adjust. You might start by simply changing your family's drink of choice: having plain water as the main thing you drink can have an enormous effect on health. A few weeks later, you might introduce an earlier dinner time and so on. You would be surprised how easy change can be when you pace yourself.

For everyone else, extending a fast is easier than you think when you understand how to do it. The list of health benefits is impressive, and I often warn my patients that time-restricted eating can act like some of their medication. If they are already on blood-pressure tablets or medication for diabetes, I suggest they monitor their blood pressure and blood sugar. After a few weeks, we might need to reduce the dose or stop it altogether because the root cause of their condition has been removed: they have reversed their insulin resistance.

Compared to calorie counting, this is a surprisingly simple concept to grasp. As I mentioned above, children often want to mimic their parents' behaviour and I am no exception. My parents had actually been doing time-restricted eating for a couple of years before I considered it myself. I had to go through my teenage-esque rebellion first and was wary of the idea, partly because *they* were the ones doing it. But one Christmas, while reading *The Diet Myth*, I was distracted in the morning as I slowly sipped black coffee. I looked up from the book and was surprised to see it was 12:30pm. As a devout breakfast lover and someone who had always been prone to 'hanger', this was a deeply thought-provoking moment. Could I keep this up?

Each day, during my holiday, I stuck to the same ritual and was surprised by how easy it was to wait for my eating window to open at noon. I wasn't counting calories or restricting myself – my meals were delicious and completely filling. The only thing that had changed was when I ate them. When I went back to work as a GP registrar, I found the pattern a little bit harder, but not much.* Remember, our stress hormone, cortisol, makes us feel hungrier and I certainly feel less stressed on holiday than I do at work. But equally, I found the pace of my morning clinic a helpful distraction – being busy stops you thinking about your appetite. I also found hunger would only last for a maximum of 30 minutes before subsiding; sipping black coffee seemed to help it pass. This is an anecdotal observation shared by many people who fast and I'm not sure why it works, but it does. I did really look forward to lunch and found myself quite hungry when it arrived but, miraculously, with time, this waned. After a few months, this pattern of eating felt like second nature – hunger became a calm feeling rather than an urgent sensation.

Going 'cold turkey' and jumping straight into a 16-hour fast worked for me but we are all unique and, according to Satchin Panda in his book *The Circadian Code*, a 14-hour fast creates exactly the same metabolic benefits as the traditional 16 hours – you need to pick the one that suits you best. You can also build up to it more slowly if that feels more comfortable, gradually delaying breakfast each week, or perhaps you would prefer an earlier dinner. Find a technique that works best for you.

When I suggest TRE to a new patient sometimes they have already tried it and given up – I find this is for one of three reasons. The first is that they didn't see any weight-loss results

---

* Registrar is the grade before you become a consultant or GP as a doctor in the UK – the final stage of training before becoming a fully trained specialist.

quickly and so they saw no point in continuing. When I tell them about all the other health benefits, they often reconsider. Importantly, how soon you lose weight depends on your level of insulin resistance and how many glycogen stores you have in your 'fridge'. If you have very high levels of fasting insulin, which many people living with obesity do, 16 hours of fasting might still not flip your metabolic switch into fat burning straight away. But with every day that goes by, your body has less and less glycogen left – it might take days or even weeks but eventually, after a 16-hour fast there will be nothing left. Finally, the body can then use the fat stores in your 'freezer' for energy and insulin levels start to drop in your bloodstream. The longer you continue this, the less insulin you are asking your body to make and, with time, you retrain the body to become sensitive to insulin. This means the insulin has a more potent effect on your cells: you need less of it to move blood sugar into them. Less insulin means less fat storing and more metabolic flexibility. This is literally the opposite of what happens in type 2 diabetes and is a huge part of why time-restricted eating promotes health so much.

The second reason patients give up quickly is that they find they're always hungry and can't stand fasting. According to Gin Stephens, author of the brilliant book *Fast. Feast. Repeat.*, this is usually because they aren't doing a 'clean fast', which simply means they have unknowingly been spiking their insulin during their fast. This could be by chewing gum, drinking calorie-free sweetened drinks or having milk in their tea/coffee. They have triggered the 'cephalic phase' (see p. 63) of their insulin spike, which often prompts a ghrelin spike. Without calories, this drops blood sugar, causing the 'dashboard' alarm that you are hangry! But, of course, this can be avoided. If you want to start prolonging your fast, only drink water, black coffee, black tea or green tea (without milk) during the fast. Nothing else.

Finally, from my point of view, the third reason why people give up is they simply aren't eating filling meals. No one teaches us how to do this and it's amazing how many traditional meals provide 'packaged hunger' but none of the building blocks for satiety. Breakfast cereal is a perfect example – with minimal fibre, fat or protein it doesn't stimulate any fullness mechanisms. Instead, it paradoxically triggers more hunger. Toast and jam, plain porridge, pasta and tomato sauce are other examples. Remember food is information for your body – you need to start sending the correct messages. Achieving this is surprisingly easy! And over the next few chapters I will show you how to apply these principles in a way that makes food both filling and enjoyable.

Eat to feel less hungry (and more full)

If you want a meal to stimulate *all* of your clever satiety mechanisms it must include three things: protein, fat and fibre. You hopefully now understand that this is so you can stimulate your fullness hormones, PYY, CCK, GLP-1, stretch the stomach and feed a healthy microbiome. (There are a few other fullness hormones, which you will also be influencing but, for simplicity, these are the most important.) Yet, it's amazing how many of us mindlessly eat culturally normalised foods which ignore this advice. Next time you buy food on the go, break it down into its parts: ready-made sandwiches, cereal bars and packets of snacks are primarily based on processed carbohydrates and refined sugars. Even with everything I know, I still struggle to find food on the go which will scientifically fill me up. It is surprisingly normal for us to eat non-filling food which behaves like 'packaged hunger'. I will address the anatomy of a good meal when we look at *what* you should eat later but for now, let's take a closer look at how to prevent an unplanned, extra ghrelin spike. It all comes down to regulating your blood sugar. Remember, blood sugar is normal and necessary for life. If it drops too low, you can go into a coma and die. I am not suggesting you need to avoid blood sugar spikes altogether.

However, you would be surprised by how dramatically you can alter *how* it spikes. The results are truly incredible.

The concept of regulating our blood sugar has become popularised in recent years even for people who don't have diabetes. As mentioned earlier, continuous glucose monitors (CGMs) are ingenious gadgets you can wear on your skin to track blood sugar for 14 days. By using them, scientists have discovered amazing tricks called 'glucose hacks' to alter our blood sugar spikes and dips. Importantly, there is a growing body of health professionals who now despair of what they believe is CGM misuse. In a way, I can see why. For anyone who is prone to perfectionism or obsession when it comes to their diet, monitoring blood sugar could be perceived as the new calorie, leaching joy away from food and simply giving people something new to agonise about. Another concern is that the data can be misinterpreted and paradoxically cause people to engage in less healthy habits. For example, exercise can spike your blood sugar while drinking vodka can drop it – obviously, even if it means a lower blood sugar, swapping a workout for alcohol is not a healthy solution. Ultimately, a blood sugar spike isn't good or bad; there is incredible *nuance* to interpreting the data and the effect it is having on your body. Therefore, I don't propose everyone should regularly wear a CGM – however, for some it can be a useful experience to learn from. Even if you never do this you can still benefit from using the glucose hacks they have unearthed.

At the time of writing this, I have worn a CGM once and found it a truly fascinating experience. What amazed me most was how my blood sugar correlated in real time with physical symptoms. One day I remember feeling famished two hours after a big lunch but, on top of my hunger, I also felt extremely fatigued and dizzy, as if I might faint. As I mentioned in the Introduction, fainting and dizziness have been a lifelong problem I have never been able to understand. My CGM finally gave me some answers: during the time of my symptoms, my blood sugar had been dancing up and down in a jittery pattern. This kept happening – whenever I felt like I was about to faint my blood sugar was erratic. Each time I looked back at the meal preceding my symptoms and, as a rule, it was very high in simple carbohydrates. I noticed particularly unpleasant symptoms in the morning if I had a lot of sugar after dinner. In fact, I would compare the experience to being hungover and now think of these symptoms as my 'sugar hangover'. If you find yourself feeling drained, lethargic, very hungry and maybe even dizzy, you could be giving yourself this sugar hangover too.*

Interestingly, the week before my period my blood sugar became much more erratic – even though I was eating the same food, my blood sugar was completely different. I'm not alone! We now know that premenstrual blood sugar spikes and dips more than at other times in the month. In hindsight, I realise the dizziness and fainting I have struggled with since childhood has often been unpredictable; however, like clockwork, it always got worse before my period. The interesting thing is that erratic blood sugar causes other symptoms too, including fatigue, irritability, anxiety, brain fog and hanger. Many women will recognise these symptoms before their period too and, for reasons they don't understand, will also develop them more often after reaching perimenopause. We now know this is because their blood sugar control simply changes around these times – as a result, learning to incorporate glucose hacks can significantly improve symptoms. In fact, erratic blood sugar can influence everything from migraines to acne – it also drives excess ghrelin production making us feel much hungrier. In short, I try to teach all of my patients about glucose hacks because they will be relevant for anyone who wants to feel well and avoid future disease.

---

* Dizziness is incredibly complex and I don't mean to imply erratic blood sugar is the only cause. There are many other causes, such as medication, a sudden drop in blood pressure, various ear, nose and throat (ENT) conditions and even neurological causes. Always see your own doctor if you have new symptoms, but if you can't get to the bottom of it, look at what you eat. The solution may well be in your own hands.

There are many different clever lifestyle tricks or 'glucose hacks' I could write a whole book about but luckily, I don't have to because Jessie Inchauspé has already done that in her incredible book *Glucose Revolution*. I ask almost all my patients to read this and, to my surprise, a lot of them actually listen to me! I highly recommend reading it if you haven't already to appreciate the full detail. Importantly, Inchauspé strongly suggests food should be *enjoyed*; she echoes my sentiment that weight loss is just a pleasant side effect where health is the goal. The tricks suggested can be used as and when it is *convenient*, but are by no means set in stone. I will briefly summarise my favourite ones, which I incorporate into my own life.

BE FRENCH

The first trick is to 'be French' which, in a roundabout way, is a memory tool for several glucose hacks in one. Without even meaning to there are a number of things French people do which conveniently stabilise their blood sugar – I suggest we copy them. However, we first need to make sure we are on the same page about what French food is: I am talking about what they eat at home, not what tourists are served. So often, I find cuisines are misinterpreted by other countries. You might think of French food as baguettes, croissants and wine. But French restaurants don't necessarily reflect the home cook's cuisine. A traditional plate of home-cooked food in France will have plenty of fibre, fat and some protein, which all stimulate fullness mechanisms, while also allowing for calm and steady blood sugar.

My idea of a French home-cooked meal starts with a big, crunchy salad, drenched in a delicious dressing which includes vinegar. This is a genius start to any meal because it embodies several glucose-controlling principles. In fact, I almost always start dinner with salad and vinegar, which I highly recommend my patients copy. As Jessie Inchauspé calls it, this 'vegetable starter hack' is a brilliant way to calm your blood sugar spike,

but it doesn't need to be a salad; it can be anything savoury with fibre, meaning some olives or a handful of nuts works just as well. Soup* can be an example, as long as it's not made up of starchy root vegetables. The key is to inject lots of fibre before you later eat some starch. If you begin a meal with savoury plants, their valuable fibre is given a head start; once they're in your intestines with the rest of your meal they create a gloopy 'net' between sugar molecules and your blood supply. The goal isn't to stop sugar getting into your blood, it just enters more slowly. These nets simply create a very *gradual* rise in blood sugar, which can calmly drop back down, thus avoiding extra insulin, a rapid drop and a subsequent spike in ghrelin.

To harness this effect further, eating food in a specific order can help but I wouldn't overthink this and only consider it when it is convenient to do so. When you can, try to eat most of the fibre, fat and protein first, before you enjoy the bulk of simple carbohydrates or sugar. My best example of this is a roast dinner: I fully intend to eat each component, but I do it with my biology in mind. First, I often order a salad with vinegar as my 'veggie starter'. Later when my main arrives, I eat most of the fibrous vegetables and protein. Once I have finished most of this I tuck into the root vegetables and simple starches, like carrots and potatoes, as well as the Yorkshire pudding. I pick a drink which isn't sweet – usually sparkling water – and save sugar for dessert. Simply by eating the fibre, fat and protein first, I slow how quickly I can absorb sugar from the rest of my meal.

Interestingly, the vinegar on the salad also helps in its own right; some people exploit this by popping 2 tablespoons in water and drinking it 20 minutes before their meal. It can reduce

---

* With soup I lean towards chunky options which still need to be chewed so that I can make use of my chewing and stomach stretching satiety cues. However, I am not a perfectionist! This does not mean puréed soup is 'bad' or that I would NEVER eat it – but when given the option I always choose food which will capitalise on my satiety mechanisms most effectively.

your blood sugar spike by an impressive 30 per cent, and this is true of any vinegar, as long as sugar hasn't been added to it. You might be wondering how on earth this happens. Remember the 2–30 types of amylase genes we all have (see p. 114) and how dramatically this can affect how we absorb energy from carbohydrates? Well, vinegar makes amylase less efficient at breaking carbs down into sugar. In other words, you slow its digestion and therefore how quickly the sugar is released into your bloodstream. Vinegar also seems to have a beneficial effect on your mitochondria. In both ways, it seems to calm your blood sugar spike but, again, I only incorporate it when it's convenient.

BEGIN THE DAY RIGHT

People always say breakfast is the most important meal of the day, but I now say 'break-fast' is the most important meal. When you choose to break your fast is up to you; as I said, I do this roughly around lunchtime and I now know my first meal will dramatically shape my blood sugar spikes for the rest of the day. For reasons discussed above, once that cycle of over-excited insulin and ghrelin starts, it is very hard to stop. The first meal of your day is like that anxiety-inducing climb to the first drop of a rollercoaster; if you start with a huge spike you get momentum to bounce up and down furiously for the rest of the ride. But if it's just a little bump there's very little momentum. Now try to picture your breakfast's effect on blood sugar: how many carbohydrates are in your first meal? More importantly, how much fibre is there? Does it actually trigger your fullness hormones with lots of healthy fat and protein? I find my patients' 'break-fast' is the easiest meal for me to change in the last 2 minutes of a rushed 10-minute consultation, especially with my diabetic patients. I ask them to swap their cereal or muesli for eggs, Greek yoghurt or any other high protein meal served with some fibre. I also ask them to cut out their sweet drinks (including artificial sweeteners) and send them

home with *Glucose Revolution* as homework. By the time I see their repeat blood sugar it has almost always dropped and sometimes, in a matter of months, they have even reversed their diabetes. Like I said, break-fast is the most important meal of the day.

EAT SWEET FOODS THOUGHTFULLY AND AT THE RIGHT TIME

I genuinely don't think you can live a good life without sugar. Food is more than a fuel source – it is what binds people. How many social occasions can you think of which don't include food? How many nostalgic memories are tied to it? I am not interested in demonising anything we eat; life is simply too short not to experience the simple pleasures in life, and sweet foods are one of them. But we are consuming more sweet flavours than ever before. Remember Ancel Key's 'Seven (*cough* 22) Countries Study', which scared us into cutting out dietary fat, while never declaring its funding from the sugar industry? Around the same time, Keys had a fierce rivalry with a Professor John Yudkin who wrote a book called *Pure, White and Deadly* (1972). In it, Yudkin pointed out that dietary-fat consumption had not changed for centuries, and he sensibly questioned how it could therefore be the cause of increasing heart disease. Instead, he noted that refined-sugar consumption had exploded in tandem with our rising heart disease and wrote, 'If only a small fraction of what we know about the effects of sugar were to be revealed in relation to any other material used as a food additive that material would promptly be banned'. He wrote this more than 50 years ago and since then, we have progressively continued to eat more and more of the stuff.

Even just in my lifetime average sugar consumption has gone up by 31.5 per cent, and the average British child gets 12.3 per cent of their calories from added sugar. Apparently, this number should be more like 5 per cent, but what does that mean and how on earth can we realistically calculate how much sugar we're consuming when it is added to everything?

For example, one tablespoon of ketchup has one teaspoon of sugar in it, but who only eats one tablespoon? A glass of fruit juice contains as much sugar as a glass of Coca-Cola – care to guess how many teaspoons that is? Eight teaspoons! If you stirred eight teaspoons of sugar into water it would be unpalatably sweet but acid and salt help to mask this in soft drinks.* Artificial sweeteners are no better and may be worse because they appear to trigger overconsumption of more calories, especially from sweet foods. This is because they cause a blood sugar dip and a ghrelin spike. Ultimately, artificial sweeteners are driving the process you want least in your body: insulin resistance. Worryingly, part of the way they also achieve this is by disrupting your valuable microbiome. Remember how much our bugs can protect us from diseases like allergy, auto-immune conditions, IBS, cancer and depression to name a few? Is artificial sweetness worth disrupting that?

But what can you do with all this information? The wellness community suggests blitzing dates and other dried fruits with several 'healthy' sugars from honey or coconut sugar. But in truth, to your body, sugar is sugar. You may get more nutrients or polyphenols with other 'natural' sources, but this won't undo the total volume you are consuming. Remember, eating refined sugar is one of the easiest ways to trigger insulin resistance. Part of how that happens is through damaging your liver with a condition called non-alcoholic fatty-liver disease (NAFLD). I see this all the time in many of my young

---

* If this is a useful visual mnemonic for you, I recommend reading how many grams of sugar are in a food you are about to consume. Divide that number by four and you have the teaspoon of sugar. However, watch out for the portion sizes suggested on the packet. Many cereal packets suggest you will eat a small handful but in reality (because cereal stimulates none of our fullness mechanisms), we can eat ten times the amount. Many sweet cereals have 13g (3.25 teaspoons) sugar per handful – ten handfuls would be *easy* to eat and would give you 32.5 teaspoons sugar. Imagine mixing that with water and drinking it. Is that something you want to consume? And, more importantly, is that something you want your child to consume?

patients and, increasingly, we are seeing it in children as well. Usually, we just monitor it, but if it progresses for long enough, it scars the liver irreversibly causing cirrhosis, which you can die from. This takes time, so if you are triggering the liver damage in childhood, it behaves like compound interest, allowing far more time to progress to life-threatening cirrhosis. NAFLD isn't something I would wish on anyone because, by definition, if you are clogging your liver up with fatty changes you are massively driving insulin resistance around the rest of the body. One of the main things driving NAFLD is a sugar molecule called fructose because, unlike other sugar molecules, it can mostly only be metabolised in the liver. Starch in potatoes, for example, is made up of a chain of glucose molecules which can be used anywhere in the body. On the other hand, sweet-tasting fruit or table sugar is made of a combination of glucose and fructose. It's not that our bodies can't tolerate *any* sugar – obviously fruit has been a delicious and healthy part of our evolution. The liver simply can't cope with the total volume of fructose we are exposing it to. So please try not to be fooled; most people with a Western diet would significantly benefit from reducing how much fructose they consume. But how can we do this intuitively without stripping the joy out of food and treating every bite like a maths calculation?

One problem is that most people don't even register how much sugar they are consuming because over time, as food companies have been sneaking sweetness into almost everything, our palates have become desensitised to it. The exact same thing happens with spicy food – the longer and more frequently someone eats it, the less their palate will register it. With practice, they can tolerate spicier food. Without realising it you might have become less sensitive to sugar, meaning you can tolerate (and even enjoy) a flavour which would once have been unpalatably sweet. Importantly, I need to repeat that I don't want to demonise food or encourage obsessive tracking of what you eat. Food can and should be something which feels intuitive to us. My advice is simple: you need to retrain your palate and resensitise it to sweet flavours. If you eat fewer sweet flavours, over time certain foods will start to taste unpalatably sweet and you simply won't enjoy them anymore. This will also open your palate up to appreciate new bitter flavours, which are often tied to an abundance of polyphenols in foods like dark chocolate or black coffee. But how can you meaningfully resensitise your palate to sweet flavours without feeling restricted?

Firstly, stop drinking sweet drinks – you don't need them in your life. Honestly, think about it: drinking plain water is not a hardship. But if you want a sweet drink as a rare treat, sip it slowly with a meal when you're spiking your insulin anyway.

Secondly, we need to talk about fruit. Again, fruit is a wonderful thing and very healthy for you, but I ask that you mostly eat it in its whole form and ideally not dried. Removing its water shrinks its volume, meaning you can eat a much bigger quantity and therefore get much more sugar than you would from the fresh version. And though I don't want to be tyrannical about this, please try to chew your fruit for reasons mentioned above; drinking it, whether as a juice or smoothie, also allows you to consume more fruit (and sugar) than you normally would. Fruit juice really only became a popular purchase after a big marketing campaign in the 1980s and soft drinks were reserved as a rare treat. Plain water deserves a marketing campaign of its own – we need to normalise hydrating ourselves with what our ancestors evolved drinking. Next, though this might sound extreme, I generally don't eat much more than two portions of fruit a day. I am not going off piste here – the 5 A Day campaign in the UK advises three portions of vegetables and two of fruit.*

---

* This is also what I was taught in nutrition lectures at medical school. Importantly, there is nuance here: some fruits like berries are actually very low in sugar so you can't directly compare them to tropical fruits – like mango, for example. I'm also not suggesting it needs to be a hard rule all of the time and, of course, some days I happen to have a little bit more. But my average is around two portions a day and this does not leave me feeling restricted in any way.

Being asked to eat *less* fruit by a doctor might sound strange but some of my patients eat *enormous* volumes. Remember that sugar is sugar – it might come from different sources, but the total volume you consume also matters. Perfectionism isn't the goal here but, for some people struggling with consequences of insulin resistance, their volume of fruit consumption is something they've never even considered.

Finally, if you are going to eat something sweet (including fruit), save it for the end of a savoury meal, after you have already released that fibre 'net' into your intestines. This will make the blood sugar rise much calmer. I don't follow this rule perfectly all the time – low-sugar fruits like berries are fine in a yoghurt bowl and don't need to be eaten separately. Equally, I sometimes like fruit in a salad. When I first learned about these techniques, I stopped 'allowing' myself fruit in salad, until I realised this was bordering on obsessive. Again, food should be delicious and enjoyable – if you are agonising about some apple slices in a salad, you're overdoing it. Please catch yourself should you do anything similar: if you are fretting about whether a healthy food is 'healthy enough', it's time to calm down. Importantly, sugar can still be part of your life. Populations with the best life expectancies and heart health *do* eat dessert, but only really once a week as a treat. How do I incorporate this into my own life? On weekdays, I have some fruit after dinner and maybe some 85 per cent dark chocolate as well – I consider this a delicious end to my meal and not a hardship or form of 'restriction'. Biscuits, cakes, ice cream and puddings are not something I eat every day. But trust me, when I do eat them as a rare treat I truly savour and enjoy every bite. A delicious homemade dessert treated as a weekly ritual feels like an event, and it's one I'm happy to wait for.

I hope the theory we covered in Part I is starting to click into place. You know now that you are heavily influenced by your hormones – but we can mould these ourselves. Understanding food is a language to your body puts the ball back in your court. By recalibrating your hunger hormone, ghrelin, to spike in a predictable and calm way, you no longer feel under the control of your appetite. Instead, you become the one guiding your body, helping to align it with a lifestyle that is convenient for you. Feeling constantly hungry isn't just inconvenient, it is uncomfortable and incredibly distracting. Learning how to appropriately stimulate your fullness mechanisms manages it even more. But the benefits are greater still: if you can train your body to become metabolically flexible, eating can become truly intuitive. Analysing, counting or restricting it in any way won't be necessary because you will be able to trust your appetite. It might ask you to eat more some days and less on others because that's what your body needs. Finally, you can stop worrying about it and eating can be what it should always have been: an incredibly enjoyable pastime. But there's more. If you follow the advice in this chapter, you will already be dramatically improving your health. Next, we need to take a closer look at the specific foods you are eating because they can also make you feel better and live longer.

How to eat: Key points

1) Your body has evolved with tightly controlled mechanisms to monitor your food requirements and communicates this with you through your appetite. Our modern lives have disrupted these messages, but it is entirely possible to recalibrate them so that you can eat intuitively.

2) The goal of any change should be health, but there is nothing wrong with wanting to lose weight – I just don't suggest you monitor this. If you trust the process, the weight will come off and this will arrive as a pleasant surprise. If you want to monitor anything, use a tape measure: it won't punish you for gaining muscle like the scales might.

3) Time-restricted eating and not snacking are not new concepts – we always used to eat this way and it's only in the last 50 years that this changed. Adopting these techniques will result in a plethora of health benefits and will also transform your experience of appetite. Like me, you might find it reduces and feels more like a predictable and calm sensation, rather than something you need to address urgently.

4) Learning how to regulate your blood sugar dramatically influences health and many daily symptoms but also helps to control ghrelin. A vegetable starter and vinegar, eating foods in the right order and leaving sweet flavours for the end of a meal are a good place to start.

5) You don't need sweet drinks. Full stop. I would reserve them as rare treats only. As much as possible, hydrate with plain water and if you want flavour, focus on drinks that have bitter flavours like plain tea/black coffee.

6) Over the last 50 years, our consumption of all sugars has jumped significantly. You need to recalibrate your palate and 'resensitise' it to sweet flavours. Dessert should be an occasional treat, not a daily custom. Finally, fruit is absolutely very healthy, as long as you eat it in the right way.

Ideally, try to consume no more than two portions of whole fruit, which needs to be chewed (i.e. not juices/smoothies), and try mostly to have it at the end of a savoury meal.

CHAPTER 8

FOOD

What should you eat?

By now it will feel like we have covered a lot: that's because we have. So far I have given you the tools to change *how* you eat to boost health but what is it you should actually be eating? How can you boost your all-important microbiome? And what approach should you take to food if you want to live a long life and protect yourself from disease? Scroll through social media and you'll see *a lot* of opinions on this. You'll find fancy-sounding names of specific food chemicals and a load of niche research. You don't really *need* to know any of this to eat well. There are many populations around the world who do all the right things without ever learning anything about nutrition. Food might be a medicine, but it doesn't need to be treated like one.

No health subject is more furiously debated than food and with social media virtually anyone can advertise their 'expertise'; even if they do have relevant credentials, it is hard to confirm them but, in truth, a nice body is worth more than any résumé. I have fallen for countless trends, convinced I was promoting health when really, I was hindering it. But how can you possibly sift through the noise when for every person who tells you to do one thing there is another telling you to do the opposite? It turns out, while the science is profoundly complex, the question of what you should eat is surprisingly easy to answer. We are the ones complicating it with academic debate but eating food doesn't need to feel like you are sitting a test. If I have convinced you simply to value the science already covered, what will follow should feel intuitive.

Intuitive food choices

Most people associate cravings with something negative and assume they should be resisted. In fact, giving into our cravings somehow feels like a personal weakness, as if it were driven by our character. But what was the original evolutionary role of these impulses? At its most extreme, we see examples of odd food cravings in something called 'pica' – a condition often seen in pregnant women who are overcome by a desire to eat things that aren't food. They find themselves eating things like soil, clay or even pebbles. Blood tests often show that they are deficient in iron or zinc – their biology has overcome social etiquette in the hunt for a nutrient they are deficient in. A similar phenomenon is seen in animals: when given a selection of nutrient sources, they will intuitively eat what they are lacking. However, if only given one food with no source of what they are deficient in, something very interesting happens: they start to furiously overeat. In his book *Ultra-Processed People* Dr Chris van Tulleken proposes we are doing the exact same thing: our Westernised food landscape has stripped the nutrient value of food beyond recognition. Many products add some vitamins back in but remember, there are 25,000 phyto-chemicals in the plants we eat, many of which we don't fully understand. No food company can compete with this which means that having replaced up to 70 per cent of our diets with ultra-processed foods (UPFs), we are malnourished beyond our wildest dreams. Our endlessly intelligent bodies will do anything they can to seek out missing nutrients, driving an evolutionary reflex to overeat.

Is it really possible for us to somehow, on a subconscious level, be guided by cravings to eat what we are lacking? The best way to examine this is to look at people who have never been exposed to food before and see how they behave – an arguably challenging feat both practically and ethically. Fortunately, scientists were less concerned about ethics 100 years ago and we actually do have a fascinating study no one would ever dare repeat today. Dr Tulleken tells the story of Dr Clara Davis, an American paediatrician who was becoming increasingly disillusioned with what her patients were being fed. 'Experts' at the time were popping up everywhere and parents were being given ever more complicated advice about what they should feed their children. Historically, kids simply ate what their parents ate – when they were younger it was mashed up for them but, on the whole, these little humans were served the same as the adults. Specially designed diets* became the 'in' thing in the 1920s, but there was one problem: children refused to eat them. Parents flocked to their doctors in desperation and were told to remain strong with the advice that these 'fussy' eaters should be left hungry, until they accepted the food. Davis considered this obscene and wanted to see what would happen if babies were left to choose their own food.

Here comes the ethically questionable part: 15 babies (under 12 months of age) who had only ever been exclusively breast-fed were admitted into a facility away from their parents for a rather abrupt weaning process. Mothers willing to hand over their babies for several months did so because they were destitute and, as a result, some of the children were malnourished and very underweight. Every day each baby was offered a variety of 34 different whole food options which, when combined, provided them with every single macro- and micronutrient they could ever need. The nurses looking after them were not allowed to prompt or encourage any of the foods – what and how they ate was entirely decided by the baby who, remember, had never eaten anything before. Interestingly, apart from two children who didn't like lettuce and one who didn't like spinach,

---

* Rather than serving infants a softened or slightly mashed portion of what the parent was eating it was declared that they needed separate 'baby food'. This could be plain sieved fruit/potatoes or different types of plain cereals. These were likely less appetising but also meant food was no longer a social interaction in which the baby was trying to copy the eating habits of their parents.

every food item was consumed happily and without coercion. The babies were not 'fussy'; on the contrary, they were noted to have very good appetites. They were independently able to consume an entirely balanced diet, getting enough fat, protein, carbohydrates and micronutrients to meet their precise needs. They even willingly ate plain salt from a dish; though it made them splutter and cry when they tried it, they still went back for more, thus meeting their salt requirements. I'm not proposing parents repeat this experiment at home with a salt dish, and I suggest they still defer to the trusted health advice they receive in this area. But it is interesting that these babies were able to self-regulate their diet so well.

The most amazing finding was seen in a particularly thin and malnourished child who had developed rickets from vitamin D deficiency. At the time, the only source of vitamin D replacement came in the form of cod-liver oil, which is just as unpalatable as it sounds. For three months, the child with rickets ate this fishy oil by choice every single day until, one day, he abruptly stopped. Though it was still offered to him, he voluntarily turned down what had been a daily ritual. When they repeated his X-rays and tests, they found his rickets had cleared: he didn't crave the oil anymore because he was no longer deficient in vitamin D. This is astounding when, really, it shouldn't be: if animals intuitively know how and what to eat without calorie counting, using vitamin supplements or diet plans from a dietician, why shouldn't we be able to do this too? The catch here is that this study was performed in 1928, the participants had never been exposed to food before and were only served 100 per cent whole food ingredients. Many of us today would struggle to respond intuitively to cravings because of how exposed we are to UPFs.

In the depths of my yo-yo dieting, I became enamoured with the idea of intuitive eating and earnestly tried to 'listen to my body', eating anything and everything I craved. In fact, it made me gain much more weight – but, in hindsight, I realise that's not because intuitive eating isn't possible. In our current food environment, if you are told to eat whatever you feel like and as much as you like, you have to remember your microbiome, insulin resistance and metabolic flexibility (or more likely inflexibility) are calling the shots. Not to mention, UPFs are cleverly designed to bypass your fullness mechanisms and also stimulate the same addictive pathways as cocaine. Also, unlike the babies in the experiment, you have obviously had some prior exposure to food which is not just a form of fuel. Food is a cultural ritual with huge subconscious emotions and memories attached to it – the meals that bring you a sense of nostalgia, for example, might bypass the ancient nutrient-seeking mechanisms within you. You will perceive this as a craving when really, it is an emotional longing. Trying to decipher the difference between these two is very difficult, especially in times of stress. But with practice – and the advice in this chapter – I think it is achievable, at least in my experience.

Another important reason why intuitive eating often doesn't work well is because, as with people suffering from pica, what many of us are eating arguably isn't actually real food. This impacts the nutrients we are (or rather, aren't) getting, which, in turn, can affect our reflex to eat. As Van Tulleken puts it, when it comes to our UPF diet, we are eating 'food-like substances'. The man-made mush we willingly consume would be completely inedible without a cocktail of largely unregulated flavourings and other chemicals. There are many environmental, ethical and even philosophical problems with how these foods are made, and they are covered beautifully in Van Tulleken's book, but, as you might have guessed, there are several health problems too.

On the simplest level, our bodies and their teams of microbiomes did not evolve alongside these products, which means our nutrient-seeking pathways didn't either. Mark Schatzker explores this in his book *The Dorito Effect* and suggests that the flavour of food isn't just needed for pleasure, it actually provides the body with vital instructions. Remember how well our bodies can track what food is coming in to influence satiety? Something similar happens with flavour and cravings – the body links it to the nutrients it is associated with; not only can it track what it is receiving, it can signal to you what it needs. Flavour is a language. You don't wake up thinking, *I could really do with some more iodine today*, but you might think: *I wouldn't mind some salmon tonight.* If you trick the body into thinking it is receiving nutrients via fake flavours it will drive you to eat more, hoping this increases your chances of stumbling across what you are missing.

As mentioned earlier, some of the longest-living populations in the world eat amazingly healthful diets without ever reading about nutrition. Food does not need to be complicated. Bizarrely, often some of the poorest people in the world can have far less disease. We already saw one example with the study comparing bowel cancer in rural Africans to African Americans (see p. 39). But my favourite example involves five pockets in the world, called the Blue Zones, where an unusual percentage of citizens live into their hundreds. Dan Buettner* has been researching them for many years and their 'secrets' are surprising. Most of these people aren't rich; if anything, they are arguably quite poor. They lead simple, meaningful and highly sociable lives, but they don't count calories, measure their macros or pop supplements. The Mediterranean diet is one of the most heavily researched diets, with ample evidence that it dramatically reduces disease, so it's no surprise that there are Blue Zones in both Italy and Greece. However, the others are in Japan, Costa Rica and the United States. A new one even seems to be emerging in Singapore. Though their cuisines are

---

* National Geographic Fellow Dan Buettner is quickly becoming a household name after his decades of research into the Blue Zones. He has written several books on the subject and, more recently, appears in the Netflix documentary *Live to 100: Secrets of the Blue Zones*, which I often set my patients as 'homework'.

all different, when it comes to what these groups eat they have one thing in common: the food is very traditional. In other words, these centenarians embrace a strong 'food culture' and are incredibly proud to cook recipes their grandparents taught them. If you speak to any Italian nonna (grandmother) and ask how she describes her food, she won't tell you that it is 'healthy', she will simply say her food is 'good'.

Places where food heritage has been displaced by ultra-processed foods don't get it – you don't need to 'behave' or 'restrict' yourself to eat 'healthy' food. You just need to know what 'good' food looks like. That's why I don't teach my patients to memorise how many grams of protein or fibre they can get from a chia seed: I simply teach them how to cook *good* food. If you know how to do this, everything else will fall into place and, with some principles, eating can really become intuitive again. Essentially, the main things you need to know are: how to feed a healthy microbiome, reach your basic dietary requirements and optimise your blood fats. If you do this, not only will you protect yourself from many diseases, you will also spend your day-to-day life genuinely feeling well. First, I will cover the principles and in the next chapter I will show you how I achieve them with the food I personally eat.

Principle number 1: Feed your microbiome what it likes

Remember Wu's gruel and how it transformed his health (see p. 18)? We can do the exact same thing ourselves if we know which foods a diverse and healthy microbiome thrives off. The wonderful thing is that a lot of this involves an attitude of abundance towards food. When thinking about what to feed your microbiome, more is more.

We now understand that different bacteria tend to thrive off different plants. The key to a healthy microbiome is diversity and to achieve this, your food also needs to be diverse. For the first time in my life, after learning about the microbiome, I started thinking, *What can I add?* rather than, *What should I restrict?* This mindset is the opposite to many classic eating disorders and felt like such a relief. Rather than denying myself foods, I always think about what microbiome-boosting foods I can squeeze on to my plate or how to mix things up. What I eat is constantly changing because I know that's how to keep my gut bugs on their toes – the novelty of a new ingredient or recipe also keeps food interesting for me. I'm not trying to 'be good' and I'm certainly not on a diet. Food is more exciting now than it's ever been before; let me show you how ...

PREBIOTICS

The term 'prebiotic' wasn't even a recognised word when I was born. It basically just means a substance our microbiomes can consume to produce beneficial health outcomes. It's the food that makes them happy, in other words.

Most soluble fibre is a prebiotic and a particularly well-documented one is called inulin, found in the allium family (onion-tasting vegetables), garlic, Jerusalem artichoke, globe artichoke, asparagus, dandelion leaves, bananas and plantains. Beta-glucans are another important soluble fibre found in barley, oats, rye, mushrooms and seaweed, to name a few. But our bugs thrive off things other than fibre and one example is something called resistant starch, which can also act like a prebiotic. When you let a cooked starch like potatoes, rice or pasta cool, the shape of the starch molecules changes, making them 'resistant' against digestion long enough for them to reach the large intestine where your microbiome can feed off them. The humble potato has never received much good press in the wellness community but, if you just let it cool, it is a cheap health hack. Salad niçoise, fried leftover potatoes and even homemade gnocchi, therefore, all have some prebiotic resistant starches.

The even more humble bean* would be an extortionately expensive 'superfood' if we discovered it now, as it is another amazing source of prebiotics. But the OG prebiotic we can be exposed to is in breastmilk in the form of something called HMO (human milk oligosaccharides), which can feed a healthy microbiome for the baby. In fact, breast milk may even be a *probiotic* too. We always used to think bodily fluids were all sterile, but breast milk contains hundreds of microbiome species, and this might be another reason why breastfed babies have better health outcomes.

PLANT VARIETY

This is the most important bit of advice but also the most uplifting because, though it might be daunting at first, challenging yourself to eat more variety is surprisingly fun. Simply put, we know people who eat at least 30 different plants a week have much healthier microbiomes. Given half of your cells are actually bugs, which have a huge impact on your health, when I say more is more, I mean more plants is more health. It is as simple as that. But let's put it into context and look at people who are getting their microbiomes just right.

A perfect example is the hunter-gatherer Hadza tribe in Tanzania. Their microbiomes are 40 per cent more diverse than the average American's. They eat around 600 different plants a year, knocking back more than 100g fibre a day. A measly 12 plants make up 75 per cent of the food we eat in the West; the average American eats 15g fibre a day and totals less than 50 different types of plants in a year. That's a sizeable difference. Bearing in mind that there are 300,000 edible plants in the world, most of us are fairly unadventurous from our guts' point of view. You may take comfort in familiarity and have a tendency to eat the same breakfast each day – perhaps you are

---

* Really, I should use the umbrella term 'legume' here – it basically encompasses all the 'beans' (including peanuts, which technically aren't a nut), peas and lentils.

prone to using the same recipes each week for other meals. But your bugs don't see that as comforting. They find it boring. Always think of your microbiome as a party: it's your job to make it a fun one.

But how can you meaningfully mix things up? It's easier than you think. Firstly, you have to understand what counts as a plant and broaden your food repertoire. Grains, legumes, nuts, seeds, spices, herbs, cocoa powder (or dark chocolate), tea, wine, coffee, fruits and vegetables all count. Better still, even another variety of the same plant or just another colour of the same plant will count as something *different*. I appreciate the idea of eating 30 different vegetables a week might be daunting, but they are only one type of plant. Let's say white rice is a staple you eat most days – that's a wasted opportunity for plant diversity. Why not mix it up? One day try pearl barley, on another, have a mixture of three potato varieties and the next day, go for a tricolour quinoa mix. Already, instead of one plant providing your carb base, you now have seven. Then throw in a side salad with four different types of leaves and four other plants each night and that's an extra eight. So just your dinner carb and side salad have got you halfway to your target for the week. The more attention you pay to variety opportunities, the more you will see how incredibly easy it is to rack up 30 a week – in fact, you might manage far more. The easiest change you can make is to look at your plate and think, *What could I add to this?* There will always be room for a sprinkle of seeds, spices, herbs, a drizzle of salsa, a side salad or anything else that is a plant. These small things all add up.

Next, become excited about food and aim *not* to become a good cook: become a brilliant one! Cultures that churn out brilliant home cooks have better health – this is something public health campaigns could capitalise on. Perhaps one day home economics will be a compulsory class in all schools, teaching kids to cook food which is as delicious for them as it is for their microbiome. For now, invest time and energy to becoming a better cook yourself. If you explore new cuisines, that's even better because that likely means using new plants you probably don't usually cook with. Foraging* or growing your own food is an excellent way to expose yourself to even more variety, especially given supermarkets sell relatively few varieties of plants. For example, there are over 7,500 different varieties of apple, which could each count as a different plant point – most supermarkets I have been to have the same five all year round.

Finally, on that note, eating the same food all year round makes no sense from an environmental point of view or from that of our bugs. With globalisation, we can now eat the same plants every day if we want, even though Mother Nature naturally provides a constant change, month on month. Why eat an apple in the middle of summer, shipped from the other side of the world, stored for months, with gradually less nutritional value, when you could eat fresh plums that are in season? As much as I can, I try to eat local, seasonal food, if not to support the environment of the planet and my gut, then at least to support local farmers who are struggling in our current food climate. We should each aim for about 30g fibre a day, but please don't feel this is something you need to meticulously calculate. I strongly believe food and calculators should have nothing to do with each other, and I have found I can easily keep a rough tally of plants in my head; remember 30 plants is a minimum sweet spot which confers huge benefit. If you get 30 or more plants in a week with hearty, wholefood recipes, you should comfortably meet your daily fibre requirements. However, you are welcome to have more, just like the Hadza tribe clearly do.

---

* Of course, foraged food should be sourced carefully and ethically – only take what you *need*, not what you *want* so you can ensure the plant is able to grow back the next year. And only ever eat food you have identified with 100 per cent confidence!

POLYPHENOLS

Put very simply, polyphenols are defence chemicals found in plants, which actually serve to protect them from harsh weather or predators. Funnily enough, as their 'predators' ourselves, we now seek these plants out for the polyphenols which were designed to deter us!

Learning more about which foods contain the most polyphenols is one of my favourite parts of Tim Spector's book *Food for Life*. Plants with vibrant colours and, in some cases, quite bitter flavours can be packed with these helpful chemicals. Very deep colours seen in foods like coffee, cocoa, black beans, plums and blackberries are a sign of exceptionally high levels of polyphenols. Sadly, many of the plants we eat have been bred not for their nutritional value, but for their shelf life. Iceberg lettuce is an excellent example of one that has almost no nutritional value when you compare it to other brightly coloured, spicy, bitter and frilly salads which perish much faster. The spicy kick you get at the back of your throat from a good-quality extra virgin olive oil is also a sign of its amazing polyphenol content – something which can vary significantly in different brands. Perhaps one day, instead of a traffic-light sign with quantities of fat and calories, food packets will specifically advertise grams of fibre and polyphenols.

But what is so great about these polyphenols and why should you consciously try to eat more of them? Firstly, if your microbiome is a calm cocktail party, polyphenols turn it into a cinematic and explosive 'part-ay'. Prebiotics might loosen our bugs' inhibitions but polyphenols positively remove them and they go absolutely wild, having the time of their lives. Next, and this particularly excites me, polyphenols look after our vital blood vessels. They significantly lower inflammation in the blood vessels, protecting them from plaques and narrowing. Downstream, this affects the vital organs at the end of those blood vessels, like your brain and heart. (Statins, a drug I often prescribe, have a very similar effect: reducing inflammation in blood vessels is part of what protects people from strokes and heart attacks.) A diet high in polyphenols can reduce cardiovascular disease risk by a whopping 46 per cent. Need I say more?

Getting lots of polyphenols means eating brightly coloured foods, lots of spices and even bitter flavours. A traditional Mediterranean diet will be teeming with polyphenols – but again, I am referring to a home cook's version, not the tourist's interpretation (see p. 168). Nutrition science is very much in its infancy as a scientific discipline, partly because promoting the benefits of simple food isn't a great way to make money. In truth, we are only now scratching the surface of what polyphenols can do for us, but can already see they also fight cancer, protect the skin from damage and signs of ageing, while also boosting cognitive performance. You don't need to pay for a prescription or supplement to harness these benefits: you just need to eat the right foods.

PROBIOTIC FOODS

As I said at the start of the book, when I mention the gut microbiome to my patients, many of them ask, 'Oh, do you just want me to take some probiotics?' It almost amuses me how quickly most of us assume health needs to come in a pill. I personally don't take probiotic capsules; without mapping my microbiome and specifically deciphering which species I am lacking, self-medicating with a random mixture in a pill doesn't feel worth my time or money. Especially when there is enormous evidence behind fermented foods, which can be exceptionally cheap, particularly when you learn to make them yourself. More than that, they usually come with beneficial nutrients alongside the bugs.

Sadly, wherever there is an opportunity to make money, the food industry will jump on it – and they have done just that with 'probiotic' foods. Legally, they aren't required to contain any actual bugs, which is convenient because, for most ferments, when left out of the fridge they continue to actively ferment the food and produce a lot of gas (exploding bottles aren't great for business). Transporting them is, therefore, expensive and so is storing them. If a container of sauerkraut, kimchi or kombucha is sold on a shelf at room temperature, it is safe to assume the bacteria have been removed. In fact, you don't need to even assume this because it will say 'pasteurised' on the packet. Kombucha (fermented tea), in particular, is often pumped with artificial chemicals making it an ultra-processed product disguised as a health drink. There are some good-quality options you can buy in the refrigerated section, but it is much cheaper (and tastier) to make your own.

That said, you don't even need to delve into the world of trendy ferments if you don't want to. Plain yoghurt is an excellent vehicle for probiotics – just make sure it isn't ultra-processed. I pick a plain-flavoured, full-fat option and make sure 'milk' is the only listed ingredient, alongside bacterial strains.* Kefir is like yoghurt's better-looking brother, cramming in far more strains of bugs; I often ask patients to take kefir with their antibiotics to mediate the damage to the microbiome. Luckily, water kefir is also an option for people who don't eat dairy. Cheese (especially unpasteurised) is also home to plenty of great bugs and may be one reason for the 'French Paradox': the observation that French people have low rates of obesity and heart disease despite the fact that they ignore wellness culture by continuing to eat 'unhealthy' fat. On average, the French each put away 24kg of cheese per year, which is almost double the amount of Brits and Americans. It turns out, when full-fat dairy products are fermented with bacteria, they have a net beneficial effect, *reducing* inflammation and obesity; boosting the microbiome is presumably one of the reasons why. Realistically, the French Paradox is multifactorial, influenced by cultural things on top of food (a month-long holiday every August probably helps). As I

---

* Yes, *full* fat. I will discuss why shortly.

mentioned earlier, populations with a strong food culture, including plenty of plants in recipes grandparents once used too, simply have better health. The French, in my opinion, don't eat 'healthy' food – they just know how to make *good* food. Interestingly, you can also expose yourself to doses of healthy bacteria simply by not being uber concerned about hygiene; I don't mean you need to go lick the street, but living with pets and gardening both boost the microbiome because of the dirt you get exposed to. Lastly, even simple whole foods can be a sort of 'probiotic': fresh fruit and vegetables are often teeming with bugs, essentially acting like probiotics. If you pick them yourself, from foraging or gardening, they're even better and won't be hindered by pesticides.

OMEGA-3

The one last shout out I will briefly make is to healthy fat in the form of omega-3, which directly boosts microbiome diversity. Many people associate it with oily fish, like sardines and mackerel, which are my personal favourites because they are cheap and not overfished. However, you can get plenty of excellent omega-3 from plant sources like chia seeds, walnuts, hempseeds and flaxseeds, which I recommend enjoying regularly.

Principle number 2: Try not to feed your microbiome what it doesn't like

I try to mostly focus on the positive attitude that a healthy microbiome is primarily driven by things you are adding, rather than subtracting. However, it is naive and stubborn to ignore what we might unknowingly be doing to harm our microbiomes. Remember my patients who were forced to wear adult nappies due to severe, chronic diarrhoea with no clear cause (see p. 5)? After invasive colonoscopies, specialist input and countless GP appointments, I was the first to ask them what they ate. I spent time teaching them about the microbiome and all the amazing things they could do to improve it; interestingly, they both only made one significant change, which is not uncommon. I find a lot of patients can be overwhelmed by the volume of information I give them and only make one or two changes to begin with. When I follow them up, with every subsequent appointment, I repeat the same advice and each time they slowly build on it. Change takes time and you don't need to transform everything all at once. The one thing my two chronic-diarrhoea patients did was to remove artificial sweeteners from their diets. Nothing else! And after half a decade of debilitating symptoms which had stopped one of them leaving the house, the diarrhoea disappeared. Remember, many of the chemical additives we have been injecting into food over the last 50 years only needed to be 'generally' regarded as safe (see p. 138). Would you take a medication which was 'generally' safe, but not formally tested in drug trials? Without realising it many of us could be experiencing debilitating symptoms partly triggered by these additives – my two patients really brought this home for me and, hopefully, serve as cautionary tales for you.

We know artificial sweeteners and other added chemicals, like emulsifiers, play havoc with your microbiome and drive leaky-gut syndrome with all the nasty diseases that entails. Worryingly, for every 10 per cent of calories you get from UPFs in your diet, overall mortality goes up by 14 per cent and cancer goes up by 10 per cent! The average British child gets 70 per cent of their calories from UPFs and adults get more than half – imagine the potential health benefits of reducing this by any amount.

UPFs increasingly sound pretty unappetising – the problem is you might be eating them without realising it. If you read the list of ingredients on a packet, ask yourself if you could buy each of them in a standard supermarket and recreate what you're about to eat. If the answer is no, it's a UPF. Most shop-bought cakes, ready meals and confectionaries quite obviously stand out as examples. However, many are easy to miss, like most supermarket breads, many yoghurts, bottled smoothies, spreads, dips and even tinned coconut milk. Do you need to completely cut them out of your life and eat 100 per cent whole ingredients? It is up to you, but I personally don't do that. As I've said already, I strongly believe life is there to be lived, and never having another scoop of my favourite ice cream is not my idea of living. I sometimes use a stock cube, which is technically a UPF, but in the context of the mountain of plants I am cooking it with, logically, I think the good outweighs the bad. Common sense must prevail here, and I am anxious not to promote another layer of orthorexia, or any other eating disorder for that matter. UPFs now make up a tiny percentage of my overall diet and I don't overthink it, but equally, they don't feel like a hard thing to resist; I share a similar sentiment to Van Tulleken's advice in *Ultra-Processed People*: I simply feel disgusted by most UPFs and honestly don't want to eat them.

A number of medications also damage the microbiome, such as NSAIDs (nonsteroidal anti-inflammatories), like naproxen or ibuprofen, and PPIs (proton-pump inhibitors), like omeprazole. I happily still prescribe these medications; in fact, omeprazole can absolutely save someone's life. But I am mindful of the impact on the microbiome and, as much as possible, point this out to patients. Some remain on PPIs for life for uncomfortable heartburn, but never try out time-restricted eating (TRE), which could reverse the cause. The Hippocratic oath doesn't begin with 'Do good', it actually starts with 'First do no harm' – but where does the microbiome fit in here? As we learn more about the microbiome, doctors and their patients will need to have more frank conversations about the potential risk-benefit of certain drugs.

The most obvious example of a medication which dramatically disrupts the microbiome is one I prescribe all the time as a GP: antibiotics. They can and do save people's lives every day, but there's no such thing as a free lunch; in payment for fighting dangerous bugs, you surrender some of your good ones, and sometimes to the extreme. You don't even need to be prescribed them because some 13 million kilograms of antibiotics are used today in agriculture (compared to just 50kg in the 1950s). This isn't because livestock get more infections than they used to; it's because in the 1960s, farmers realised animals gained weight faster if they were given antibiotics. This meant more money and faster. Just like mice and human studies, if you kill off their healthy microbiome, weight gain becomes much easier. Farmed fish are also pumped with antibiotics for the same reason and, tragically, these seep into our oceans and rivers, meaning up to 75 per cent of wild fish also contain them. Being vegan doesn't afford protection from unwanted antibiotics either because fields are fertilised with antibiotic-laden manure. And even our water has trace antibiotics. This background exposure to medication designed to kill bacteria may be but one of many changes driving worse health over the last 60 years.

Sounds pretty gloomy, but what can we do about it? As an individual you can't change agriculture where you live, but you can be mindful of what you put into your own body. Pesticides are a whole other matter, and I don't have a long enough word count for that, but yes, they do damage your microbiome. Some foods contain more pesticides than others – PAN (Pesticide Action Network) monitor levels on British foods and publish a list to avoid on their website.* Examples of foods worth buying organic include oats, citrus, berries, apples, pears, peaches, parsnips, asparagus and apricots.

Importantly, I don't want to scaremonger or stop people taking prescribed antibiotics – again, they can save your life. But many courses are given for minor illnesses which would clear if you allowed your immune system time to do its thing. If you have another option, like an antibacterial cream for a superficial infection, try that first if you can. If you are prone

---

* This 'dirty dozen' list of foods to avoid can be found on www.pan-uk.org

to recurrent infections, like urinary tract infections (UTIs), ask why. Anecdotally, I have heard 'microbiome-enthusiastic' GPs tell patients to cut out foods with emulsifiers (i.e. UPFs) and the recurrent UTIs eventually stop. This is more of a problem in women because they have important microbiomes within their vulva, vagina and urethra. For peri- and postmenopausal patients with recurrent UTIs I usually prescribe vaginal oestrogen cream, which helps prevent them happening in the first place. I also ask all women to only use plain water when cleaning – *any* soap can disrupt the delicate ecosystem of micro-organisms living in the vagina. By using preventative tactics, you can cleverly reduce your total use of antibiotics in future.

A healthy lifestyle which supports your immune system is also a powerful way to prevent infections. I constantly come into close contact with viral vectors (AKA patients) who cough and splutter all over me but don't often get ill myself. Why? I take infection-preventing measures every day with the food I eat and the way I live my life. For many people, I fully acknowledge it will be much more complicated, and sometimes long-term antibiotics are their only option. My advice is always to consider the least invasive option with any treatment – sometimes this means a lifestyle change first or combining that with a drug. It doesn't need to be either/or, but equally, if your GP asks you to engage in a lifestyle change first, they are not fobbing you off: they are trying to exercise their duty of care and *first do no harm*.

Principle number 3: Confront constipation

This might seem like a slight diversion from the topic at hand but I promise you it is a very relevant one. Discussing one's bowel movements has never been part of polite conversation but I think this might need to change. Patients are often surprised by how often I want to know about this intimate part of their lives and are even more taken aback by the level of detail I need. Before becoming a doctor I could never have imagined how much this bodily function can impact health and disease. Increasingly, though, I see it as a vital measure of health and now take my own 'activity' in this area rather seriously. You see constipation really isn't good for you and many of my patients serve as a vital reminder of this fact.

During the Covid-19 pandemic, I was completing my hospital posts as part of my GP training and happened to spend a lot of this time on the Covid wards. It was a fugue-state experience: both my life and work felt absurd, chaotic and a bit unreal. In an attempt to siphon off wards with Covid outbreaks, the hospital took to moving specialists and their patients around the building like an odd game of musical chairs. Every few days or so, you would turn up to one ward assuming that's where, say, cardiology lived, only to discover gastroenterology had just moved in. One day managers decided to move the respiratory department to my ward but forgot to bring the patients, which meant, to their huge surprise, a group of lung doctors and nurses were left manning a dementia ward. Their new patients technically all had Covid so bed managers reasoned it was still *sort of* respiratory anyway and so the arrangement stuck until the next move.

Of all the patients on that ward, I specifically remember a lovely lady whom I will call Betty. She had fairly severe dementia but of the very happy sort and would usually spend all day in bed singing. She could communicate her basic needs and always had a smile on her face. After a few days off work, I returned to find her completely changed: she couldn't speak anymore and was lying in bed *constantly* wailing. None of my colleagues knew what her baseline was – they were all brand new to the ward – so I was the only person to realise this was *not* normal for her. I couldn't find any obvious medical cause, but then I remembered something my colleagues hadn't checked: her stool chart.* In geriatrics, this is just as important as a

---

* The stool chart lists in precise detail every time a patient has a bowel movement, what it looked like and roughly how much was there.

blood test because the very moment an elderly person becomes constipated, they can develop something devastating called delirium. In many ways, it's a fascinating condition, which can present in different ways: patients become completely disorientated, confused and sometimes even psychotic with visual hallucinations. The condition can be caused by all kinds of things, including infections, a low blood sodium and medications, but, in my experience, one of the most common causes is constipation. I immediately prescribed Betty some laxatives and the next morning she was a new woman, busy flirting with two strapping physiotherapists who were helping her walk. My consultant was baffled and delighted, joking with her, 'You will be doing the can-can next.' To the physios' amazement, she responded by doing the can-can, laughing happily. They clung on to her, terrified she might fall over. It is my most cherished memory from the wards and a constant reminder never to forget the value of a good bowel movement.

Betty's case is only one example of constipation's potential complications. It can also be the trigger for a sudden deterioration in Parkinson's and liver cirrhosis patients – in both cases, they can become incredibly unwell. Bizarre as it sounds, getting their bowels moving can also miraculously improve symptoms! I fear many people have grown so used to constipation that they don't even know what a normal bowel movement should feel like. I have also seen examples of adults and children who have had such severe constipation that their bowel and rectum distend too much, damaging the nerve signals to their brains. The sensation and desire to empty your bowels comes from these nerves, so people simply become incontinent, soiling themselves because they can't help it. What is desperately sad is that this could have been avoided with a change in lifestyle.

It is safe to assume your bowel movements are a very important sign of your overall health. In fact, not only is a faster transit time generally associated with better health outcomes, the size of your stool is too: bigger is very much better.* This is something we have known for a long time; a man named Denis Burkitt researched African tribes in the 20th century, noting that they had almost no modern diseases compared to African Americans. The main difference he discovered was in their poo: the average African stool weighed 900g, while Americans' were a measly 115g. This all makes so much more sense now that we have discovered the microbiome: both a faster transit time and larger stools are associated with better microbiome diversity. A sizeable and regular bowel movement is therefore very much a life hack. I wonder if fitfluencers will one day start weighing their stools and gloat happily about their size.

If I could rid my patients of even mild constipation, I genuinely think that would resolve a huge chunk of non-specific abdominal pain and, based on what happens in delirium, I wonder if we all experience a watered-down version of that earlier in life too. Could brain fog, forgetfulness and fatigue somehow be linked to constipation? We know the microbiome sends chemicals which can cross the blood–brain barrier; perhaps constipation is them ringing the alarm to say they're not happy and need some help.

But what can you do to really optimise your bowel movements to achieve a regular and hefty stool? Well, let's not forget African tribes eat up to 600 plants a year and 100g of fibre a day – you don't need to reach these levels, but you can certainly aim to eat 30 different plants a week. As we have already covered, respecting the circadian rhythm of your bowel pushes its contents down with a timed, rhythmic wave of electricity

---

* Transit time is how long it takes your food to travel through your gut. People who have a quick transit time with soft, more regular bowel movements have better health. The best time seems to be around 24 hours, but for some people it's five days. A shorter time is associated with less type 2 diabetes, better blood-sugar control and less internal fat, probably because it is also associated with a more diverse microbiome. The caveat is that if it is too short, resulting in diarrhoea, this is not associated with better health.

called the migratory motor complex (MMC – see p. 98), which takes three to four hours to complete. Eating interrupts this cycle and it needs to start from the top each time you do so. As I mentioned in the last chapter, if we go back to how people ate in the 1950s, our MMC would have time to do its thing.

A surprising trick I picked up from general surgeons is to replace magnesium. If you are running low, your bowels become sluggish, driving constipation. In its most extreme form, this can cause a 'pseudo bowel obstruction': an impenetrable traffic jam caused simply by densely packed stool. During my surgical job, rather than scalpels, we turned to magnesium replacements, which often solved the problem! I now suspect many chronically constipated people just don't get enough magnesium in their diets from things like nuts, legumes/beans, seeds, wholegrains and leafy greens. They can take magnesium tablets or they could simply just improve their diet. In the last one-minute spiel of a consultation, when I'm in a rush, I ask patients to drink plenty of water and eat more chia seeds, flaxseeds, plums and kiwis to get things going. In fact, in New Zealand, I hear paediatricians don't bother with laxatives – they just suggest parents feed their children puréed kiwis (with the skin left on) and it works a treat! Food clearly can be medicine. Treating and preventing constipation is the condition I use it for most often.

Principle 4: Simple tricks
for other gut symptoms

As mentioned at the start of the book, the advice I share here is not a replacement for a doctor's appointment, so if you have any new symptoms, particularly stomach pains, *any* change in your bowels, bloating, unexplained weight loss or blood in your stool, get it checked. But if tests are all normal, many non-specific gut symptoms can improve if you feed a healthy microbiome. Briefly, I find diarrhoea often improves dramatically by significantly reducing UPFs and, as I have demonstrated earlier in this chapter, especially by removing artificial sweeteners. Another trick most people seem completely unaware of is to try a six-week period off dairy – you would be surprised at how many people spend decades living with fluctuating diarrhoea, never realising they are just lactose intolerant.

Importantly, if you have dysbiosis – an unhelpful mixture of gut bacteria – changing your diet can initially be uncomfortable. You might enthusiastically challenge yourself with a very-high-fibre diet and find you develop painful, even debilitating bloating and stomach cramps. This generally isn't because your human cells are intolerant to the food; it's simply that you don't have the microbiome or gut transit time to support the fibre *yet*. Respecting your MMC and allowing your gut time to rest with some TRE will make this much easier by boosting your microbiome and calming down leaky-gut syndrome. Then start low and go slow: gradually increase small amounts of fibre as you can tolerate it. If your symptoms are very uncomfortable, it might be worth sticking to cooked plants first because these are easier to digest. Later, after a few weeks, you can start to experiment eating them raw.

Finally, though I personally don't suggest randomly removing things from your diet, one thing I have found helpful is to take a break from bread specifically – this is something I have anecdotally found very helpful for me and my patients. However, let me be clear: if you aren't coeliac, you don't need to cut gluten out of your diet. In fact, a gluten-free diet in non-coeliacs has been found to worsen the microbiome. This is, in part, because many gluten-free products are ultra-processed, but also because many gluten-containing foods are rich in valuable prebiotics. There are other niche gluten or wheat intolerances, but I would advise seeking specialist input before you start cutting food groups out of your diet. On the whole, most people will benefit from *adding* to what they eat, rather than blindly subtracting from their diets. However, temporarily taking a break from bread might ease bloating while you are taking time to improve your microbiome. I personally don't eat bread very often anymore, partly because I find using the exact same carbohydrate every day is a missed opportunity for plant variety. Quinoa, bulgar wheat, pearl barley, spelt, different-coloured rice, beans/legumes and different types of potato often fill in the gap where bread used to sit. When I occasionally do eat it, as one of *many* carbohydrate sources, I just make sure it isn't a UPF. I enjoy every bite largely because, by increasing the variety of what I eat, each food feels like a novelty, rather than something I have every day.

Food doesn't need to be complicated

As I keep saying food has turned into an uber-academic debate when really it doesn't need to be so complicated. If you stop overthinking it and focus heavily on cooking traditional cuisines, while copying our historical eating patterns, you will be incorporating most of the new science by default. We need to unlearn the flawed science of our elders, retrace our history and eat the way we used to. Blue Zone centenarians haven't read nutrition books; they just eat *good* food. Their definition of good food just happens to be one their microbiomes agree with: minimal UPFs, lots of plants and loads of polyphenols. Whenever I look at something I am about to eat, I imagine serving it to a feisty Italian nonna (grandmother): if she replies, 'Eh, it's okay,' I eat it. (Note: Italians have exceptionally high standards when it comes to food and this increases with age.) But if she replies with hands gesticulating (in ways only Italian hands do) and the corners of her lips turned down in disdain, no words are required: this is not 'real food' and it certainly isn't 'good food'. I know fitfluencers' pseudo-healthy dessert recipes would elicit some furious swearing from even the most placid of said nonnas. I don't eat them. Food is a cultural ritual, a bonding experience and a nostalgic well of emotion. It is more than fuel and should be something we cherish, not something we endure.

Eat real, good food. If you use this Italian nonna test yourself and eat to feel full, my work will be done! In fact, I believe I have told you everything you need to know already. But, briefly, allow me to peruse protein and fat for completeness ...

PROTEIN

Nothing divides people more than protein – who knew one food group could drive so much stress and anxiety? Contrary to what you might have been told, you are probably eating more than enough protein without even trying. Elite athletes, the elderly and patients with malabsorption conditions might need more specific advice but, in the developed world, insufficient protein genuinely isn't a problem. That is because most things we eat are made up of various carbohydrates, fats *and* proteins. There are some food sources which are particularly high in especially 'bioavailable' (easy for our body to absorb and use) proteins, but the body breaks down their building blocks (amino acids) from meats, fish, eggs, dairy and plants: they all add up. Importantly, when it comes to eating a filling meal, stimulating PYY (fullness hormone) with a source of protein *is* very important. But as I keep saying, food should not be a tortured ritual of analysing and then reanalysing the precise quantities of each macronutrient you are consuming – this obsession strips the joy out of eating and fuels a disordered attitude to food, if not a full-blown eating disorder. Simply put, I just ask that you are always able to identify a source of protein on your plate, whether that is a decent portion of beans/legumes, yoghurt, cottage cheese, eggs, tofu, tempeh, meat or fish. Look for the portion but don't overthink it beyond that – if you eat traditional food, just like our grandparents, you won't become protein deficient.

As for where you should get your protein from, answering this requires a very complex and nuanced debate about ethics, the environment and our health. Doing this subject justice would need a whole extra book and goes beyond the scope covered by mine. However, Tim Spector's books *Spoon Fed* and *Food for Life* delve into it beautifully. Ultimately, it is a very personal decision and I don't tell my patients what they should do here. It is worth being mindful that quality really does matter; remember fish and meat are an excellent vehicle for unprescribed antibiotics. If they are organic/wild and have been raised eating a diverse range of plants the phytochemicals from their diet will influence the quality of the meat. As Dr Mark Hyman puts it, you aren't what you eat, you are 'what you eat eats'. Highly processed meats like bacon, hot dogs and ham are a recognised carcinogen according to the World Health Organization and I personally tend to avoid them. I make an exception for good-quality Italian cured meats as a rare treat because they don't contain chemicals which damage the microbiome like ultra-processed meats do. When it comes to increasing risk of heart disease and cancer from consuming meat not all studies show the same results. Interestingly, there seems to be a clear link in European studies, but this isn't the case in Asian epidemiological studies. Again, health isn't as black or white as it may seem and there is nuance in the meat debate which is partly explained by our microbiome. Our bugs also ferment meat resulting in an unhelpful by-product called 'TMAO', which increases heart disease.

You could choose to become vegan or vegetarian, or alternatively, a 'flexitarian', largely behaving like a vegetarian most days with the occasional meat and fish treat. Both would boost your microbiome and manage levels of TMAO. Eating less meat will also improve the microbiome because of what you replace it with; if it's displaced by eating more legumes and other plants you are simply providing your healthy bugs with more food they enjoy. Do you know who else eats like this? Our centenarian friends in the Blue Zones: apart from the vegetarian Adventists in California, all the other longest-living people *do* eat meat, just not often. Remember, they came from poor backgrounds and so could only really afford meat as a rare treat and in small amounts. Legumes feature heavily every day and, though they supplement with organic nutrient-rich animal products, they are largely 'plant based' – a term which is colloquially interchangeable with veganism, but when used in scientific literature just means plants are the star of the show.

How often you eat fish or meat is up to you; in a way, I try to be intuitive. Since learning about the microbiome, without thinking about it, I migrated to a heavily vegetarian diet because I was enthused by everything I was feeding my microbiome. When I periodically get a craving for fish or meat, I treat myself to good-quality sources. It might take a month before I crave meat or fish; other times I want it more often. Perhaps, now that I don't have many UPFs and have spent a long time improving my microbiome, I am just responding to internal cues like Clara Davis's babies (see p. 181). Blue Zone centenarians probably vary their frequency too, but don't seem to have meat more than a few times a month. I suggest you find what works best for you, but if fish and meat are something you eat every day, it might be worth reducing this.

CHOLESTEROL AND DIETARY FAT

I repeat: I've already told you everything you need to know. If you do some form of TRE (even if it's only 12 hours), boost your microbiome, regulate your blood sugar and eat traditional recipes, your blood cholesterol will improve. I wish I could put this into a meaningful soundbite for my patients, but the context would be missed.

Frustratingly, whenever I talk to my patients about cholesterol, often the only thing they are interested in is a low-fat diet. They don't realise that this government advice from the 1980s was based on flawed research. By scapegoating dietary fat, we have ignored the real players, like fibre – its role in cholesterol, heart disease and health in general is impossible to overstate! As many as 90 per cent of us aren't getting enough fibre and *this* is the subject we should be focusing on. Amazingly, even eating just an extra 7 grams of fibre per day can reduce your overall risk of future heart disease by 10 per cent. That's half a cup of beans – believe me, if drug companies could harness such amazing results they would make a fortune.

What most of my patients don't realise is that their gut microbiome plays a huge role in optimising blood cholesterol. The medicinal SCFAs they produce directly influence how the liver produces cholesterol. They also act directly on our cholesterol-containing bile acid. You might recall that TRE improves cholesterol by helping us to clear more through our bile acid, but some of our bacteria help too, almost acting like mops for excess cholesterol. Hopefully, as well as prescribing life-saving medications, one day cardiologists will send their patients high-fibre recipes like I do.

Cholesterol has actually been very misunderstood and over-simplified; unfortunately, it will probably be some time before current medical guidelines catch up with our new understanding of it. Firstly, the cholesterol you eat has a negligible effect on your blood cholesterol, which is actually mostly made in the liver. Secondly, cholesterol as a whole isn't a 'bad' thing – in fact, it plays a vital role in the body and contributes to the immune system and production of vitamin D, bile acid and hormones. Part of why it is misunderstood is because we have oversimplified one type of cholesterol called LDL, which is a bit of a Jekyll and Hyde. What I mean by that is that LDL comes in two types: type A is big and bouncy and type B is small and dense. Imagine big soft balloons and small hard bullets bouncing around your home – which would you prefer? The small type-B particles do more damage because they penetrate the lining of our arteries more.* Believe it or not, being insulin resistant is an excellent way to increase these harmful bullets. Remember how we become insulin resistant? Constantly spiking insulin throughout

---

* This is referred to as 'apoB' (apolipoprotein) in medical literature. These terms refer to structures which transport cholesterol but for simplicity we often just refer to them as 'types' of cholesterol.

the day is a good start, but lots of sugar and simple starches will really get the job done. Read that again! Most patients with an unhealthy cholesterol panel are never taught that the sugar they eat might be the cause. Why don't chocolate bars come with warnings like: 'Will increase harmful cholesterol, heart disease, stroke, diabetes and dementia if consumed to excess'?

It gets more complicated because you also have something colloquially called 'good' cholesterol or HDL. If this is raised, it's protective against heart disease but, rather confusingly, the main number people worry about is their *total* cholesterol, which you get by adding LDL (types A + B) to HDL. Remember, type B is the one we should be worried about, and a high HDL might be a good thing: even if maths isn't your strong suit, can you see why adding all these numbers together isn't particularly helpful? There are specialist calculations and tests which can help to analyse your level of type B. However, the point of this book is not to bog you down with academia. All you need to know is how to eat in a way that will raise your HDL and lower your type-B LDL. Believe it or not, I've already taught you how to do that: a traditional, plant-heavy, microbiome-boosting diet that controls insulin, eaten in the right way, won't guarantee a good *total* cholesterol, but it doesn't need to. It will give you an optimised cholesterol profile with more HDL and less type B, which will protect you from the diseases we all dread. The centenarians in Blue Zones already do this effortlessly without studying the subject at all: they simply eat good food.

So does this mean you can you eat as much dietary fat as you like? Honestly, this question is complicated by the fact that we don't all respond to food in the same way. Some people are especially good at clearing fat from their blood quickly after a meal, while others are much slower. This means dietary fat can have two very different effects, depending on who is eating it. As I have mentioned before, we see the same thing with simple carbohydrates – how we break food down is influenced by our

genes and our highly unique microbiomes. We call this personalised nutrition, which is something people can already pay for
to tailor their diet. This is an exciting area of research, and I
suspect personalised nutrition advice will become increasingly
available to us over the next few years. But in the meantime,
there are some simple things about dietary fat you should know.

Importantly, not all fat is created equal, and we should eat
different amounts of certain types. In truth, I suggest leaving
the details to scientists who are performing research – it is of
academic interest, but not something you need to analyse if
you want to eat my definition of good food. I have memorised
the minutia of dietary fat for exams and learned the precise
chemical structure of trans, saturated, monounsaturated and
polyunsaturated fats, but this never changed what I ate at the
time. Translating my flash-card facts into actual food was too
confusing for me. I also promptly forgot the details after said
exam. For the same reason, asking my patients to memorise
subtypes of fats isn't especially practical. Applying this information to what you eat is hard to do because many foods have
a combination of fat types, and we have been vilifying some
more than is necessary.

For example, for many years, the general advice has been to
avoid saturated fats to protect heart health. However, there is
some saturated fat in extra virgin olive oil (EVOO) and we now
recognise this oil to be incredibly healthy for us and our microbiomes, partly because it has amazing polyphenols. To label a
food as 'bad' just because it contains saturated fats is, like so
many of our previous beliefs, a complete oversimplification of
the facts. My favourite heart health study is called PREDIMED
(published in 2013): it assigned Spanish people to three different diets. They all had a generally Mediterranean diet, but one
group included up to 4 tablespoons EVOO a day; the second
had 30g mixed nuts a day and the third had neither. They had
to stop the study early because the benefits of both EVOO and
nuts were so profound it was considered unethical to withhold

these clear medicines from the third group. It turns out eating these fats was good for their hearts, not bad. So unlike Ancel Keys's smudged and cherry-picked data suggested, dietary fat looks like it can protect against heart disease. This is especially true in the form of extra virgin olive oil, nuts, seeds, avocado and oily fish.

These discoveries are turning our previous beliefs on their heads, but the plot thickens. Remember the dietary fat omega-3? Well, it has a friend called omega-6* and enormous debate surrounds how they both affect our health. Some argue we are simply getting too many omega-6 fats in our diet and not enough omega-3s. One famous study, called the Lyon Diet Heart Study, achieved what some describe as an ideal omega-6: omega-3 ratio of 1:4 by using a Mediterranean diet. In contrast, many diets in the West achieve a ratio closer to 25:1. The Lyon Diet Heart Study did manage to reduce the risk of heart disease complications by 70 per cent compared to those eating an American Heart Association (AHA) diet. However, implying the only difference between these two diets was their omega ratio is misleading. Importantly, omega-6 isn't a villain here – it's an 'essential fatty acid', which means we do still need it in our diets. More recent data suggests that, as long as you are getting enough omega-3 in your diet, the overall ratio doesn't actually matter. This is a huge relief to me because I have abso-lutely no idea how to meaningfully calculate my own ratio! At least not in a way that would be practical on a day-to-day basis.

Ultimately, it is an oversimplification to imply a type of dietary fat is completely 'bad'. The one exception is 'industrial trans fat' – this *should* be avoided. It is made by chemically altering vegetable oils to make them solid – for example, butter replacements in the 1970s. We now know they reduce our HDL and increase our type-B LDL, while also increasing

---

* Examples of omega-6 fats we get in our diet are canola, soybean, sunflower, corn, grapeseed, rice bran and safflower oils.

inflammation in the body. Just 4g trans fats a day can increase your risk of heart disease by 25 per cent! Fortunately, this is something we recognised a few decades ago and these industrial trans fats have mostly been removed from our foods and are actually illegal in the US. Except for this rare example, dietary fat actually isn't bad for you, and we can let go of aiming for low-fat diets.

So how can you apply this information to your health without turning eating into a highly cerebral, academic endeavour? Well, again, I've already told you everything you need to know! If you eat in a way that is delicious for you *and* your microbiome, you'll be eating the right dietary fats already. A plant-heavy, fibre-rich, whole food base with sources of omega-3s in the form of chia seeds, flax seeds, walnuts and occasional oily fish should do the trick.

If you carefully break down every meal into its calories, macronutrients, micronutrients and types of fat, you can successfully strip your food of any joy. Again, the Blue Zone centenarians don't think about any of this – instead, they are intuitively guided by an inherited wisdom. They don't have nutrition degrees: they have culture. Food remains a joyous and bonding experience for them, not something they need to analyse. That's precisely why I have invited patients into my own kitchen – they say a picture is worth a thousand words, and I'd argue a recipe is worth even more. But you don't need to overhaul your entire diet overnight. Change takes time. To begin with, just remember you aren't eating for one – you're eating for 38 trillion bugs too. If you value these critters, feeding them what they like won't feel like a hardship.

Secondly, always do the 'nonna test' – imagine a stern, highly opinionated grandmother sitting next to you and how she would react to your food. Perfection isn't the goal here – just keep a smile on her face *most* of the time. Importantly, this nonna doesn't need to be Italian – maybe she's Greek, Japanese,

Costa Rican or Nigerian. In truth, many cuisines align with our microbiomes' idea of good food. Often, they are traditional, simple, fairly cheap, packed with plants and generally made with whole ingredients. Rather than worrying about your food, simply invest time in finding traditional recipes your bugs will like. Everything else will work itself out from there. Although I can't cover every possible recipe which fits this description, in the next chapter I will give you the general gist. I hope some tips and example recipes will inspire you to find many more. Really, food is a wonderful and expansive thing – when you realise that, cooking it won't feel like a chore!

Food: Key points

1) We have inbuilt nutrient-sensing pathways in our bodies which are informed by the flavours we eat. By consuming artificial flavours, we are sending false information to the body, which responds by driving an urge to overeat as a reflex to compensate for nutrient deficiencies. By displacing whole foods with UPFs, many of us are malnourished and an increased appetite is only one of the consequences.

2) Blue Zones around the world provide amazing insight into diets and lifestyles which can prolong our lives and prevent disease. We don't need to medicalise food to achieve this: we need to focus on nourishing a healthy 'food culture', which doesn't perceive food as 'healthy', but simply defines what 'good food' is. Delicious and healthy are not mutually exclusive.

3) Learn to feed your microbiome what it likes: at least 30 different types of plants a week which frequently vary; brightly/deeply coloured, spiced or bitter foods; fermented foods like kefir, yoghurt and kombucha (to name a few); and foods rich in omega-3s like flaxseeds, chia seeds, walnuts and oily fish.

4) When possible, learn not to feed your microbiome what it doesn't like: antibiotics, NSAIDs, PPIs, UPFs and excessive meat/fish.

5) Our bowel movements are an important sign of health, and constipation can be a well-recognised trigger for various conditions like delirium and non-specific abdominal pains. A large and regular bowel movement is synonymous with a healthy microbiome and is something we should all be aiming for.

6) Where you get protein from is a personal decision, but you don't need to agonise about or calculate it. Just aim to eat a portion of protein-rich food with every meal and try to move to a more plant-heavy diet wherever possible. I suggest eating whole food sources and not falling for UPF supplements.

7) Cholesterol and dietary fat have both been massively over-simplified. TRE, a healthy microbiome and avoiding insulin resistance are the best ways to optimise your cholesterol. Avoiding too many UPFs and focusing on omega-3 rich fats will improve it even more.

CHAPTER 9

RECIPES

What your doctor eats

When I first learned everything in this book, I was incredibly excited to share it with my patients. However, I quickly realised it was impossible to explain it all in ten minutes – even an hour wouldn't have felt long enough. Instead, as mentioned in my introduction, I reasoned the easiest thing to do would be to simply *show* them what I ate myself. I set up an Instagram account called @whatyourdoctoreats and still use this as a food diary today. Inviting patients into my kitchen changed everything, and would eventually lead me to a book deal of all things. But at its heart it was just meant to be a time-saving tool to meaningfully help my patients.

So what do I actually eat? Remember, it is one thing to understand something in theory, but it is quite another thing to apply it in practice. Many of us will listen to long podcasts, watch documentaries and read many books but end up feeling like a deer in headlights. It can be so much to take in and the sheer volume of information makes each meal feel like a battlefield. Should you carry a notebook around with you and fill out a checklist before every mouthful? No, of course not. With time, and practice, the principles will come as second nature, and my hope is that food will no longer be something you worry about. It will simply be an important aspect of life that you enjoy – just like the French and Italians. What they eat is a proud cultural celebration – they don't *think* they eat good food – they *know* they do. And I want you to feel quietly confident in this assertion too. Let me explain what I think 'good food' looks like.

Firstly, I want to stress that food culture is unique to each of us, and I think it would be horrible to dismantle this. We are all influenced by our own backgrounds and, as we have seen with the Blue Zones (see p. 184), more than one type of cuisine can confer the same benefits. A traditional rural African diet has the power to make rates of chronic disease and bowel cancer plummet. Equally, homecooked food in France, Italy, Singapore and Japan is incredibly good for us. In my opinion, exploring another culture's cuisine is the greatest compliment you can pay and I do this regularly. My own childhood was characterised largely by a Mediterranean approach, which is one of the most studied diets and comes with incredible health benefits. As a general rule, every day will include lots of leafy green vegetables, a portion of legumes, fruit, coffee, nuts, wholegrains and generous glugs of extra virgin olive oil. I see eggs as a quick, healthy and delicious protein, which I enjoy several times a week. As I mentioned earlier, I do eat seafood and meat, but not very often. Like my great-grandmother, a bowl of salad is always on my dinner table. Sweet food is something I eat at the end of meals, usually in the form of whole fruit and often some 85 per cent dark chocolate. I do enjoy traditional desserts, but see them as a treat, not a daily ritual. UPFs still feature in my life, but they make up less than 20 per cent of my diet. Very importantly, I make a conscious effort to eat fermented food every day but don't agonise about this. I know having three to five portions a day is ideal, and whenever I can, I try to incorporate different types throughout my day. This also includes fermented dairy, like plain Greek yoghurt, kefir and cheese. Finally, the fluids I drink mostly serve to hydrate me and I usually don't drink things that will spike my insulin – at least not in between meals or while I'm fasting. Plain water and good-quality black coffee are my main drinks, day to day. I also like green and redbush tea and will often have homemade kombucha with a meal. Any other type of drink is seen as a treat and, again, not a daily ritual.

Now very importantly, I absolutely don't see food as some-thing I should restrict in any way. I am not a psychologist, but I suspect our attitudes to food can significantly affect our eating behaviours in ways that are beyond my expertise. But more than that, I now understand my evolutionary biology and how intel-ligent my body is: I can't bypass or fool its clever mechanisms. For that reason, I am not interested in forcing myself to feel hungry all day and then trying to pretend it doesn't bother me. I did this for years and, like the men in the Minnesota Starvation experiment (see p. 141), it made me miserable. However, I now know how to alter my body's experience of appetite. By chore-ographing my eating in a predictable way, using time-restricted eating, optimising my microbiome and carefully stimulating my fullness mechanism, I genuinely feel full. I'm not forcing myself to 'be good'; rather, like a breastfed baby, I can simply eat when I'm hungry and stop when I'm full. After years of being under the spell of diet culture and many fitfluencers, I can't begin to explain what a relief this approach has been.

A note on alcohol

As I've mentioned, I had a very European childhood and suspect this influenced my approach to alcohol. Growing up, adults almost always had wine with dinner – it was enjoyed slowly, as part of the meal. When I moved to the UK, attitudes around alcohol were my biggest culture shock. Peers taught me I didn't need to enjoy the flavour of what I was drinking but should focus on the pace at which I could drink it. Many people now look to pockets of the Mediterranean, including those in Blue Zones, as evidence that alcohol is somehow a longevity tonic. This is an incredibly complex debate but let's get one thing straight: the centenarians in those places don't down their drinks in a quest to get 'hammered'.

The science coming out about alcohol and its effects on our health is pretty damning. Some declare with absolute certainty that the only safe amount to consume is none at all. We now know alcohol consumption costs the NHS £3.5 billion a year and 75 per cent of that is from people who aren't classed as alcohol dependent. In comparison, tobacco costs the NHS 1 billion less a year. Most people are well versed in the consequences of cigarettes, but did you know that even less than 2 units of alcohol a day is associated with an increase in breast, mouth, throat and oesophagus cancer? Alcohol can also cause detrimental brain changes, increasing risk of cognitive impairment and dementia. On top of that, it's linked to abnormal heart rhythms, worsens diabetes and, as a drug itself, can interact with plenty of medications. However, having said all that, it is true that some very long-living populations enjoy alcohol in moderation. Teasing apart the confounding factors contributing to this is very difficult. Is it the polyphenols in the red wine making their microbiome happy? Or is it the genuine human connection this social lubricant often fosters? I try not to overthink the cause and effect because – though this may be controversial to say – not everything I do in life is for my health.

Being a doctor has often given me a stark reminder of how fickle and unpredictable life can be. Aiming for perfection and longevity at all costs doesn't make sense to me. Whether short or very long, what is the point in life if you didn't actually *enjoy* it? A savoured glass of wine in good company is a simple pleasure I still cherish, not because I think it is a health hack, but because I want to. I usually easily have *less* than 14 units a week, as per UK drinking guidelines. For celebrations or holidays, I will sometimes have more. I am not perfect and don't aim to be! I would never suggest someone take up drinking alcohol – realistically, the most cautious approach would be to have nothing at all. But if, on reflection, you think small amounts of alcohol make life a bit sweeter, then it is worth remembering we only get one (life, that is). I take a similar approach to other indulgences – in my opinion, balance wins over perfection in most cases.

Next, let's look at some of the tips and tricks to make all the principles we have covered feel easy and intuitive.

What can you add?

It would be impossible to share absolutely everything I eat in one chapter. If you want an insight into my daily eating habits, you are welcome to take a look at my Instagram account @whatyourdoctoreats. However, I think it is empowering to understand the techniques I follow to optimise my own microbiome and health. Of course, we all have unique lives, schedules and food cultures. Copying my every meal might not suit you, but I do hope it gives you a rough framework and some inspiration.

The first trick is simply an attitude: when you look at any plate or bowl of food, always think, *What could I add to this?* Variety and abundance in the plants you eat is the most powerful way to achieve a diverse and healthy microbiome. Remember, many things we eat count as plants, including different grains, seeds, nuts, herbs, spices, fruits and vegetables to name a few. Here are some examples of what you can add:

SPRINKLE:
- sesame seeds, sliced kefir lime leaves or coriander on to Asian dishes
- other fresh herbs on to anything savoury (mint works well on sweet dishes too)
- nigella/pumpkin/sunflower seeds into salads
- dried herbs (oregano on to Greek-inspired salads, basil/rosemary/za'atar on to grilled vegetables)
- dukkah (a crunchy spice mix including nuts, sesame seeds, fennel seeds, salt and various spices) on top of chicken, dips, eggs, Middle Eastern dishes
- sumac – a citrus-flavoured spice, often pinched out of a bowl on the dinner table in Middle Eastern countries and

sprinkled on anything; it's especially lovely in marinated/pickled red onions or any other salad

- ras el hanout or baharat spice blend – Middle Eastern bombs of flavour, lovely on roasted vegetables (especially aubergine or sweet potato) or any fish/meat dish
- cumin seeds – surprisingly delicious sprinkled on anything from boiled eggs to salad
- cinnamon – into coffee and yoghurt bowls
- chia/flax/hemp seeds – into yoghurt bowls
- pomegranate seeds – the tart flavour will elevate most savoury or sweet dishes (my family have a huge bowl on the table for most dinners, including Christmas dinner)
- nuts – either on top of yoghurt bowls, added to salads or just enjoyed as a handful on the side; I try to eat two handfuls of different nuts each day (remember their heart-healthy benefits from the PREDIMED study (see p. 209)).

SPOON OVER:

- houmous, muhammara, tzatziki, romesco, chimichurri, fresh pestos, tahini dressing, basil vinaigrette
- salsa
- guacamole
- pickles (I especially love pickled red onions or quick pickled red cabbage)
- fermented food (for example, sauerkraut, kimchi, cheese, kefir).

ADD A SIDE DISH OF:

- a handful of salad leaves (whichever you have – every dinner has room for a salad, so be like my great-grandmother and serve a bowl with every meal)
- quickly blanched green vegetables like peas, green beans, broccoli with some extra virgin olive oil and salt
- a spoonful or two of beans/lentils/peas – you can usually squeeze these on to any plate.

DRINK:

Could you add some plant variety to your meal with what you are drinking?

- Kombucha
- Even wine counts (but drinking 30 different types of wine is not a loophole I am suggesting!)
- Coffee
- Different teas

As before, be mindful of choreographing your insulin spikes. Ask yourself if you are drinking for hydration versus pleasure – the latter is fine as a treat, ideally alongside your meals. I maintain that plain or sparkling water should be your main source of hydration. I also generally ask all my patients to stop sweetening their hot beverages – with time your palate will readjust and you will eventually find going back to the sweet option actually becomes unappetising.

Reassess your staples

Look carefully at your weekly eating patterns and work out which foods appear often. Are you eating the same bread every day? Maybe rice, potatoes, pasta or oats are other ingredients you eat almost daily. The point is not to ban a food you enjoy, but it is important to remember you are trying to keep a potentially bored microbiome entertained. Repeatedly exposing them to the same ingredient base, day after day, is a missed opportunity for variety. Our carbohydrate base is often the aspect of a meal we don't change, but there are many other options which could provide more bang for your microbiome. Mix things up! Consider swapping your usual carbohydrate base to another and alternate them regularly.

Consider options like different types of rice (which are each *different* plants); also, different types of:

- potato
- bread grains (maybe try rye or spelt some days); mixing several types of flour into one bread is another clever way to boost variety. Avoid shop-bought UPF breads as much as you can
- flatbread (lentil, sweet potato, etc. – recipes to follow)
- grains (bulgur wheat, pearl barley, quinoa, freekeh, etc.)
- mash (mashed beans, celeriac, swede, etc.)
- legumes – these can often provide a nice replacement for a carbohydrate base (for example, butter beans instead of pasta/gnocchi, cannellini beans instead of rice to make a risotto into a 'beanotto').

Eat with the seasons

Hello, everyone, my name is Camilla, and I am an apple-holic. I grew up with a strange obsession with apples and used to have one or two 365 days of the year. Since learning about the microbiome, I realised this was probably great for my apple-loving bugs, but unfair for all the other fruit bugs. In hindsight, it's also not great for the environment because when they're not in season they have to be shipped from abroad, even if that is literally from the other side of the world (many of my favourite varieties come from New Zealand). What a silly thing to do when many apples can be grown within walking distance of my house. I now try to eat foods that are in season and, as much as possible, support my most local farms by visiting farmers' markets and farm shops. I still love apples and try to eat as many different varieties as I can find, but only in the autumn/winter months. I treat spring/summer as my apple break, giving my microbiome a chance to mingle with fresh berries, stone fruits, grapes, figs and melon. Another example is asparagus; it has a very short season in the spring which is when I eat it. I then take an asparagus holiday for the rest of the year, meaning I really enjoy it when the season is back.

Learning to eat with the seasons isn't that hard and, in some countries I used to live in, it took no effort because seasonal produce was all that was available. If you generally try to eat what is in season, you will naturally vary your diet as the year goes by. Perhaps you have an apple-eating habit like I did, or maybe you eat fresh strawberries all year round – by ignoring the seasons you are keeping one group of bugs very happy, while neglecting the others. Remember, your microbiome is like a party – I suggest inviting more guests if you want it to be a good one.

If eating with the seasons is a new concept to you, I recommend a quick internet search – there are countless websites listing what is in season in each country. I even have a beautifully illustrated calendar hanging on my kitchen wall to help me keep track. With time, it will become easy – more than that, it will be fun. When I turn the page of my calendar to a new month, I get excited and inspired to come up with recipes for a new list of ingredients.

Forage or grow your own food

I mentioned this in Chapter 8, and I take my own advice here. I grow some of my own vegetables/herbs/fruits and also love foraging sloes, blackberries, wild garlic, elderflower and magnolia blossom among other things. I don't claim to be an expert and hope to learn more about foraging all the incredible edible plants readily available to any of us. They can keep all of our microbiomes on their toes and also inject some new bugs into the mix, much like natural probiotics.

Of course, we all have unique lives and access to different environments. If you have no outdoor space, you can still grow herbs on a windowsill or even try out sprouting in a jar. Learning how to forage is easy with all the free education we have access to online. There are many websites and YouTube accounts dedicated just to this particular art. Again, it goes without saying you should only ever eat a foraged ingredient when you are 100% sure it is edible. Once you get into the swing of it, you'll be surprised by how fun this activity can be. It's also a lovely way to spend more time outside, which many of us would benefit from.

Ultra-processed swaps

The more time you spend thinking about your microbiome and health in general, the less you'll find the idea of UPFs appealing. As I mentioned in the previous chapter, I have certainly started to feel disgusted by them after reading Van Tulleken's *Ultra-Processed People*. The only way to slowly phase these foods out of your diet is to start reading ingredient lists when you go food shopping. There are other options on the shelves which aren't UPFs, but often, just cooking food yourself is the easiest way to avoid them. The following are some simple swaps:

- Crackers – try Ryvita crispbread instead.
- Supermarket bread – seeded rye often isn't UPF; otherwise, go to a trusted bakery or bake the bread yourself.
- Wraps/flatbreads – as above or, again, consider making these yourself (see recipe, p. 241–2).
- Granola – not my idea of a glucose-steady 'break-fast'; instead, use nuts; toasted, shaved coconut; and seeds. Cocoa nibs also provide a nice chocolate flavour.
- Sweet yoghurt – buy plain yoghurt and mix with frozen berries or other fruit
- Dips/sauces – make these yourself (see recipes, pp. 233–8).
- Cereal bars or energy balls – I'm not a fan and would treat sweet foods like this as a dessert; if you really love them, cook them yourself and eat them as a treat at the end of a savoury meal.
- Cakes/biscuits/chocolate bars – as I've said before, life is there to be lived and completely banning 'junk food' isn't my personal approach; they are a very rare treat, but whenever

possible I like to bake my own sweet treats, which usually taste better than shop-bought versions and aren't UPF.

- Protein bars/supplements – I get protein from the same whole foods my grandparents ate: Greek yoghurt, cottage cheese, eggs, pulses and tofu are cheaper and better for you. I also occasionally eat fish/meat in moderation. These whole foods will stimulate more of your satiety mechanisms and have nothing to do with the wellness/fitfluencer culture I now desperately try to avoid.

How to build a meal

This might seem incredibly obvious, but it's amazing how many people eat a plate of food which doesn't stimulate their satiety mechanisms. I suggest all meals should have a source of protein, fat and fibre. Carbohydrates aren't the enemy, but you can choose how many you want to incorporate into each meal in a way that feels intuitive to you. You will see some of the recipes below don't necessarily have that many carbohydrates, but I naturally compensate throughout the day with other meals that do. Here are the steps to take:

1) Think of your protein source and build the rest of the meal around it. This does not mean becoming obsessive about protein or measuring it. Just serve a portion that looks right to you. This could include:
    - any type of legume (split peas, lentils, edamame, black beans, etc.)
    - full-fat Greek yoghurt
    - cottage cheese (other cheeses have a much higher percentage of fat so I would use these as small portions of fat, rather than see them as my main source of protein on a plate)
    - eggs
    - meat/seafood
    - tofu/tempeh.

2) Now think about your microbiomes and what they want – that means fibre, plant variety, colourful foods, spice or bitter flavours, fermented food and prebiotics (inulin, beta-glucans and resistant starches). Different vegetables, fruits, nuts, herbs and just about any other plant you can eat are all examples. Your choice to include a starchy carbohydrate will also apply here – plenty of grains, potatoes and sourdough will also give your microbiome something to feast on.

3) Ensure there is a source of fat – if there is plenty in your protein source (eggs, yoghurt, cottage cheese, meat/seafood), you might not need more. But if there isn't (e.g. with legumes or lean meat), consider adding:
   - avocado
   - nuts and seeds
   - extra virgin olive oil
   - a bit of yoghurt/crème fraîche/cheese.

With just these three steps, you should be able to see your food as a language which will correctly translate into a filling and healthy meal.

RECIPES

As a rule, I tend not to follow recipes when I cook and am usually guided by inspiration. Nevertheless, I have tried to translate these rough guides into some recipes below. If you also prefer not to follow recipes perfectly, I fully encourage you to make these dishes your own, tweaking them in whichever way you see fit.

'Break-fast'

As we have touched on before, the first meal of your day is really very important. It sets the tone for your blood-sugar trajectory for the rest of the day and is such an easy thing to change, producing quite amazing results. Again, just like with any meal, it needs a decent source of protein, fat and fibre. I repeat this here because many traditional breakfasts don't achieve that! Portion sizes need to be adjusted to your own appetite – the goal is to stop eating when you genuinely feel full. When you break your fast is up to you, as is your overall pattern of eating. I usually only eat twice a day (my 'break-fast' at noon and dinner before 8pm), so my portions are fairly large, but please be guided by your own appetite. I often also have a handful of nuts and a bit of fruit after these dishes if I am still hungry. Many of these meals are things I bring with me in Tupperware to work as my packed 'work brunch'. I often tend to break my fast with leftovers from the night before, but if I am specifically preparing something, these are my go-to dishes:

CHIA PUDDING

You can create a thousand varieties of this dish, depending on which topping or flavouring you want to put in. Instead of vanilla paste, you could use lemon or lime zest; I also love adding a teaspoon of turmeric with black pepper and topping it with pomegranate seeds. But the basic recipe is as follows:

Serves 1
2 tbsp chia seeds
Half tin coconut milk **
4–6 heaped tbsp full-fat Greek yoghurt
½ tsp vanilla paste (or a bit more to taste)
*½ tsp local honey (optional – often not needed because the
    fruit topping makes this sweet enough)*
Fruit and nuts of your choice, for topping

Mix the chia seeds, coconut milk, yoghurt, vanilla paste and honey, if using, in a container and leave for an hour in the fridge or, ideally, overnight.

Top with low-sugar fruits like berries, shaved coconut, flaked almonds or any other nuts you like.

BIRCHER MUESLI A THOUSAND WAYS

With a healthy dose of full-fat Greek yoghurt providing both protein and fat, this will regulate your blood sugar and also stimulate your fullness hormones. I make endless variations of this without following a recipe. I just mix a decent portion of yoghurt with berries, flaxseeds, cinnamon, organic jumbo oats and a variety of nuts. Sometimes I'll put a tiny bit of locally sourced honey in too. The potential combinations are infinite, but I recommend not going overboard with the fruit volume and still trying to focus mostly on low-sugar fruits like berries –

---

* Note: most coconut milk is ultra-processed with some emulsifiers. I don't aim for complete perfection in my diet and this is one UPF I still use – there are, rarely, non-UPF versions available, or you could try creamed coconut instead (for example, in curries), which usually isn't a UPF.

remember, you want the first meal of the day to provide a calm blood sugar spike. Here is one of my favourite recipes inspired by the bircher muesli served in the Sprüngli café in Zurich, where I spent a very happy chunk of my childhood.

Sprüngli bircher muesli

This is something you can make ahead and enjoy over the next two to three days, but I often just prepare it on the spot and eat it straight away. If you're going to leave it in the fridge overnight, you could also add a tablespoon of chia seeds. Half a grated apple or pear is also a nice addition and can provide sweetness instead of honey. It's also lovely topped with some chopped pistachios, shaved coconut or flaked almonds.

Serves 1
1 serving full-fat Greek yoghurt (4–6 heaped tbsp)
Small drizzle of plain kefir
Organic jumbo oats (approx. 30–40g)
2 tbsp ground flaxseeds
1–2 handfuls frozen mixed berries (raspberry, blackberry,
*   redcurrant, blackcurrant) **
Zest and juice of half a lemon (start with less juice and
*   adjust to taste)*
1 tsp locally sourced honey (optional)

To prepare I just defrost the berries in the microwave and then add all of the ingredients into the same dish. If you don't mind the texture of raw oats, you can eat this straight away. Otherwise leave to sit for 30 minutes or overnight in the fridge.

---

* If there are any sneaky strawberries in the mix, remove them immediately! I feel quite strongly about this; I don't want to discriminate against strawberries but if you want to achieve the correct level of tartness, they absolutely must be removed. The currants are very much the star of this dish.

NOT-SO-TURKISH EGGS

I love ordering Turkish eggs in restaurants to break my fast, but can never be bothered to make them, and am also not hugely keen on the flavour of melted butter. I still enjoy small amounts of butter in moderation, but prefer to really taste it, cold on bread or on warm leaves of globe artichoke with a pinch of salt. I like to serve these eggs with something crisp and crunchy, like pea shoots. You might also like a slice of good-quality bread but, to be honest, it is filling enough without.

Serves 1
Full-fat Greek yoghurt (adjust this to your own appetite –
  I use around 4 heaped tbsp)
1–2 tsp harissa paste
2 fried eggs
Roughly 1 tsp dukkah spice blend (or if unavailable cumin
  seeds would also be nice)
Sea salt

Spoon the Greek yoghurt across a shallow dish, then swirl the harissa paste through it to create a beautiful pattern. Top with your fried eggs, then sprinkle over some salt and the dukkah.

COTTAGE-CHEESE BOWL

You can make this in a thousand ways with the ingredients you like most or have in the house. Aim for different textures, flavours and colours – I like lots of fresh crunchy vegetables and often include tangy flavours from pickles or ferments. These are my favourites:

Serves 1
1–2 soft-boiled eggs (medium-sized)
Big handful mixed radishes
Handful sliced fennel
Big handful rocket or pea shoots
150–300g serving cottage cheese

Pinch of cumin seeds
Sea salt

Bring a pan of water to the boil, then submerge the egg(s) into the simmering water. Leave for 7 minutes precisely, then remove and submerge in ice-cold water (including some ice cubes). Leave to cool for about 1 minute, then tap the top of the egg(s) on a surface, followed by a tap to the bottom. Next, tap around the sides and gently peel off the shell – it should come away effortlessly. Cut the egg(s) in half to reveal a soft, golden and perfectly cooked jammy egg.

Put the cottage cheese in a shallow bowl and add all of the listed ingredients on top. Sprinkle over some salt and the cumin seeds and enjoy!

OBSCENELY GOOD AVOCADO TOAST

I borrowed this idea and changed it slightly from something I saw posted on Instagram. It is heavenly beyond words and puts most other avocado toast recipes to shame! You could add other things on top of your toast, like smoked salmon, sliced (very ripe) tomatoes or even just some finely sliced red chilli – it's up to you.

Since leaving my 20s behind, I have come to realise the mojito muddler I was sold was misbranded. It may well be good for muddling cocktails, but it's much better at generally shmooshing all sorts of things that need to be shmooshed. Avocados are the perfect example! However, if you don't own a mojito muddler feel free to use a fork instead.

Serves 1
1 small or ½ large avocado
Half tin cannellini beans
3–4 artichoke hearts, chopped (from a jar)
Zest of ½ or 1 lemon
Juice of ½ lemon
Small handful dill, chopped

Small handful parsley, chopped
Good-quality sourdough (or 100 per cent seeded
*   rye bread)*
Extra virgin olive oil, for drizzling
Sea salt to taste

Mash the avocado in a bowl and then semi-mash the beans into it, leaving some of them whole. Add the chopped artichoke hearts, lemon zest and juice, chopped dill and parsley. Please be cautious adding the lemon juice – so many dishes are quickly ruined by adding too much! Start with less than you think you need and taste before adding more. Now add salt to taste. Toast the bread, then drizzle some extra virgin olive oil over it before spooning over the avocado and bean topping.

GREEN FRITTATA OF DREAMS

I was inspired by a Persian egg dish called kuku sabzi, which I saw someone else make on Instagram. Though I love trying new things, I hate following recipes, so usually run with a rough idea and make the dish my own. I clearly got distracted by dreams of Greek spanakopita while making this, so it has turned into a Persian-Greek fusion dish.

This frittata is lovely and, while very much not a kuku sabzi, delicious all the same. You can prepare it ahead of time and I personally also think it would make a lovely centrepiece for dinner too. Any frittata would be a great break-fast because of the protein/fat from the eggs and fibre from the other ingredients. You can make many varieties and don't need to follow a recipe – this just happens to be one of my favourites:

Provides 3 large servings
1 leek, finely chopped (and washed carerfully!)
Extra virgin olive oil, for frying
6 large eggs
1 200g packet feta, crumbled finely
2–4 large handfuls cavolo nero (and/or spinach), chopped

*1 **huge** handful of both fresh dill and parsley, chopped,
   plus extra dill, to serve*
1 tsp dried oregano

Preheat the oven to 190°C. In an oven-safe frying pan, slowly fry down the leek, until beautifully soft and sweet. Just before it reaches this point, add in the cavolo nero and/or spinach. Let the ingredients cook down and slowly get to know each other until softened. Meanwhile, in a medium bowl, mix the eggs, two thirds of the feta, the chopped herbs and dried oregano. No salt is needed here because the feta is salty enough. When the veg have cooked down and are completely soft, turn off the heat and add the egg mixture. Combine the eggs with the veg, then throw the pan in the oven, until the frittata is firm and fully cooked through. This should take about 10 minutes. Serve, topped with the remaining feta and some dill to garnish.

What can you add?

Mastering a few sides and sauces to easily throw on to any dish is a genius way to elevate your food, while effortlessly boosting your microbiome. You can generally keep these in your fridge and reach for them as and when needed.

ROMESCO-ISH SAUCE

In recent years, I have developed what I would describe as a perfectly healthy obsession with anything that reminds me of a romesco sauce. Classically, this is made by blitzing roasted peppers, basil, garlic, extra virgin olive oil, paprika, vinegar, salt and almonds. However, I have found that you can mix things up and alter the recipe to suit your needs. I use jarred peppers, rather than roasting my own because this saves time, but also provides a lovely hint of vinegar which the sauce also needs (if you do roast your own, I suggest a little dash of red wine vinegar to compensate).

I use this sauce in countless ways. It is a perfect salad (or anything else) dressing, but I just leave out the nuts if I want it to be very loose. It's also lovely as a replacement for tomato sauce. One of my favourite ways to use it is as a base for a spectacular centrepiece: place a thick layer on a serving dish and then serve any roasted vegetables on top, perhaps with a sprinkling of herbs and pomegranate seeds.

Here is a rough basic recipe, but please adjust according to your own palate:

1 jar roasted peppers (I quite like mixed colours)
1 huge handful fresh basil
1 handful almonds (skin on)
1 tsp paprika
Glug of extra virgin olive oil (about 2 tbsp)
Garlic (debatable – I don't always like the harsh taste
    and would prefer a clove of roasted or confit garlic,
    but if you enjoy a stronger garlic flavour, go ahead
    and include a raw clove)

I just throw all of these ingredients into a bullet blender, blitz and then taste. It's usually perfect but if it needs anything else like salt or more basil, for example, I add and keep adjusting until it tastes just right.

MUHAMMARA-GANOUSH DIP

Sorry, Syria, I was going to make a traditional muhammara dip but got confused with baba ganoush and created this delicious monster of a dip instead. This is a wonderful addition to any meat, fish or roasted veg. It's also lovely as a dip and great as a base in a wrap or sandwich.

2–3 large red peppers, roughly chopped
1 aubergine (leave the skin on, why lose the fibre and
    polyphenols?), roughly chopped
3–4 (or more) whole garlic cloves (depending on how
    much you like garlic), skin on

1–2 handfuls walnuts
Generous glug extra virgin olive oil
Lemon juice (start with less and adjust to taste)
1 tsp ground cumin
1 tsp Aleppo pepper flakes (or use smoked, sweet paprika)
1 tbsp pomegranate molasses
1 tsp red wine vinegar (optional, if you feel it would
*   benefit from a sharper flavour after tasting)*
Sea salt

For topping
Extra virgin olive oil
Pomegranate seeds
Fresh mint
Chopped walnuts

Preheat the oven to 200°C. Roast the red peppers, aubergine and garlic cloves with olive oil and a generous pinch of salt, until completely soft. This should take about 15–20 minutes but monitor to make sure they don't burn. Squeeze the garlic out of its skin, then blitz with the peppers, aubergine and remaining ingredients, either in a food processor or with a hand-held blender. When combined, taste it and adjust to your own palate – you might like extra salt, pomegranate molasses or vinegar at this stage. Feeling confident to adjust a recipe to a flavour profile you enjoy most is the best way to become a truly good cook! To serve as a spectacular dip, spread it out on a dish and drizzle over extra virgin olive oil with a sprinkling of pomegranate seeds, fresh mint and some chopped walnuts. You could also serve it with a pitta and more roasted vegetables, cheese or falafel.

CHIMICHURRI

This vibrant green salsa-cum-sauce is completely delicious over any seafood, meat or vegetable dish. I love to keep a jar of this in my fridge. Just pour some olive oil on the top to seal it and it will stay fresh to use for days and days.

1–2 big handfuls fresh parsley and coriander
1 garlic clove
1–2 tsp dried oregano
Lemon juice, to taste (approx. ½ lemon)
1 small red and 1 small green chilli (I remove seeds
    because I'm not a huge fan of spice)
Extra virgin olive oil (enough to get the consistency you
    like – at least 4–6 tbsp)

You make this either by blitzing the ingredients or just chopping them up finely. If I blitz them, I prefer to chop the peppers separately and then add them to the blitzed ingredients to provide texture and manage the heat. But if you prefer, you can just throw all of it into a blender.

PESTO

By definition I don't think you can really have just one recipe for pesto because 'pesto' literally just means 'to pound'. So any combination of ingredients pounded together can be a type of pesto. I was taught to make it as a child by measuring everything by eye and repeatedly tasting and adjusting, until the taste was just right. Please note the measurements given are very rough and can be adjusted to your own palate.

I purposefully don't include garlic in this one because I think it allows the toasted flavour of the pine nuts to really come through. Another delicious alternative uses wild garlic leaves instead of basil (just don't add more garlic). You'll get plenty of garlic flavour already from these foraged leaves. You can also swap the pine nuts out for walnuts, which are cheaper and much more nutrient dense.

2–3 very large handfuls basil leaves
1 large handful baby spinach (makes it greener)
1 large handful toasted pine nuts
2–3 tbsp Parmesan (or more according to your palate)

*Extra-virgin olive oil (start with 4 tbsp, adding more,
    as needed, to achieve desired consistency)*
Pinch of salt

Blitz all the ingredients together, until completely smooth. To make it really good use a blitz-taste-adjust-blitz-taste-again method. Only you know what really tastes good to you!

TAHINI DRESSING

If you don't regularly serve your food with a concoction of different tahini dressings, you are missing out – and so are your microbiome bugs. Tahini provides an amazing source of healthy fat, fibre, magnesium and B vitamins; it's also just genuinely delicious when you know what you're doing. There are a million variations of a tahini dressing – you can blitz it with water, salt, garlic, lemon juice and any green herb you like to come up with a delicious 'green goddess' type dressing. But my favourite thing to do is to slowly whisk small amounts of water into it, watching an interesting and slightly confusing transformation unfold. Initially, it will dry up and clump together, so you think you have ruined it. But gradually, if you just persist with whisking more and more drops of water into it, it forms a silky, smooth and luscious consistency. The stunning metamorphosis never ceases to amaze me. From here, you can mix in all sorts of things: maybe some kefir with lemon zest and juice. I also love gochujang and a bit of teriyaki sauce or a big spoon of harissa. The combinations are endless and I encourage you to explore you own favourites.

Harissa tahini dressing
    5 tbsp (approx.) good-quality tahini
    Pinch of sea salt
    Water (enough to form the right consistency)
    *2 tsp harissa paste (I usually buy rose harissa,
        but any will do)*

Pour the tahini into a bowl (I measure this by eye but it's roughly 5 tablespoons). Add the salt and then slowly whisk in the water, a tablespoon or two at a time. When it turns a pale colour and is silky smooth, with a consistency you like, you can stop adding water. Now just add the harissa paste and enjoy. It's lovely on roasted vegetables or as a salad dressing.

BASIL VINAIGRETTE

This is lovely drizzled over a tomato salad or in a sandwich with other Mediterranean flavours – for example, mozzarella and roasted courgettes/aubergine. It should keep in the fridge for a week or two.

> *2 large handfuls basil*
> *Extra virgin olive oil (at least 4 tbsp, but enough for the right consistency)*
> *1 tsp red wine vinegar*
> *Pinch of salt*

Blitz the ingredients together, adding the olive oil by eye for the consistency you want. Start with 4 tbsp and adjust as necessary. Store in a jar, covered with a layer of olive oil to keep it fresh for longer.

QUICK PICKLED ('QUICKLED') RED ONIONS

I refer to these as my marinated onions, but someone on Instagram joked I should really call them my 'quickles', which I love. I love adding bright pink, zingy red onions to wraps, sandwiches, salads and even on top of some curries. These are super speedy and create a similar result to traditional pickles, which need to sit in the fridge for much longer.

> *1 red onion*
> *Pinch of salt*
> *Red wine vinegar (enough to mostly cover)*
> *1–2 tbsp extra virgin olive oil*

1 tsp sumac (optional)
1 tsp cumin seeds (optional)

Finely slice the red onion and submerge in boiling water for about a minute. Drain and submerge in cold water to cool, then drain again. Mix in the salt, then pour over a decent amount of red wine vinegar, until mostly covered. Pour over the extra virgin olive oil and spices, if using. You can then carry on with whatever else you are cooking and the onions will be ready to enjoy by the time you are done. (They need at least 20 minutes of marinating but last well in the fridge as a wonderful leftover.)

'QUICKLED' RED CABBAGE

This is a lovely idea for a side for any Mexican or Asian dish. It's also delicious inside a wrap or salad and keeps for a few days in the fridge.

Red cabbage (however much you want to serve)
Salt
Lime juice (to taste)

Finely slice the red cabbage, sprinkle it with salt and massage this in with your hands, until the cabbage is soft. Squeeze over the lime juice, then set aside while you prepare the rest of your meal. Serve it as a lovely side or incorporate it into salads. It keeps well for several days in the fridge so you can add it to lots of different dishes throughout the week.

Reassess your staples

Again, a lot of carbohydrate bases are a missed opportunity for more microbiome-boosting options. Perhaps you tend to eat pasta, rice or potatoes most days of the week. That might be convenient for you, but boring for your microbiome! Here are some simple examples of alternative carbohydrate bases to try.

MICROBIOME-BOOSTING SODA BREAD

I was inspired by sourdough expert Dr Vanessa Kimbell's approach to bread here because she argues, rightly, that it can serve as an excellent vehicle for amazing plant variety if you combine different flours. Wherever possible when I bake, I try to incorporate a handful of different flours, so that even this simple component is keeping the microbiome interested. This recipe hardly counts as proper baking and genuinely requires no skill to make (I should know because even I can successfully make it!).

100g rye flour
250g other flours (combine your own favourites here –
    I often just use a mixture of wholemeal, spelt and
    Khorasan)
50g organic jumbo oats
1 tsp bicarbonate of soda
Mixed seeds (as many as you like – I throw in about 4–6
    tbsp)
Pinch of salt
1 egg
300ml buttermilk (or kefir)

Mix all the dry ingredients together in a bowl, then form a well in the middle. In a separate bowl, beat the egg into the buttermilk and then pour this mixture into the well, gently combining it with your dry ingredients. You don't need to really knead this dough – just make sure it is well combined. Shape the dough into a ball and cut a deep cross (about a third of the depth) with a wet knife. Bake at 190°C for 40–45 minutes. Remove from the oven and wrap in a clean tea towel to keep the crust soft. You can enjoy this bread with all kinds of toppings – I love a bit of butter (on warm bread), locally sourced honey and a sprinkling of cinnamon as a sweet treat. Whatever you choose to eat it with, don't forget the role of glucose hacks – if it is the first meal of the day include more fat and protein, e.g. eggs. If it is a sweet treat, have it at the end of a savoury meal. In both scenarios, your blood sugar rise will be calmed by moving your body after eating – this could be a 10-minute walk or just some housework.

LENTIL PANCAKES/WRAPS

These are exquisitely easy to make, as long as you have a decent non-stick frying pan. They are also surprisingly delicious, and pack in a hefty dose of fibre compared to other wraps. This recipe uses equal volumes of lentils and water – if you don't have cup measures you can use a standard mug instead.

Makes 3–4 wraps
1 cup red lentils (washed)
1 cup water
Pinch of salt
1 tbsp nigella seeds
Extra virgin olive oil, for greasing

Pour the lentils and water into a blender or food processer, then set aside for about an hour. Later, add the salt before blitzing to a fine batter. Transfer to a bowl or jug and mix in the nigella seeds and maybe slightly more water, until you have a loose consistency, similar to that of a crepe batter. Pour a ladleful of batter and gently swirl across the surface of an oiled frying pan. Cook for about 1–2 minutes on each side until the surface firms enough to flip. Serve as you would any wrap with whatever fillings you like. A number of the sauces/dips and 'quickles' in this section are lovely ideas for delicious fillings.

YOGHURT FLATBREAD

This is a quick and tasty alternative to buying UPF wraps/flatbreads, lovely served with any dip or curry and also nice as a wrap with sandwich fillers. With the yoghurt and chickpea flour, they will be more filling and produce a calmer blood-sugar response compared to traditional flatbreads.

Makes around 4–5 flatbreads

150g self-raising flour

50g chickpea flour

200g plain yoghurt (not Greek, as this will be too thick)

Pinch of salt

1½ tbsp nigella seeds (alternatively, you could throw in some roasted garlic and finely chopped rosemary or any other flavour enhancers you like)

Combine the ingredients and separate into 4–5 little balls. Roll them out to a size that works well for you, then dry fry in a frying pan, until slightly brown on either side.

PEAS PUDDING

This is a lovely, hearty alternative to mashed potatoes to serve as your carbohydrate base for any meal. One serving packs in more than 10g of fibre which is impressive, considering we are aiming for 30g a day. I have only ever made it using green split peas but Google tells me it can also be made with the yellow ones. Who knew?

500g green split peas

1 stock cube

1 litre water

1 large red onion (roughly chopped into quarters)

2 bay leaves (if you happen to have them)

Extra virgin olive oil

Sea salt and freshly ground black pepper

Throw the ingredients into a slow cooker/crockpot or just into a pot on the stove and let them simmer away gently while you're busy doing something else. I tend to mostly forget about them and just intermittently taste them. Once the ingredients are completely soft, remove from the heat. You may need to top up the liquid if it is drying out. It should probably take about an hour to get the right consistency. Remove the bay leaves and blitz with a hand-held mixer, until you have a smooth purée. Taste and season as needed. Add a glug of extra virgin olive oil, until it has a flavour you like.

I love serving this in place of mashed potatoes or just as an extra side. It has a subtle pea-like flavour I completely adore. My favourite way to use it is simply serving a generous portion in a bowl, with beautifully caramelised slices of winter squash on top, followed by crumbled feta and an extra glug of extra virgin olive oil on top. Heavenly!

CELERIAC AND BUTTER-BEAN MASH

If you like the taste of celeriac, you will love this creamy, luxurious alternative to mashed potatoes.

1 medium celeriac, peeled and chopped
1 tin butter beans, drained
Extra virgin olive oil
2–4 garlic cloves (ideally, roasted or confit garlic)
Fresh thyme (optional – fresh parsley or chives would also work)
Sea salt

Place the celeriac in salted boiling water and cook, until very soft. Drain completely, then add the butter beans, a good drizzle of extra virgin olive oil and a pinch of sea salt. I also include 2–4 cloves roasted garlic/confit garlic, but if you don't have this to hand, just throw the cloves into the boiling water raw. Blitz until smooth and adjust with salt to taste. I like stirring through some fresh thyme, but I imagine parsley or chives would be just as nice.

Spectacular mains

My approach to specific meals is now very fluid – in all honesty, my 'break-fast' and dinner are often interchangeable. However, here are some examples of mains I really love.

ROMESCO AUBERGINE PARMIGIANA

Many people think they don't like aubergine, but that's usually because they don't know how to cook it properly. I often find cooking it twice is what creates the nicest texture.

> 2 large aubergines, sliced into rounds
> Large pinch of sea salt
> Extra virgin olive oil, for roasting and greasing
> 1 large batch of romesco (see p. 234)
> 250g mozzarella (2 balls), chopped
> 2 large handfuls grated Parmesan

Preheat the oven to 200°C. Place the aubergine rounds on a baking sheet (or you might need two, to allow enough space). Sprinkle over a large pinch of sea salt and a generous glug of extra virgin olive oil, mix to combine. Roast, until the aubergine slices have a silky, soft texture. This usually takes around 15–20 minutes. Oil the base of a deep baking dish, then add layers of the roasted aubergine, alternating with the romesco sauce and chopped mozzarella, finishing with a layer of aubergine. Sprinkle the Parmesan on top and return to the oven, until the cheese has melted and the dish looks bubbly and delicious. Serve with another protein source and maybe some salad.

COURGETTE, BUTTER-BEAN AND ZA'ATAR FRY-UP

I made this in a rush as a last-minute fridge raid and struck gold. It is honestly so quick and delicious. I use jarred beans here because they have a truly superior texture and flavour. (However, I do still use tinned ones when the texture isn't as important – for example, when blending them into a mash.)

1 garlic clove, sliced
A glug of extra virgin olive oil
1 courgette, roughly diced
½ large jar (700g) of butter beans, drained
1–2 tsp za'atar spice blend
125g burrata cheese (1 ball)
2–3 tsp basil vinaigrette (see p. 238)
Sea salt

Gently fry the sliced garlic in the olive oil, shortly followed by the roughly diced courgette. Cook down, until soft, then add the beans and allow them to warm through. Add a sprinkle of salt and the za'atar. Serve up on a plate with a ball of burrata nestled on top. Spoon over the basil vinaigrette and tuck in. You might want to add even more vinaigrette because it is so delicious. This is a fairly high-fat meal – I just compensate by eating less fat in my other meals but find it all evens out. You can replace the burrata with dollops of soft goat's cheese, which is also delicious.

SWEET POTATO 'NACHOS'

This is a real crowd pleaser and one of my most popular Instagram recipes. You are essentially borrowing the flavours of nachos but replacing the chips with deliciously caramelised sweet potatoes.

1–2 large sweet potatoes (enough to fill the base of your
  roasting tin of choice)
Extra virgin olive oil, for roasting
Large pinch of sea salt
2 tsp paprika
2 tsp garlic granules
1 tin black beans, drained
1 tin kidney beans, drained
2 large handfuls grated mature Cheddar

To serve
Sour cream or crème fraîche
Fresh coriander
Pickled red onions (or my 'quickled' onions on pp. 238–9)
Pickled jalapeños

Preheat the oven to 200°C. Wash/scrub the sweet potatoes, keeping the skin on. Slice into rounds and place in a roasting tin, so they completely cover the base. Pour over a generous glug of extra virgin olive oil, then sprinkle over the salt, paprika and garlic. Mix to combine well, then roast until completely squidgy, soft and a bit browned – this should take 15–20 minutes, but keep an eye on them, so they don't burn. Remove from the oven, then pour over the drained beans, distributing them evenly. Follow with a generous sprinkling of cheese, then return to the oven long enough for the cheese to melt (5 minutes should be more than enough). Serve with dollops of sour cream and a sprinkling of coriander and the pickles. Tuck in and enjoy.

Anatomy of a good salad

There are thousands of salad recipes out there and obviously I can't do them all justice in a paragraph. But given the enormous variety of ingredient combinations, they do really serve as an amazing way to boost your microbiome. I generally eat a salad with dinner most days or turn at least one meal into a huge and filling salad. Many people think they don't like salad, but that is simply because they have never tried a good one before. Here are some basic principles:

1) **The quality of the ingredients used will decide how good the salad is.** For example, an outrageously sweet beef tomato with salt and extra virgin olive oil on its own is delicious.
2) **A delicious dressing using good-quality ingredients can win over anyone.** The romesco and tahini recipes (see pp. 234

and 237) are just some examples. Being able to master a very basic French vinaigrette can also elevate any vegetable. To be honest, I often just enjoy pouring good-quality extra virgin olive oil and tangy balsamic vinegar on my salads. It almost doesn't matter what dressing you use, but it shouldn't be UPF.

3) **Mix up your salad base.** If you use mixed leaves, each different leaf counts as another plant, thus adding to your microbiome diversity. I like buying a seasonal mix from my local farm shop which often includes edible flowers too. Be brave and try bitter leaves like radicchio and rocket – they have more polyphenols, which your bugs will love. Even if you don't like them now, once you've reduced the amount of sweet food you eat and built up a healthy microbiome, your palate will adjust to enjoy them. After washing, make sure they are bone dry, so the dressing coats each leaf properly.

4) **Add texture.** When we eat crunchy things, we get a pleasure response in the brain (this is a trick food companies use heavily in a lot of their UPF products; advertisements for these foods even make a big fuss about just how crunchy they are). Adding in different crunchy ingredients like fennel, raw carrot, radishes, red cabbage and many other things will make a salad more appealing to your brain. This is complemented by opposite textures, like creamy avocado or goat's cheese.

5) **Bulk it out.** This isn't so necessary if it's just a side dish, but if the salad is the main event, bulk it out with roasted vegetables (sweet potatoes are my favourites) or some legumes.

6) **Add protein.** Again, if the salad is the whole meal, it needs to spike your PYY (satiety hormone) with protein which you can get from meat, fish, legumes and boiled eggs. Some cheese and nuts can also add to the protein content.

7) **Sprinkle.** Don't forget the previous microbiome-boosting principles. Most salads benefit from an extra sprinkle of nuts, seeds or fresh herbs.

8) **Mix up the flavours.** Just like surprising your palate with different textures, a mixture of different types of flavours will make the salad a genuinely enjoyable thing to eat. I love a hit of sourness from ingredients like pickled onions or even some sauerkraut; bitter flavours from olives or salad leaves; salty flavours from capers or feta cheese; sweet flavours from pomegranate seeds or other fruits; and sometimes even umami flavours from meat or fish.

MY FAVOURITE SALAD COMBINATIONS

Most salads really don't need a recipe per se – it is really hard to get these wrong! But as a rough guide these are some of the ingredients I like to combine:

- Rocket, grated carrot and drained kidney beans with plenty of extra virgin olive oil, salt, pepper and balsamic vinegar.
- Rocket, radicchio, fruit (either pear, apples or figs), crumbled Stilton cheese and walnuts. Dressed in olive oil and balsamic vinegar.
- Red cabbage (massaged in salt), fennel slices, shaved carrot, apple slices, pomegranate seeds, nigella seeds, olive oil, balsamic vinegar and pomegranate molasses.
- Mixed leaves (including some bitter ones), roasted beetroot, segments of blood orange (or normal orange, if blood orange is not in season), mozzarella. Dressed with a squeeze of orange juice, extra virgin olive oil, salt and pomegranate molasses.
- Mixed leaves, roasted sweet potatoes and chickpeas (using ras el hanout or just paprika/salt/garlic granules) and feta. Dressed in romesco sauce.
- Classic Greek salad flavours with salad leaves of choice, good quality mixed tomatoes, feta, olives, cucumber, 'quickled' onions, extra virgin olive oil and lots of dried oregano.

The list of combinations is endless and many more can be found on my Instagram account @whatyourdoctoreats.

With all the cuisines and flavour combinations out there, the options for helpful recipes are truly endless. However, by understanding the science and core principles, you should feel released from the need to follow a meal plan. Given that the babies in Dr Davis's experiment (see p. 181) were able to intuitively select the foods they needed according to their precise nutrient requirements, it would be odd for me to suggest a structured approach with precise advice on what you should eat. You should be allowed to be guided by your own cravings and appetite to make the experience of eating feel truly intuitive and enjoyable. Seeing each meal as an opportunity to feed your microbiome will hopefully feel like an uplifting change from an often restrictive attitude to food.

By now, food should feel like an art form you can use creatively yourself. However, there is one character from Part I we haven't really addressed yet. He can influence your health and appetite in a plethora of ways, independent of the food you are eating. This book is called *What Your Doctor Eats*, but to ignore the outside forces that influence our eating habits is naive. If I am really to help you achieve long-lasting health, I can't ignore the role of an important 'associate' we all have. I am talking about your stress hormone, cortisol. Next, let me show you how to stay on his good side.

What your doctor eats: Key points

1) Many cuisines can achieve incredible health outcomes. The goal isn't to all eat the same thing. Instead, we can simply be guided by principles which naturally support health.

2) Your choice to drink alcohol is a personal decision. Although most people are aware of the ways smoking can cause disease, most of us are ignorant of alcohol's effects. If you do drink, I strongly encourage you do so in moderation and make sure you only drink things you genuinely enjoy – otherwise, what's the point in this indulgence?

3) How you break your fast is very important – there are many recipes which promote satiety and a very stable blood sugar. Familiarising yourself with the need for a protein-rich break-fast can dramatically improve how you feel on the day, while also helping to shape health outcomes.

4) Seeing your meals as an opportunity to keep your microbiome entertained is a positive and fun way to eat. Swapping carb bases, thinking of things you can add and trying to eat with the seasons are some simple techniques to use.

CHAPTER 10

CONTROL STRESS

The bridge between mind and body

I hope I have convinced you that food is an incredibly important part, not just of good health, but of life itself. To imply it is just fuel is simply not true: your microbiome, hormones, appetite, energy levels and risk of disease are all directly affected by it. But more than that, it's not fair to detach people from their culture or the simple pleasure we all get from food. So often it can be a source of comfort or even, for some, a type of love language.

However, our relationship with food isn't as clear as it may seem. So many of my patients come back to me and feel frustrated because they are doing 'all the right things'. They have already learned how to choreograph meals in a way that regulates their appetite and stabilises their blood sugar. I sit with them and pick apart what they eat and it sounds like food any microbiome would love. So why then are they still not feeling well? If they're trying to lose weight, how can it possibly plateau when everything they seem to be doing is apparently perfect? In my experience, there is one last puzzle piece: cortisol.

Remember, I can stimulate weight gain in any patient simply by prescribing a steroid called prednisolone, which is a synthetic form of cortisol. It won't be my patient's fault or a reflection of their willpower but they will *absolutely* gain weight. This is partly because it increases appetite (which I hope you now see isn't something we can simply ignore), but it also directly increases insulin, thus driving more fat storing. Without realising it, many of my patients are triggering the exact same process in their bodies: they are living lives that facilitate chronic levels of raised cortisol. But if you think back to how this 'associate' can influence disease, weight loss should be the least of your worries. To truly optimise your health, you need to understand how to manage what we colloquially refer to as 'stress'. This isn't a fluffy, wishy-washy concept: it is a serious risk factor for disease and a shortened life. I want you to take it very seriously and, over the next chapter, I will show you some surprising new science so you know how.

First, though, allow me to refresh your memory and remind you of the 'mafia' in your body. As you have seen, insulin is very much the 'godfather' – he exerts enormous control over your health. But he doesn't work alone. Cortisol is his second in command and, together, they can drive all the insulin-resistance complications you don't want. I'm talking about heart disease, stroke, type 2 diabetes and an increased risk of cancer. Remember, cortisol also speaks directly to the mitochondria who are responsible for your energy and also behave like an hourglass: amazingly, they are part of what predicts how short or long your life will be. That's a morbid image but with new longevity and lifestyle research we can finally understand one invaluable fact: we don't age at the same rate. How you treat your mitochondria matters. Constantly exposing them to high cortisol and raised blood sugar will make the sand run much faster in that hourglass. It can trigger chronic fatigue and seems to partly explain previously misunderstood conditions like fibromyalgia. If a condition is linked to trauma or stress, for some reason many take it less seriously. But our mitochondria are where the mind and body meet – finally, we are starting to understand these conditions. Boosting the health of your mitochondria with a diet that keeps blood sugar well controlled is a valuable technique, but managing stress is just as important.

Change your perception of what stress says about you

When I ask my patients about their levels of stress most of them do something strange: they laugh. It's a snorting kind of knowing laugh, as if to say, 'Well, yes, of course I'm stressed.' In some it comes across as something they are almost proud of. Stress is apparently a marker of success, responsibility or importance for all manner of people. I see it in my pot-bellied lawyers, sleepless university students and anyone who is a parent. The latter will always mention the child's age to express a higher level of stress, but ultimately, babies, toddlers, prepubescents, teenagers or 20-somethings will all be cited as stress-inducing ages. I don't want to undermine the overwhelming stress of being a parent – it is a blessed curse: in payment for having someone in your life for whom you will feel almost unbearable love, you will endure a never-ending worry. Love is by definition painful because of the fear of loss it brings.

However, I do want you to think about society's celebration of stress. Have you unknowingly been celebrating your own? Does it feel like someone has pressed the fast-forward button on your life, making it fast paced? Are you in a frantic rush, juggling a million things, hustling and striving for … what? I am not suggesting achievement and purpose aren't important in life. But many of us feel rushed to do something without knowing what it is. I often confront my patients with big questions: why are you doing this? Is it what you *really* want? Sometimes they have amazing epiphanies and even completely change their careers as a result. That won't be the right answer for most of us but many people never ask themselves these two vital questions. Philosopher Eckhart Tolle famously said, 'The secret to life is to die before you die.' He was referring to people who have had near-death experiences: it was only when they were about to die that they realised what life was all about. Then, having survived, they saw the world through fresh eyes and could finally appreciate the things that *really* matter. People who recover following a dreaded diagnosis like cancer often have a similar experience. In a way, they died before they actually died: the first death just opened their eyes. If you are to truly tackle stress, I invite you to have this same epiphany and think carefully about what and who really matters to you. Pressing fast-forward on your life will only make it feel shorter – if you slow down, you might savour the people and things you care about most.

I appreciate this has been a gloomy start to what is meant to be an uplifting chapter on happiness. Who even gave me the right to waffle on about this philosophical stuff? Believe it or not, this is a huge part of my job as a GP. People go to their doctors for guidance all the time. They tell us they want to kill themselves, are hopeless, lost and don't know what to do. I have long conversations about why I think someone shouldn't end their life more often than you want to know. Teaching my patients how to become happy again is part of my bread and butter; I talk about it every single day. It also comes up when we discuss their physical health because countless autoimmune and skin conditions are triggered by severe stress. It can also cause periods to stop, subfertility, recurrent infections, insomnia, high blood pressure, headaches and even hair loss. In its most severe form, acute stress can even cause a heart-attack-like condition called 'takotsubo' or 'broken-heart syndrome' which I saw once when working in cardiology. A heart scan will show no blockage; instead, the cause is a huge surge of stress chemicals in the body.

Once again, tackling stress is not a wishy-washy undertaking. This is serious stuff. However, I have come to realise most people have never actually been taught the scientific theory of happiness. In fact, most of my patients look bemused when I mention it. Surely, happiness isn't a science? But it actually is. A whole field of research is entirely dedicated to picking apart what makes humans most happy. You can even get a PhD in happiness! Sadly, many of the concepts are tucked away in academia and, for some reason, aren't something most of us are ever taught about.

Having researched this myself, I incorporate it into many of my appointments whether we are talking about mental health or not. Here are some of the questions I ask:

- Who do you live with?
- How are things at home?
- What do you do (career)? How is it going?
- Do you have local family/friends? How often do you see them?
- How much exercise do you do?
- How is your sleep?
- What do you eat?
- How do you spend your time when you're not working/ what are your hobbies?
- What do you feel passionate about in life?

If I am to help patients, I need to understand their lives, so I can work out how they've ended up where they are. Many have their own theories but occasionally, some have no idea why they feel low and can't identify an obvious trigger. I once spoke to a man in his late 40s who had never struggled with his mental health before but one day randomly developed new anxiety attacks. We both tried to pick apart his life and work out what could possibly have changed. Eventually, I asked: have you recently been bereaved? It turned out a lifelong family friend had recently died but, as he talked about this man, he realised he had always seen him as a father figure. It had never occurred to him that this event could trigger anxiety attacks three months later but grief often has a delayed effect. I told him, 'Well, this all makes sense now. You don't have depression: in your mind you have just lost a father. You are grieving.' He burst into tears, overcome by the permission I had given him to grieve. For other patients, the trigger can be insidious, multi-factorial or a combination of classic life stressors, as follows:

- Loss of any kind (even pets – for many these genuinely feel like family)
- Divorce or any breakdown in a relationship (romantic or not)
- Change/loss of a job
- Moving house
- Major illness or injury

These five are also the classic triggers for suicidal thoughts, but when it comes to assessing the impact of life events on stress, there are many others. Take a look at the 'Life Change Index Scale' on p. 257 to see where you sit.*(I find it almost amusing that 'Christmas approaching' counts as a life stress but, ironically, many of us will concede this 'happy' time can be anxiety inducing for several reasons.) But why list all these life stressors? I am not proposing that anyone can remove these events from their life – that would be naive. And we wouldn't want to because there are several 'happy' events (besides Christmas) which come with a stress score: getting married, going on holiday or retiring for example. Many of life's greatest adventures are coupled with some stress – a cautious reaction to change is embedded in our evolution and makes perfect sense. In other words, it is possible to be excited and stressed at the same time and this isn't a bad thing. What I want is for you to have *insight* into this because when you understand what is driving your life stress and therefore your cortisol, you will be better placed to manage it. Equally, it won't come as a surprise, nor will you

---

* This scale is based on the Holmes and Rahe stress scale which was shown to correlate with a risk of disease in the following two years. It is by no means a perfect measure of an individual's experience of stress because we are all unique. Everything from our genes, environment, personalities and hormones can influence how we respond to stressful life events. However, it is a simple and useful illustration of how 'total stress' is influenced by several factors: they can add up and compound to produce a feeling of extreme stress in ways we might not be able to recognise in the moment. It has been criticised for not differentiating between positive and negative stress, but the scores adjust for this and, if anything, it is interesting to acknowledge that positive changes in life can still bring an element of stress.

feel misplaced guilt for your emotions. The key takeaway here is that by learning how to *anticipate* our cortisol spikes, we can prophylactically begin to *mitigate* them. Let me explain how.

LIFE CHANGE INDEX SCALE (THE STRESS TEST)

Event	Impact score	My score
Death of spouse	100	
Divorce	73	
Marital separation	65	
Jail term	63	
Death of close family member	63	
Personal injury or illness	53	
Marriage	50	
Fired at work	47	
Marital reconciliation	45	
Retirement	45	
Change in health of family member	44	
Pregnancy	40	
Sex difficulties	39	
Gain of a new family member	39	
Business readjustment	39	
Change in financial state	38	
Death of close friend	37	
Change to different line of work	36	
Change in number of arguments with spouse	35	
Mortgage over $20,000	31	
Foreclosure of mortgage or loan	30	
Change in responsibilities at work	29	
Son or daughter leaving home	29	
Trouble with in-laws	29	
Outstanding personal achievement	28	
Spouse begins or stops work	26	
Begin or end school	26	
Change in living conditions	25	
Revisions of personal habits	24	
Trouble with boss	23	
Change in work hours or conditions	20	

Event	Impact score	My score
Change in residence	20	
Change in schools	20	
Change in recreations	19	
Change in church activities	19	
Change in social activities	19	
Mortgage or loan less than $20,000	17	
Change in sleeping habits	16	
Change in number of family get-togethers	15	
Change in eating habits	15	
Vacation	13	
Christmas approaching	12	
Minor violation of the law	11	
Total		

- 150pts or less means a relatively low amount of life change and a low susceptibility to stress-induced health problems.
- 150 to 300pts implies about a 50 per cent chance of a major stress-induced health problem in the next two years.
- 300pts or more raises the odds to about 80 per cent, according to the Holmes-Rahe prediction model.

Flow

I teach my patients what I believe to be the five pillars of human happiness, inspired by a lecture I attended as a GP trainee. They are: nature, community, sleep, movement and charity, and I will delve into them shortly. However, one important concept was not mentioned in this talk, even though it influences every pillar in one way or another. It is the concept of 'flow state' – a term coined by Hungarian–American psychologist Mihaly Csikszentmihalyi in 1990. To date, when I mention this groundbreaking psychological theory to my patients, absolutely none of them have ever heard of it.

We now know that if you peruse the world for its happiest people, they will have several things in common. One of these is that they spend a decent chunk of their time in flow state. But what does this mean? As I explain it to my patients, it is the experience of engaging in an activity where, if someone tapped you on the shoulder and asked 'How long have you been doing that?' you genuinely wouldn't have a clue. It could have been ten minutes or four hours – time seems to completely disappear as you almost disassociate into an exquisite level of concentration. By definition, you aren't thinking about your childhood trauma or your fears for the future; you can't analyse your insecurities or have racing thoughts about all the things that are going wrong in your life. Your mind is locked into the task at hand and the experience almost feels like being in a trance. It is no surprise that in this state productivity increases by up to 500 per cent: if you can calibrate and streamline your mental energy like this, what you can achieve almost feels superhuman. It should also be no surprise that the experience of flow state is tied to human happiness – you aren't bored, you aren't overwhelmed and you absolutely can't feel self-conscious. Of course, this is an amazing recipe for simple, unreserved contentment.

There are many theories about what happens in the brain in flow state and scientists have played around with fancy gadgets like EEGs* and functional MRI scans to explore what is actually going on. One theory is that, just like alcohol, flow state seems to inhibit your prefrontal cortex: this is the centre of your personality and is where a lot of your 'executive function' takes place. It is the last part of the brain to finish developing which is why armies like their soldiers nice and young: without a fully developed prefrontal cortex, they experience less fear and are far less conscious of their mortality. This might make them seem 'braver' than older soldiers but really they just have an underdeveloped fear response. This part of the brain is also heavily involved in our ability to self-regulate our emotions, especially in social situations; to anyone who spends time with a teenager, it might not be a surprise to learn that the prefrontal cortex

---

* An electroencephalogram (EEG) measures the electrical activity of the brain.

doesn't finish developing until the age of 25. If flow some-how calms activity in this part of your brain, it makes sense that it inhibits feelings of insecurity. Other theories suggest flow influences our automatic processes in parts of the brain like the cerebellum and basal ganglia, making a behaviour feel both intuitive and effortless. Whether playing tennis, skiing or juggling, you aren't even thinking about what you are doing – it feels like your body and mind are in perfect sync. If you have ever experienced this, you know how wonderful it can feel!

One of my favourite examples of flow state is surfing – even just watching this entrancing act makes me feel some level of calm. Surfers aren't thinking about what they need to make for dinner or the rude driver who cut them off earlier that morn-ing: they are completely engrossed in analysing the waves, synchronising their fine-tuned movements and balancing on the board. I even have a theory that flow state is the main reason why Hawaii is ranked as the happiest state in America: these beautiful islands are where surfing was invented and it still serves as an ancient Polynesian ritual, as well as a way of life. If you drive to the suburbs, you will find whole commu-nities of people who live to surf all day, every day and choose to do this instead of investing in careers. You could argue they are financially poor, some living in tents and just making do, but I suspect they don't feel poor. They are willing to forgo societal norms because the flow surfing brings them is clearly intoxicating – even sharks in hotspots like 'Leftovers Beach' won't deter them from this cherished pursuit. Of course, this is an extreme example, and I'm not proposing my patients throw their lives or responsibilities out the window in the hunt for an equivalent pastime. However, very often, many of them are unable to give me even one example of a flow-state activity they regularly engage in. It doesn't matter what it is: baking, gardening, rock-climbing, writing, painting, dancing – I don't care what they choose, but I ask that they find some form of flow and incorporate it into their life.

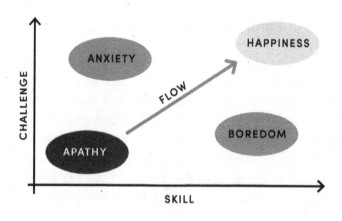

Figure 3: Flow state

As you can see in Figure 3, a flow state requires two things: challenge and skill. In other words, not only should it be an activity you've learned and mastered, you also need to put conscious effort into it. In contrast, spending time on a skill which requires no challenge is a recipe for boredom. On the other hand, an activity that requires no actual skill but extreme challenge might cause anxiety. When you find *just* the right balance of both you'll elicit flow state, calming your prefrontal cortex and increasing your overall ability to feel happy. The strange thing is that many of us unwind by doing the precise opposite of this: watching TV or mindlessly doom scrolling require no challenge or skill. People might think it is making them feel happy but really, all it does is stop them from feeling anything at all. Without realising it, your pastime is actually igniting apathy. Of course, you don't need to completely give up these passive forms of pleasure in your life – I certainly haven't. But when it comes to whiling away the hours, I consciously spend more time doing this in flow state and you should too. Of course, happiness, like health, is complex and finding a new hobby won't be the only way to achieve it. Let's explore the five core pillars which are heavily influencing your cortisol and experience of stress.

Pillar number 1: Nature

The research coming out about nature's impact on health is truly mesmerising when, in a way, it shouldn't be. Beneath the surface, we are all simply animals who, for about 6–7 million years, evolved in a natural environment. Being surrounded by greenery and areas of natural beauty should be our natural habitat, but since the 18th century, when cities started to grow, we have opted more and more to live in quite the opposite. Concrete jungles, unnatural light and confined spaces now block out birdsong and outshine the night sky. Children don't lie in the grass, waiting to wish on shooting stars. With tablets and smartphones, how often do they look at the sky at all? For countless reasons, the man-made environment we now find ourselves in does not serve our biology; if anything, it does the opposite.

However, when you inject nature back into urban communities, amazing things start to happen. Health inequalities between the rich and poor start to flatten out if both groups live surrounded by nature. In fact, even putting patients in hospital beds with a view of nature speeds up their recovery. This was seen in 1984, when a study measured how quickly people bounced back from having their gallbladders removed – those with a window facing a brick wall performed worse than those looking at a garden. If you inject even a smidge of greenery into high-crime areas, violence plummets. A famous example was seen in Chicago in an area where, on average, there was one murder a day. Two high-rise buildings were investigated: when they were built a drainage problem meant the grass around one of them died and was replaced with concrete, while the second was unaffected and so had a lawn, bushes and even a few trees. Researchers noticed people living in the 'green' building would stop and chat outside, creating a community of friendships. Strangely, the opposite happened where there was concrete: when leaving or arriving, neighbours kept their heads down and didn't talk to each other.

Crime rates plummeted where there was greenery. Why? Because being in nature relaxes us, opens us up and promotes prosocial behaviour. We see this in traumatised children too: if their education is taken outside to a place of natural beauty, this helps them to build trust in their teachers and peers. There are many other examples of prosocial behaviour in nature; simply put, if we are in our natural environment, this promotes a positive mood and we can't help but feel more sociable.

Some of the most famous research into health and nature comes out of Japan, where people are actively encouraged to engage in 'shinrin-yoku' or 'forest bathing'. Walking through a forest seems to have profoundly positive consequences for your health, including: reduced blood pressure, cortisol and blood sugar, improved symptoms of depression, better sleep, optimised memory and even an enhanced immune system. If you could sell that in a pill, you would make millions; being free doesn't mean it's not powerful and that's why the Japanese government actively encourages its citizens to partake. There are probably many reasons for the benefits but some experts argue it is partly down to essential oils called phytoncides, emitted by trees. If you think how much our subconscious is influenced by pheromones, it is no surprise that other smells we don't even notice can affect us.

Being in nature seems to affect every stage of life, even before you are born. We know mothers who spend a decent chunk of their pregnancy out in nature have healthier children. If those children then grow up playing outside, they will develop a larger hippocampus in their brains, improving learning and reducing their risk of depression. The research exploring the calming pathways in our physiology and even in functional MRI scans is extensive; covering it fully would surpass my word count enormously but that in itself should impress upon you its value. Now imagine the opposite: concrete jungles, clinical spaces and harsh artificial lighting. Dr Rangan Chatterjee argues straight lines are the opposite of what we experience in nature and so if your surroundings, whether in the city or suburbs, are built up of rectangular shapes without any softening from nature you are missing out on this powerful stress-relieving tool. When our homes are cluttered and messy he believes this instils the opposite of nature's calm, so taking out time to prioritise the appearance of your home matters. If you ever feel overwhelmed by life I suggest looking closely at your home – organise and declutter your things, add some houseplants and soft lighting with candles and lamps. For reasons you can't really explain to yourself, the weight of the world will immediately feel lighter.

For those fortunate enough to be near nature's beauty, whether a park or garden, I suggest actively seeking this space out and consciously seeing what you are looking at. Lying in the grass gazing at the light flickering through leaves in a tree or blades of grass is not unproductive or lazy: actively choosing to rest and 'bathe' in nature genuinely stimulates a calming explosion of chemicals and nerve signals which enormously benefit your current and future health.

No mention of nature can go without acknowledging our recently discovered 'organ': the microbiome. As we have discussed, we evolved intimately with these micro-organisms, so it should be no surprise that spending time in the environment where that took place is good for them too. When we come into contact with flecks of dirt which we then happen to ingest, we are exposing our microbiome to new strains of bacteria. This is a big part of why gardeners tend to have healthier microbiomes. The calming effect of nature will also help because anything that is good for you will be good for your microbiome too. Of course, whether you are weeding, hiking or surfing, being outside will give you many opportunities to enter flow state as well.

Pillar number 2: Community

Coming back to what I said before, as human beings we are simply animals who depend on feeling safe. We evolved in tribes of about 150 people and belonging to this intimate network of kin was not for fun; amid tribal warfare and many very real predators, we needed to stick together to survive. It is therefore completely logical that to feel content we need to feel that we are safe, valued and that we belong: our modern-day 'tribes' subconsciously signal these most basic needs have been met, but serious problems will arise if they haven't. This is why research predicting longevity and health outcomes has singled out a surprising risk factor we never used to think about: a lack of community.

One of the longest studies on human health ever performed is called the Grant and Glueck study.* In 1938, researchers looked at men from two very different worlds: one was a group of Harvard alumni and the second was from a poor part of Boston. The researchers checked in with the men regularly for over 70 years, asking them all about their lives, in a quest to understand what predicted a happy and long life. The answer wasn't about food, exercise or money. It turned out the best predictor of a long life was the people in it: those who had the most meaningful social connections lived longer than anyone else. Importantly, a strong marriage was only one of these important relationships, but every social interaction contributed, including friends.

We know that people who are lonely are 30 per cent more likely to die from a heart attack or stroke but why? In our evolution, if we were shunned or kicked out of our tribe and were forced to spend time alone, this was life-threatening. And our brains still perceive being alone as a threat, which drives chronically raised cortisol and chronic inflammation. In 2019, the World Health Organization declared that loneliness was a

---

* AKA the 'Study of Adult Development'.

public-health epidemic, just as serious as obesity, smoking and sedentary lifestyles. They went on to urge governments to tackle this genuine health risk with as much gusto as they would any of the others and, as a GP, I can fully understand why. Remember, I specifically quiz my patients about their living situation, colleagues, friends and loved ones. I do it for a reason: to help them I need to understand them and to understand them I need to build up a picture of their lives. I am always surprised by how many people have no one they feel they can turn to: most of their free time is spent alone. To me, this is a dangerous behaviour that needs to change.

But what is so beneficial about social interaction? Well, put simply, we can see positive social engagement translate in the chemistry of your brain. If someone smiles at you – or, better than that, you manage to make them laugh – your brain becomes flooded with the feelgood chemical dopamine. Even thinking back fondly to that as a positive memory will also trigger a little wave of dopamine. This is perceived as a reward in your brain, meaning that, in a way, receiving someone's approval through their laughter acts like a neural currency: they have paid you in dopamine. Negative social interactions obviously do not have this effect; if your 'tribe' bullies, shuns or dismisses you, this is a danger signal in your brain which will drive all the unwanted consequences of chronic stress. That's because we have 'mirror cells' in our brains – this might sound absurd, but these cells make you experience the same emotions you are witnessing in someone else. In our evolution this was brilliant for social connection and is essentially the biology of our empathy: seeing someone cry changes your facial expression and demeanour immediately. It also changes your own emotions and allows you to console the person in front of you. Sadly, if you witness anxiety or aggression, the same effect happens. Have you ever wondered why some people automatically make you feel tense when you are around them? Mirror cells! Without meaning to, you are taking on their emotions.

Now think about the people you surround yourself with: how do they stimulate your mirror cells and what neural currency are they giving you? It is said that you are essentially a summary of the people you surround yourself with and this is true: your friends, colleagues and loved ones directly affect your risk of disease through tangible chemical signals in your body. Given how short life is, I would argue you should feel empowered to think very carefully about who you let into your tribe. Many of us continue relationships with fake friends and hostile colleagues; we pretend to ignore their subtle digs and backhanded compliments. Maybe you have a history with that person – ending the relationship might feel socially awkward or inconvenient. But remember, you are *giving* your finite time to people in your life – you won't get it back. Hand it out wisely and try not to give it to people who flood your brain with a negative neural currency.

Now, what has changed so drastically in our society that the big guns (WHO) are declaring loneliness a new epidemic? In my opinion, there is one very big player: (un)social media and smartphones in general. I am infinitely grateful to be the last generation who can still remember a childhood without smartphones or social media. But I have stopped telling my teenage patients about 'days gone by' back 'when I was your age' because they immediately roll their eyes. To them, it is an unimaginable time and certainly doesn't feel like an age of innocence they would pine for. They don't realise time spent on their phone displaces the time they would have spent sitting in a park with friends, climbing trees, flirting, dancing and much more. They can't compare these social interactions to their own because even when they 'socialise' IRL (in real life) they are still looking at their phones. There is, in fact, a new disorder called nomophobia, which is the discomfort you feel when your phone isn't near by (never mind if it is lost). People now reach for their phones after a stressful event to self-soothe, much like children use their comfort blankets or toys. But why?

WHAT YOUR DOCTOR EATS

It's all about dopamine. Only, unlike a giggle from a friend, the dopamine hits you get from checking your phone are more of a punch; instead of a gentle wave, you get an overwhelming tsunami. As with insulin, your body can't help but dampen down its response to this extreme volume of dopamine; over time you become resistant, meaning you need more and more to get the same effect. This is the exact same pathway triggered by addiction, whether to sugar or cocaine. It is why we now 'pleasure-stack' our behaviours: watching a film is no longer enough to get a decent dopamine hit, so most people, without even thinking about it, reach for their phone at the same time. Engaging in one activity – reading a book, pensively listening to a song, flicking through a magazine, baking a cake or doing any other hobby – isn't enough, which means people lose the ability to feel any real pleasure from anything that once could have brought them joy. We have dysregulated our dopamine-reward pathways such that we have become incapable of experiencing simple, unfiltered contentment from any one thing.

As a result of our virtual personas, curating idealised online versions of ourselves, many of us are losing the art of socialising. During any mental health chat, I often ask teenage patients to check the average daily screen time on their phone – it can be as much as eight hours! Smartphones have become full-time jobs for them but, remember, just one generation ago much of that time was spent in flow state. We are now willing to hand over our finite time for apathy. It feels easy because it *is* easy – but don't confuse that with happiness. You just aren't feeling anything at all. Of course, adults of all ages are also spending more and more time on their phones, often not realising quite how much. Conversation is a skill and, arguably, an art which takes hours upon hours to master. In my opinion, we are allowing young people to forgo this life skill and replace it with texting, tweets and hashtags. But the mental stimulation is not the same. If you never learn how to have a meaningful conversation or portray yourself authentically, people can't know you – not really. This is explored in one of my favourite books, *The Top Five Regrets of the Dying*. Having worked as a palliative carer, the author, Bronnie Ware, summarised the most common deathbed conversations she had. One of the regrets most frequently expressed by people was not spending time with anyone who *truly* knew them. When it was too late, her dying clients understood a new definition of loneliness: that you can be surrounded by people and still feel lonely if none of them really knows *you* as you know yourself.

My fear for our youngest generations is that they will spend a lifetime feeling alone in the company of many because they simply won't know how to connect with anyone in a meaningful way. They will live in an alternative online community enduring the online-disinhibition effect – a phenomenon where, shielded by anonymity, people feel brave enough to spew negative and devastatingly rude comments they would never dare say in person. And they may learn that this is what it is to connect and so their real-life relationships become channels for passive-aggressive or just aggressive-aggressive exchanges. Missing out on the medicinal effects of positive relationships, their health will simply pay the price.

Still, as with so many aspects of health, our loneliness epidemic is a complex topic influenced by many other things besides social media. For example, it is no longer unusual to move away from your childhood home. Historically, villages and communities remained constant – we didn't stray far from where we grew up. Being nearby to your parents, siblings and extended family meant you automatically had a readily available support network. This was especially important when raising children, which was something the family unit did together, not apart. The childhood friends you had known all your life also didn't leave. Life was simpler, which doesn't automatically mean better, but at least it was easier to spend time with people who *really* knew you. Whether it is to progress our careers or education, many of us now move around the country or even the world. I am not suggesting we should stop doing this, but it may be one change which could be contributing to loneliness. Also, since the pandemic working from home has become much easier. Although this brings with it many advantages, it also involves less time spent around colleagues who often become our friends.

What can we do with this information? In a way, the most important thing is to acknowledge the value of social connection. It directly affects health and longevity which is a trend we see clearly throughout all the Blue Zones where people live the longest (see p. 184). They lead simple lives focused heavily on nurturing a sense of community. The family unit is strong, as are their ties to long-term friends. Importantly, I think we need to change our relationship with our phones and social media, especially for children and teenagers. Admittedly, I've sometimes felt addicted to my phone myself and have needed to consciously reduce the time I spend on it with inbuilt reminders to time out. Ultimately, I know that time spent alone with a screen adds up to less meaningful time spent with others. Read that again. So many people complain that they don't have time for all manner of things, but time is an illusion. Really, you make time for the things that are important to you – screens are not one of those things but, somehow, we let them displace time we could have spent socialising. Finally, let's not forget that genuine social connection is another perfect example of flow state – I often think I have been at a party for about 40 minutes only to realise it has been 4 hours! If spent in the company of people you really like, is it ever possible to waste time? Clearly, the same cannot be said for doom scrolling. We need to stop isolating ourselves with screens and honour what we evolved to do: spending time with other people.

Pillar number 3: Sleep

We all know that not getting enough sleep can affect how we feel, and we can see this translated in our hormones. Every parent has experienced a day of endless tantrums after their child has had a disturbed night – but what makes us think adults are any different? You've probably noticed that you become more irritable when you're not sleeping well. Maybe you feel low in mood, overwhelmed or snap at people in ways you normally wouldn't? That's because you spiked your cortisol. Importantly, good sleep does much more than calm our cortisol and boost mood: its health benefits are truly astounding and to skim over them would be negligent of me. After all, I am writing this book as a manual on health and want to do the subject justice. Just like food, I now need to convince you to value the truly medicinal impact of good sleep. Once you understand its effects, you will do everything you can to get it!

Insomnia is one of the most common things patients come to me about. Now, anyone who knows me will say I am a chronic people pleaser which, as a doctor, is terrible news. Often, I feel torn between what I know is best for my patient and a strong desire to appease them. However, there is one topic that triggers an amazing metamorphosis in my character: sleeping pills. I usually find it uncomfortable to refuse my patients things they want but not with these – if a patient asks for a sleeping pill, 9.5 times out of 10, my answer is no.* During my GP training I remember a man twice my size sitting in front of me who had very recently been released from prison and, in the politest way, he didn't *not* look like a criminal. He got straight to the point and told me he wanted sleeping pills and if I didn't give him a

---

* My rare exceptions are driven by compassion, not good medicine: for example, in the case of someone who is dying and can't sleep or someone who is acutely stressed after a catastrophic bereavement. It is humane to give these people false sleep in a pill because the agony of not sleeping in these extreme situations is simply cruel. For everyone else, I need to treat the cause if I am to truly help them.

prescription, he would 'just get them on the street'. It felt like some kind of threat but I didn't flinch. When he received my answer his face went red and a vein on the side of his forehead started to bulge. I held eye contact with a poker face I imagined read 'You want summa dis?' but in reality probably just made me look constipated. He wasn't happy. I broke the silence tactfully: my demeanour shifted, and I widened my sympathetic blue eyes before explaining my logic. 'I want to help you, but I want to do it properly.' Cue slow head tilt. 'Why don't you tell me *why* you think you're not sleeping?' Boom! Out of nowhere he burst into tears and offloaded a lifetime of pent-up traumas which were haunting him every night. By the end of the appointment, he left empowered with the latest sleep science, as well as evidence-based theories of happiness. Among other things he wanted to change, he told me he would start volunteering for an animal charity. Having struggled with his mental health before, volunteering had once brought him a sense of purpose years ago, before he was incarcerated. Now that he was out, he wanted to start giving back again. It was a turn of events I could never have predicted and proof you should never judge a book by its cover.

But why am I so against sleeping pills? In short, it's because of the Hippocratic oath: first do no harm. These pills don't simulate true sleep; rather, they act like an anaesthetic which sedates you but, if you look at its electrical activity, the brain isn't actually asleep. It turns out sleep is a pretty important bodily function; in fact, very rare case reports show that if people don't sleep at all, they simply die. Cruel animal experiments demonstrate this too; sleep deprivation basically switches off the immune system and the subjects rapidly die from overwhelming infection. So if you give a person weeks, months or even years of fake sleep, it should be no surprise this causes serious health problems. Over just two and a half years, regular sleeping-pill users are 4.6 times more likely to die. If they take 132 pills a year (just under half the days of the year) this goes up to 5.3 times – they also increase their overall risk of cancer by 30–40 per cent, but if they take the more old-fashioned pills, like temazepam, the risk goes up to 60 per cent! Take that in for a moment: giving yourself 'fake sleep' in a pill significantly increases your risk of cancer. Sleeping pills also make you groggy in the day, meaning you drink more caffeine, can't sleep again and then need more sleeping pills. By sedating the brain, patients are also much more likely to fall over and hurt themselves or have fatal car accidents, hurting others while they're at it. It is difficult to tease apart how much damage is directly caused by the sleeping pill and how much comes from missing out on true sleep, the powers of which are completely astounding. But either way, a sleeping pill does nothing to treat the *cause* of poor sleep which is itself terrible for health – this is the real crux of my concern: by putting a plaster on the problem rather than actually addressing it, you are allowing a damaging process to brew disease.

So what is the cause of insomnia? On the whole, it is caused by an overreactive sympathetic nervous system – our fight-or-flight response. In other words, it is caused by chronic stress and lots of chronically raised cortisol which, by now, you should know is very bad for you. The impact of inadequate sleep is worrying; for example, if an average person usually sleeps fewer than seven hours a night, their risk of death goes up by as much as 24 per cent. There is some important nuance here though – we don't all have the exact same sleep requirements. This can vary with our genes and our age. Take a look at Figure 4 for more details on this.

Good-quality sleep is important too. The World Health Organization has classed all shift work as a potential carcinogen; in other words, my job as a hospital doctor was increasing my risk of cancer simply by disrupting my sleep. Shift work also increases your risk of obesity, diabetes, cardiovascular and gastrointestinal diseases. Why? Because asking people to flip flop their sleeping patterns negatively disrupts their biology dramatically. As we have seen, sleep directly impacts your

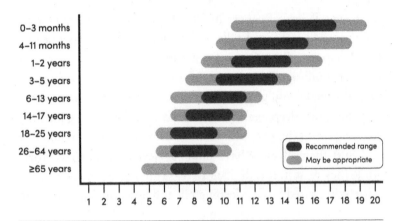

Figure 4: Recommended sleep duration in 24 hours by age, according to the National Sleep Foundation

immune system so it is not a surprise that shift workers can be more vulnerable to infections. Sleep also affects cancer risk via the immune system which, you may recall from the example of AIDS patients (see p. 38), is heavily involved in protecting us from cancer. As such, women who simply sleep at their preferred bedtime actually have better breast-cancer survival rates. Importantly, many people who don't work shifts still incur the same damage through what's known as 'social jetlag'*: staying up late partying or just watching TV with random sleeping patterns is no better for you.

One of sleep's most important roles is to consolidate memory and 'clean' the brain, removing waste products. Disrupting this process regularly will increase your risk of dementia, PTSD, anxiety, severe migraines, epilepsy and other forms of seizures. I can't stress enough how important optimising your quality of sleep is for maintaining good mental health. In fact, we know suicide rates increase in winter because of seasonal affective disorder (SAD). Many of my

---

* Social jetlag is a term I have borrowed from Satchin Panda, author of the must-read book *The Circadian Code*.

patients already have insight into this pattern – come October, I suddenly have far more depression consultations. Many of my patients tell me this is part of their normal pattern – their moods dip as soon as the days start to shorten and they always need to increase the dose of their antidepressant. But why? The answer is simple. Light! Just as food serves as information, so does light and this is especially true first thing in the morning. Your drive to fall asleep is not random – it is carefully choreographed, and daylight is what tells you when to be awake and asleep. The light you see in the morning sets a predictable internal timer – when it's done you feel tired. By being exposed to less daylight and having very dark mornings, something in our brain chemistry changes, altering this vital circadian rhythm. The quality of our sleep deteriorates which means we miss out on the mood-boosting benefits of good sleep.

We can't stop winter arriving but many of us actually create an abnormal pattern of light ourselves – for example, working in an environment with no windows and a constant stream of artificial light. Or rather than experiencing nature's naturally reduced evening light, we choose to use artificial light late into the night. If you spend your evenings in brightly lit rooms looking at lights on screens, you are telling the brain nighttime hasn't arrived yet. There is nuance to some of this but, on the whole, by winding down before bed with cosy lighting and less time on screens, you might find the quality of your sleep improves dramatically. Your mental health will benefit from the sleep itself but, if you are also consciously swapping apathy for flow state in the quest for good sleep, this will independently improve mood too.

How else does poor sleep affect us? Most people will concede that they gain weight when they get less sleep – where do you think 'Dad bods' come from? Part of this is due to our friend cortisol: inadequate sleep pushes him up, mimicking the symptoms of Cushing's disease. Not only will you lay down more fat (especially belly fat), you will also lose muscle mass.

As we have discussed, chronically raised cortisol also spikes your ghrelin, but this won't just make you hungry. No, no – we know your brain chemistry is altered to make you *famished* specifically for junk food. And as if all the above wasn't bad enough, your microbiome plays along too. As I mentioned a few chapters ago, if you transplant a stool sample from a shift worker or someone who is jetlagged into a sterile mouse it will become obese. Microbiomes have their own circadian rhythm – if you change yours, they respond by becoming obesogenic bugs. On an unrelated note, sleep is a topic I also bring up with couples who are struggling to conceive. I was inspired after hearing sleep expert Professor Russell Foster speak at a conference where he explored the vital role of good sleep for both male and female fertility. He shared anecdotal stories of 'infertile' couples suddenly conceiving after he told them to do two things: both prioritise good-quality sleep and have more sex in the morning. It turns out testosterone spikes early in the morning and with it so does a man's sperm count.

Optimising sleep is clearly vital for health and sleeping pills aren't the answer. But what is? The National Sleep Foundation recommends adults generally aim for at least seven hours of sleep, while children need at least nine. In reality, most adults simply need to aim for seven to nine hours of 'sleep opportunity'.* As long as you are within the suggested limits in Figure 4 (see page 273), you are getting good sleep if you don't struggle to fall asleep and wake up feeling refreshed and energised.

But how do we actually fall and stay asleep? Without getting into too much detail, we need two things to sleep: 'sleep pressure' and a well-timed circadian release of our sleepy hormone, melatonin. From the moment we wake up a chemical called adenosine builds in the brain, driving our desire to sleep through 'sleep pressure'. Caffeine blocks it, exercise promotes

---

* Sleep opportunity means what it says – if you go to bed at 10pm knowing you have to wake up at 7am you have given yourself 9 hours of sleep opportunity.

it. Again, like with so many things there is nuance here too, partly because we don't all respond to caffeine in the same way; however, if you are struggling to sleep, it is worth only having caffeine before 12pm. If you are very sensitive to it, your cut-off may need to be earlier and if you are still struggling with sleep, trying to come off it altogether may be necessary. On the whole, exercise is a potent catalyst for good sleep but a high-intensity workout late at night might have the opposite effect. Trying to time this earlier in the day and focusing on low-energy, relaxing movement in the evening will likely be better for your sleep. Interestingly, when we exercise our muscles produce lots of amazing chemical signals; one of them is called IL-15, which also directly supports sleep.

Next, you need to get your melatonin into a predictable rhythm; simply put, this requires a predictable life. Melatonin release behaves like clockwork and your life is what sets the tempo – ideally, you should go to bed at the same time each night and wake up at the same time each morning (even on the weekend). In fact, for people struggling with their sleep, the latter is more important. But for this to work, you need to do something specific when you wake up: get daylight into your eyes (as mentioned above). Many of us simply don't get enough real light into our eyes, which we know massively affects mental health. Daylight varies from 1,000 lux (a standard measure of light) on a cloudy day to 200,000 lux in full sun. By comparison, an office without windows offers 80–100 lux and an overhead light can produce as little as 50 lux. Wearing sunglasses dampens outdoor light to the level of being indoors. Here's the shocking thing: we spend 87 per cent of our time inside – compared to our ancestors, we are completely starving ourselves of light. This is one of the other reasons why time in nature is so paramount for our wellbeing. My advice is to wake at roughly the same time each day and, without sunglasses, quickly get as much daylight into your eyes as you can (20–30 minutes is ideal). Again, use winding down in the evening as an opportunity to get less light in your eyes and, while you're at it, try to finish all your eating 2–3 hours before bed. With some exercise in the day and a sensible approach to caffeine, you will be harnessing clever science to optimise not just your sleep, but your health too!

I can't do the complexity of recent sleep research justice in a few paragraphs, but I hope I have given a glimpse into why the question, 'While I'm here, could you just prescribe me some sleeping tablets?' is met with a hard no. For those suffering from true insomnia* the first-line treatment is CBTI (cognitive behavioural therapy for insomnia), which can be hard to access unless you go privately. To learn more, take a look at Appendix 2 on p. 304 or read Matthew Walker's brilliant book *Why We Sleep*. Instead of prescribing a sleeping tablet I teach my patients the principles discussed here and invite them back for another appointment to address their mental health. Addressing the root cause of chronic stress is complex and unique to the individual – I don't want to undermine that. Psychological therapy and other treatments may be necessary. But if you take a look at the use of flow state and my five pillars of happiness, you will see they feed into each other in a cycle. Better sleep will drive less stress which will cause even better sleep and so on. Now that you understand the medicinal effect of sleep and the harm of chronic cortisol, you should recognise the knock-on effect this can have on your risk of every disease from cancer to depression.

Pillar number 4: Movement

I remember citing being a 'lifelong student' as a reason for why I wanted to be a doctor in my application to medical school. A decade later, sitting in a lecture theatre as a GP trainee,

---

* To have a diagnosis of true insomnia you: are dissatisfied with your sleep; find lack of sleep distressing and experience daytime impairment; have experienced insomnia at least 3 nights a week for more than 3 months; and you do *not* have a co-existing mental disorder or medical condition that could otherwise cause insomnia, e.g. Parkinson's or depression.

I questioned my logic. The novelty of adult education had worn off and, in all honesty, I didn't enjoy my GP teaching sessions. This wasn't because they weren't good – I was just burnt out and tired of still feeling like a student. But that was before I met Mary.*

Mary and I met in a class led by a consultant who specialised in Parkinson's, although rather than deliver the lecture himself, he had invited 'expert patients' to teach us instead. This is commonplace in medicine – patients who have lived with a disease for years know it better than anyone else. This makes them invaluable teachers. The consultant started with a few basic slides on Parkinson's to refresh our memories; he listed various drugs and, to my surprise, ended with a blunt statement – 'In recent years, we've realised exercise is as effective as Parkinson's medications' – before handing the mic over to his patient. Mary spent the rest of the session telling us her story: she had been diagnosed with Parkinson's disease (PD) aged 52 and after just five years had morphed into an elderly woman: she was constantly tired and too weak to even stand up from the sofa. How could this be happening? At just 57 she felt like she was in her 90s. Desperate, Mary began reading and came across the work of specialist neurological physiotherapist Dr Melissa McConaghy, who had developed an exercise programme called PD Warrior. Amazingly, her patients appeared to be reversing the disease with exercise. Mary brought this information to her consultant who advised her that, though there was no current evidence that exercise significantly affected PD, she had nothing to lose. He was right.

Mary had never been particularly 'fit'. Before having children she did play hockey but, at 32, her marriage ended and time was no longer on her side. Other than walking her dogs, Mary didn't engage in any other exercise for the next few decades. At 57, she was understandably worried by her

---

* With permission, I have changed Mary's name to protect her identity.

rapidly increasing frailty and decided to join a body-balance class, which combined tai chi, yoga and Pilates. After talking to her consultant and buoyed by the PD warriors' results, she approached her body-balance teacher and said, 'I want you to stop going easy on me. Push me as hard as you can.' Now, at 68, Mary was addressing the room of young doctors and confidently declared, 'I challenge any of you to do more exercise than me', before pressing play on a video compilation of her workouts. With bulging biceps, she was lifting weights, holding effortless planks, running 5ks and getting into complex yoga poses I still struggle with. Over time, her exercise regime has progressively grown. Here is an average week:

- 1–2 dog walks a day
- 2 kettlebell workouts a week
- 1 weight class a week
- 2 PD Warrior classes a week
- 1 yoga class a week

After a few weeks of increased exercise Mary could no longer recognise herself: her posture straightened, her energy soared and her balance was better than it had ever been. One of the most exciting changes was that, despite being on medication for four years, it was only after she started exercising that her tremor disappeared.* More telling still is what happened if Mary ever stopped exercising: once, after taking a week off for a holiday abroad, the tremor came back, she became tired, her mood felt low and she developed severe constipation, which is one of the core symptoms of Parkinson's. Since then, she has learned her lesson and now packs her kettlebells for holiday, no matter what. Exercise is like a pill she can't live without. Mary doesn't claim to be more disciplined than anyone else,

---

* It is important to note that Mary would never claim that exercise alone improved her symptoms. Getting the right medications along with enough exercise is how she improved symptom control.

nor is she a natural-born athlete. But is anyone really 'born' to do extreme exercise? There is an interesting perspective on why many of us don't move enough: it is because we are responding to our evolution. If you look at our ancestors we did not evolve to do 'exercise', which was arguably a costly waste of precious calories we once struggled to acquire. Evolutionary biologist Daniel Lieberman explores this eloquently in his book *Exercised*, and points out movement was only done when it was either necessary, fun or both. For most, to choose to exercise is neither of these things and actually goes against our instincts, but there are ways to work around this. For example, Mary chooses to book exercise classes and admits she probably wouldn't be bothered to exercise if she did it alone. The social element makes it fun but, more than that, the peer pressure of having people expect her to turn up also makes it feel necessary. Seeing the results of not exercising and the genuine symptoms this triggers also makes exercise a genuine priority in her eyes.

Though many of us also experience symptoms in the absence of exercise, because we don't connect the two, we lack this insight into *why* it is specifically necessary for us. Poor sleep, fatigue, low mood, anxiety, irritability and a low libido are just some symptoms you might be experiencing yourself. The moment you notice these lift with exercise, believe me, it won't feel like something you *should* do but, instead, something you need to do. Sixteen years after her diagnosis, Mary is not completely symptom free: she can feel 'off' for two hours a day and periodically 'freezes', which is a horrible PD symptom, literally turning patients into human statues. But compared to her non-exercising counterparts, at this stage of the disease she should be housebound, if not bedbound. Instead, for most of the day she looks nothing like a 'patient' and leads a full life.

Unfortunately, for many people the main motivation to exercise is often the desire for a thin body – when we don't quickly get this result (for all the complex reasons covered before) motivation wanes. When it comes to human behaviour, simply willing yourself to do something because you vaguely think you should usually doesn't work. But do you actually know all the reasons why you should exercise? As a doctor, I find most of my patients are completely unaware of how dramatically it can impact health. The facts are jaw dropping! For example, research consistently shows that exercise is not just as effective, but often *more* effective than most antidepressants. Read that again: regular movement can work better than an antidepressant. Amazingly, despite this overwhelming evidence, only 20 per cent of psychiatrists recommend exercise to their patients. I now fondly remember following a man up after starting an antidepressant and being very surprised to hear it 'worked immediately'. I initially assumed this must be a placebo effect, fully aware that antidepressants usually take several weeks to kick in. However, at the end of the appointment he said, 'Oh – and I took your advice ...' After our first consultation he'd immediately put on his trainers and started running every morning before work. It turned out he *was* taking an immediately effective antidepressant, after all. It just wasn't in the form of a pill.

Why does exercise affect mood so dramatically? Well, our muscles serve more functions than we ever realised and are actually like mini pharmacies, churning out happiness chemicals like dopamine and serotonin. They also release our bodies' morphine-like 'opioids', marijuana-like endocannabinoids and calming chemicals like GABA, while also reducing stress hormones like cortisol. Together, this explosion of brain chemicals makes you feel elated and zen all at the same time. Importantly, I don't say any of this to undermine the vital role antidepressants can play – mental health is enormously complicated. But the vast majority of doctors aren't prescribing an equally effective treatment first: movement is a powerful drug with many beneficial 'side effects' we should all want.

Just like sleep, movement does much more for you than just improve mental health. You now know that healthy mitochondria are vital for a long life and less disease. Several conditions including heart disease, chronic fatigue and even Parkinson's are linked to mitochondrial dysfunction. It turns out exercise directly improves the quality and quantity of these mitochondria! As Lieberman puts it, 'the fountain of youth runs with sweat', and our mitochondria are a big part of this – they protect us from things like cancer and diabetes, but when they stop working properly the body ages and accumulates illnesses. If movement can keep these mitochondria healthy, that should give you motivation like nothing else to do it. It is just one more example of how you can positively change your own biology and the very trajectory of your life.

Exercise also reduces visceral fat – a dangerous type of fat you can't see because it sits around your organs. This explains why TOFIs (people who are Thin on the Outside but Fat on the Inside) can have terrible health outcomes; they might have minimal subcutaneous fat but their invisible internal fat has the power to drive chronic inflammation. Being thin is not an excuse not to move. Exercise also strengthens bones, revs up your metabolism, strengthens your cardiovascular system and improves cholesterol levels, but my favourite effect is on sugar and insulin. Most people believe exercise works by increasing their calorie expenditure but, as *The Biggest Loser* and Minnesota Starvation studies clearly demonstrate (see pp. 83 and 141), our bodies are more complicated than calculators. They simply adjust energy lost according to our internal 'thermostats', aiming to keep the status quo. We know when we eat, insulin flies into the bloodstream, putting us into a fat-storing state but, as it turns out, sugar actually has a 'back door' into the cells which sneaks past our insulin signal: muscle. When activated, muscles act like sponges soaking up sugar from the bloodstream *without* the need for insulin. That's why moving after a meal significantly reduces the blood-sugar rise and subsequent insulin spike from what you just ate. Just a ten-minute postprandial stroll can trick your body into spiking insulin less. It's also why building muscle mass is a genius way to prevent or even reverse insulin resistance: if you have a bigger sponge, you become more efficient at soaking sugar up without spiking insulin. So, as well as asking my type 2 diabetes patients to change their diets and way of eating, I ask them to start resistance training: building muscle helps to reverse the cause of their disease.

The enormous health consequences of regular movement are impossible to list in a few paragraphs. I could start by telling you moderate exercise reduces the risk of breast cancer by 30–40 per cent and colon cancer by 40–50 per cent but I won't have space to list all the other cancers it will also protect you from. It is the best-known protection from dementia, reducing your risk by 45 per cent and it also boosts your microbiome for reasons we don't fully understand. Interestingly, exercise can be a surprisingly inefficient weight-loss tool, again, because the body can compensate for energy expenditure. Either way, weight isn't exactly a useful marker of health here because gaining muscle can keep weight the same, even when you are losing fat. A scale also won't show you how much you have dropped your visceral fat or fasting insulin levels. Nor will it measure how dramatically your chronic cortisol levels have dropped too. Finally, a scale can't measure the years of added life you will gain from movement but, better than this, more of those years will be spent in good health. In other words, the main (and most important) thing exercise will do is directly increase your 'health span' – something far more valuable than a long life spent in poor health.

As a GP, I see many people living very long lives thanks to modern medicine but the last few decades are spent sick, immobile, frail and with little independence or dignity. I was lucky enough to visit Mary in her home and interview her about her experience – we realised we shared a love of hiking and compared notes on our adventures. She still regularly hikes in the alps and, like me, was lucky enough to hike around Machu Picchu, even though this was seven years after her Parkinson's diagnosis. To behold breathtaking views like these is a luxury reserved only for people fit enough to get to them. In truth, life's simplest pleasures often require some level of fitness which many forgo as they age, even though they don't have to. Lieberman argues we evolved to remain active throughout our lives because 'active grandparents' were vital for the survival of our highly dependent children. If you look at foraging populations from Australia to South America they never stop moving until they die. Centenarians in the Blue Zones are the same – chopping firewood, gardening and walking up hills is something they continue doing throughout their lives. The notion that you need to 'take it easy' because you are 'getting old' is a modern, Westernised one which ironically prevents us from engaging in the behaviours which protect against ageing and disease. Many people 'take it easy' long before they are even chronologically old, speeding up the ageing process more than they could ever know. I constantly nag my patients to exercise and specifically ask that they work on maintaining their muscle mass – the oldest recipient of this advice was 103 years old. I emailed him a video with modified resistance training and told him, 'The oldest person to live was in her 120s – you have no excuse to stop now.' Ultimately, my patients have taught me that I don't want a long life: I just want a good one and it won't happen unless I exercise.

Pillar number 5: Charity

Put bluntly, people who engage in charitable acts live longer. In fact, in 2003 a study in Michigan found those who did not provide support to others were twice as likely to die over a five-year period. Unnecessary acts of kindness flood our brains with the same endorphins we get from exercise and there are evolutionary reasons behind this. We are social creatures who depended on our tribe for survival; without the fangs or speed of our predators, we needed something else: cooperation. Ancient humans didn't just survive, they clearly thrived and part of the reason for this was their ability to look out for each other. Being in a position to receive or give this cooperation was a sign that we were safe.

Fast forward to our modern lives – if you are taking the time to do something unnecessarily kind for someone or something, by definition, you are probably relatively safe in that moment. There are, of course, exceptional acts of bravery which put the do-gooder in danger themselves. Dying trying to save a complete stranger's life isn't as rare as you might think – a fact which, in itself, suggests doing good is an evolutionary instinct we can't explain in the moment because we've already done it before thinking. But, aside from these exceptions, most acts of kindness happen in moments when we ourselves feel safe. Now remember our fight-or-flight response is what drives a sudden surge in cortisol – if the cause is short-lived, this is protective. We become hyper-vigilant, primed to effectively deal with a threat. But if chronic life stress persistently drives this reflex, you will have a chronically raised cortisol. In contrast, anything that primes your subconscious mind to automatically feel safe will achieve the opposite effect. In our evolution, sleep, socialising and leisurely time in nature were things we did when we felt safe. Just like acts of charity, engaging in any of these ancestral needs will still make you feel safe now, helping to bring down your chronic cortisol.

As I mentioned earlier, I spent a decent chunk of my GP training working on the Covid wards during the first two waves of the pandemic. The human suffering I witnessed was unfathomable for patients, relatives and staff alike. Seeing countless people die from a novel virus, in the full knowledge that you were very vulnerable to contracting it yourself, was deeply unsettling. To say staff morale was low would be an enormous understatement. Any sense of teamwork or cama-raderie was lost due to the fact that colleagues kept going off sick – one by one, many us became infected. Most days, the team I was working with were all strangers. Even the staff I did know weren't behaving normally – tempers were frayed and, though this might sound insignificant, no one was telling jokes anymore. Humour (often of a dark variety) is a ubiquitous tonic to all medical staff – when doctors and nurses stop cracking jokes, you know something is gravely wrong.

In truth, I had always been a bit of a charity sceptic, cynically assuming it was something most people did to fluff up their CVs or self-image. But when the jokes stopped, I felt strangely compelled to inject morale back into our wards and quickly started fundraising to do just that. My tactics were blunt and direct. Rather than running a marathon or campaigning enthusiastically I took more of a give-me-your-money approach. Social media helped me to raise a small sum, but it was nothing compared to the power of my hospital itself. I simply typed a heartfelt-cum-witty email explaining my plan and pressed send to every consultant in the area. The outcome still shocks me now: a dramatic outpouring of support erupted and in no time I had £16k which the hospital's charity then offered to double. I quickly set to work on a mission to cheer people up. My house turned into something of a care package warehouse which local businesses donated towards too. Once a week, I spent my day off hand-delivering these to each of our many Covid wards – Bluetooth radios, mini-Proseccos, coffee machines, hot chocolate, bubble bath and all sorts of other treats descended on the staff to enjoy. Next, I bought iPads for the Covid patients to use so they could video-call their loved ones. Tragically, many relatives weren't always able or allowed to come say their goodbyes when a patient was about to die. Staff had taken to filming a little conference call goodbye session on their own phones but this wasn't always feasible. I reasoned iPads could give family time with their loved one, whether this was to say hello or even goodbye.

My Christmas care package is the one I remember most fondly. A few decades earlier it had been customary to serve each inpatient a Christmas tipple. Given alcohol technically isn't a medical necessity or cost effective, this tradition died long ago, but I decided to bring it back for the Covid patients.

Smuggling alcohol into hospital isn't something I would usually consider but I reasoned exceptional circumstances were warranted because, if you can't do it at Christmas in the middle of a global pandemic, then when can you? I briefly considered asking the hospital's permission in advance, but it occurred to me that if I did, they might say no! So I took my chances and arrived on Christmas Day with a clinking garden trolley of sherry, port and whisky, wheeling it through every corner of the hospital to reach ITU and all the Covid wards. Long story short, the senior nurse in charge did catch me but, luckily, was more than happy to reignite the tradition this one last time.

Years later, long after my training, I still hadn't spent most of the money I raised. As a result, I worked with the hospital to build a Covid memorial garden outside the dementia ward I had worked in. We made sure it was designed with easy access for hospital beds so that, like in hospice, end-of-life patients could be wheeled out to enjoy it too. I also stocked it with gardening equipment so that dementia patients could use the space for garden therapy. But mostly, my hope was to recreate the outcome of the gallbladder operation study which showed having a view of a garden sped up recovery. Knowing it can be medicinal for patients, surely the same will hopefully be true for the staff too.

The experience removed any cynicism I once had about charity because my efforts worked. Most staff had no idea who the gifts were from, but the arrival of thoughtful care packages cheered them up. I put countless hours into doing this for them and obviously wasn't asked or paid to do so. But, in hindsight, the thing is I now realise that the person who was probably affected most by this spontaneous initiative was me. What none of the staff knew was that, while orchestrating all of this, I was having suicidal thoughts. They weren't plans or something I wanted to act on at all, but they were there. Amazingly, in my earnest efforts to lift the spirits of others I didn't realise I would be lifting my own. By channelling energy and time into something outside myself, I became completely distracted from what I now realise was a clinical depression. Of course, I won't suggest acts of unnecessary kindness are somehow a cure for suicidal ideation or depression! But even as a previous charity sceptic, I now see the theory and science behind this valuable part of life isn't just an academic notion. It actually works. I'm not surprised Blue Zone centenarians often engage in some form of charity, not out of necessity but choice – it isn't to show off or gain anything, it's just a way of life. But you don't need to sign up to volunteer for hours on end to reap the rewards. It doesn't even need to be organised charity or anything formal. Checking in on an elderly neighbour or cooking food for a friend in need both count. And if it is an *unnecessary* act of kindness, it will probably do you the same good, if not more, as the person (or creature) you are choosing to help.

Sickness behaviour

It is impossible to avoid stress in life and that isn't a bad thing! We wouldn't want to give up all the wonderful things in life that certainly come with stress, like having children, organising weddings or celebrating Christmas. In reality, stress actually serves a vital evolutionary purpose, but we simply haven't evolved in the modern world we now live in. For many, the source of stress isn't actually the problem; it's their response to it that is. Interestingly, we see similar evolutionary reactions play out in animals in something called 'sickness behaviour'.

Farmers are highly attuned to this sickness behaviour: the first sign that livestock are unwell with an infection is that they withdraw from the herd. They become lethargic, spending most of their time resting, and they go off their food and stop grooming. If you have a pet you might also recognise this pattern and know to ring the vet pronto. Here's the surprising thing: psychological trauma causes the same effect! If you separate an animal from its offspring or expose it to another stressful event, you will notice the same symptoms. Remember, the mind and body aren't separate: a spike in stress from physical infection or psychological stress will have the same result.

But what was the evolutionary advantage of this? In the case of infection or other illnesses, separating yourself from the tribe or herd prevents spreading infection. Resting conserves energy while you lose hard-won calories to mounting an immune response. When you think about it, you might remember these symptoms when you last had a cold – perhaps you skipped your shower and instead slumped on the sofa, seemingly unable to muster motivation to do anything else. You weren't being lazy or grubby; you were experiencing a sickness behaviour reflex. Once the infection resolves so do the symptoms, but that's not the case with chronic cortisol – because, if you don't remove the source, the symptoms will simply persist. Of course, we did not evolve to live with chronically raised cortisol and so this reflex is no longer protective – if anything, it exacerbates the problem.

During a time of great psychological stress, evolution dictates we would all benefit from being cocooned by our tribe, spending time outside and moving. Instead, you might notice an indescribable urge to be alone, groom less, rest and simply do nothing. This reflex was only ever designed to be a response to a temporary insult but, if a source of chronic stress doesn't quickly disappear, neither does the sickness behaviour. Instead of making you better, it feeds into a vicious cycle, stopping you from engaging in all the cortisol-lowering activities we've covered. The trick is simply to have insight and recognise when this is happening to you – then it is your job to consciously oppose it. Force yourself to see friends, do exercise, go outside and engage in flow – the vicious cycle will break and, as a rule, your mood will lift.

Pillars for life

What I eat is a valuable part of my health and I hope I have convinced you of food's amazing impact on yours too. However, to assume it is the only thing you should change to feel energised, happy and healthy is clearly missing a trick. Our stress hormone plays an integral role in so many aspects of health; it also directly alters appetite and weight gain. When I mention stress to my patients it's not because I am dismissing their symptoms or trying to undermine their experience in any way. I now fully understand the astounding impact it can have on health, exacerbating everything from heart disease to rashes like psoriasis. Importantly, to assume the body and mind are somehow separate from each other is a gross oversimplification of our biology. Triggering too much cortisol, no matter the reason, will absolutely shorten your life. So again, if I ask my patients to work on reducing their stress it isn't because I am dismissing their problems or not taking them seriously: it's because I genuinely *am* taking their health very seriously.

I have walked you through my five pillars of happiness, but you may have noticed a trend: their effects go far beyond improving mental health. Whether it's sleep's amazing ability to reduce your risk of cancer or movement's mind-blowing effect on everything from Parkinson's to longevity, the effects of each pillar are wide-reaching. In truth, happiness and health walk side by side – trying to tease them apart makes no sense. That's why, though it may be strange that a GP spends so much time teaching patients how to feel happy, in truth, it is an obvious medical intervention. Of course, mental health is an incredibly complex subject and there are many psychological and pharmacological treatment options we can also use. Harnessing a change in lifestyle is just one tool and has nothing to do with assigning blame – feeling empowered to improve your own health alongside traditional medicine can only be a good thing. Sometimes this means asking yourself the hard questions: are you giving your time to the right people? And, on that note, are you spending it on the right things? Is it leached by social media and ego, or do you give it to the things which really matter to you? When you honestly confront yourself with these questions, you will be surprised how easy it is to let go of life's chronic stressors.

Controlling stress: Key points

1) Stress is not just a subjective feeling – it translates into your very biology through hormones like cortisol. This has an enormous effect on health, and managing stress is a vital part of preventing disease and feeling well.

2) The happiest people in the world regularly engage in flow state – an activity which makes time stand still. Doing this yourself can significantly improve stress.

3) Spending time in nature reflects the natural environment in which we evolved. The research around this is amazing with clear evidence that it significantly improves stress and other health outcomes.

4) Feeling you belong to a community is the best predictor of a long life. We are in the middle of a loneliness epidemic – there are likely many causes but our overreliance on smartphones and social media is a big part of the problem.

5) Good-quality sleep directly affects mental health, immunity, brain function and even your risk of cancer. Honouring your circadian rhythm and being mindful of light exposure, caffeine, exercise and chronic stress are all vital aspects of achieving good sleep.

6) Exercise is not something we evolved to do – instead, movement is something we engaged in when it was necessary, fun or both. Trying to find ways to incorporate this in your life is vital for health because it has the power to prolong your health-span, boost your mental health and significantly reduce your risk of disease.

7) Acts of earnest charity are part of our human behaviour and again, are tied strongly to our evolution. By engaging in unnecessary acts of kindness, you can reduce stress and optimise your mental health.

8) Sickness behaviour is an evolutionary reflex which is helpful for overcoming infections but harmful for overcoming
stress! The trick is to recognise when you are engaging in it
and force yourself to do the opposite.

FINAL WORDS

As I said at the outset, I maintain that *now* is the perfect time to be alive: what we understand about health, longevity and happiness is changing beyond recognition. It turns out we are each born with a unique vessel which is not just home to our microbiomes, but centuries of clever evolution. How this vessel – or body – interacts with its environment is much more complicated than a maths equation: what you put into it isn't just a number. Rather, food is irrefutably a medicine, serving the body a vital set of instructions on whether to acquire health or disease. The good news is that we can harness this information to manipulate our very biology. Acknowledging the pivotal role you can play in your own health has nothing to do with blame – it should only empower you.

Key takeaways

I hope you will agree that, when you understand the true complexity of the body, much of health isn't as it seems. So many principles have been oversimplified: how, what and why you should eat is one of them. By getting to grips with the immaculate web that is your health and understanding what appetite is, so much stigma and misinformation falls flat on its face. We have covered an enormous amount so here is a quick recap:

- **Microbiome** – If modern medicine has had one plot twist it is our amazing microbiomes. They finally answer so many questions but, really, we've only just begun to scratch the surface. What we do know is that these bugs influence the brain, immune system, heart health, skin, hormones, cancer, gut health, weight, diabetes, how we metabolise food and many other things. We evolved with these bugs and they are very much part of us – a healthy microbiome is, therefore, inextricably linked to all round better health. Luckily, achieving this is surprisingly simple if we retrace our steps and eat what our great grandparents once ate. Expensive supplements might spike your dopamine but humble, unassuming whole foods – such as vegetables, fruits, wholegrains, pulses, nuts, seeds and fermented foods – are the real ticket to a strong microbiome.

- **Appetite** – The only reason our ancestors didn't become extinct is because they were able to experience hunger. Our appetite is not the enemy at all, and it's not something we should fight – we have simply misunderstood it. As we have now seen, our modern lifestyles don't reflect our evolution and, as a result, many of us have abnormal appetites. Part of the reason for this is that we no longer eat food which stimulates our fullness mechanisms. Many of us are also paradoxically malnourished – to compensate, our appetite increases in the hunt for nutrients we are lacking.

  I have learned not to fight my appetite and now cherish eating the diet I grew up on – hearty, humble whole foods. I now understand that hunger and fullness signals are vital messages from my body, guiding me when to start and stop eating. When you learn to work with, rather than against, this drive, food finally becomes something you can truly enjoy.

- **Timing matters** – Every system in the body runs to an internal tempo, all aligned together to optimise the ingenious engineering of our bodies. That includes when insulin and saliva are most efficiently released, our sleep hormones and even the rhythmic Mexican wave of our intestines or 'MMC'. It is not boring to offer your body and microbiome a predictable life: it is what they thrive off. Sleeping and eating at predictable times each day – crucially, ensuring your 'eating window' allows plenty of time for your digestive system to rest – can have flabbergasting results on health. But rather than feel you are restricting food, imagine you are choreographing it: simply having a routine gives your body enough notice to anticipate what is needed. This can influence everything from your risk of metabolic disease to cancer, as well as non-specific symptoms like indigestion.

- **Insulin resistance** – We have been fretting about obesity and weight gain for centuries; however, really we have been distracted by the wrong issue. Many of us are insulin resistant but it just manifests in different ways. Each person has a unique subcutaneous fat capacity – some are more able to store external fat, while others have internal signs of insulin resistance like visceral fat. In other words, being thin on the outside does not necessarily mean you are metabolically healthy.

  Instead of concentrating on weight, we should all be paying attention to our insulin resistance because it will drive most of the chronic diseases we die from. In future, I hope medicine will take a more preventative approach, priming doctors to warn patients when they are showing signs of insulin resistance (without causing offence). For example, perhaps one day a fasting insulin blood test will become a normal screening tool. But like I said at the start of the book, I don't tell anyone they should lose weight. My advice is the same for everyone, no matter their size: they need to optimise their insulin sensitivity and their microbiome. When health is the goal, weight loss can be a pleasant side effect, but the reverse isn't necessarily true!

- **Start young** – Importantly, we know insulin resistance is time-dependent: the longer you have been exposed to high insulin levels, the more resistant you become. This can begin in the womb and build in childhood – overcoming this as an adult is incredibly challenging. But that does not mean food should be restricted or scrutinised before or during pregnancy, nor should children be encouraged to over-analyse their food. Everyone, young and old, should simply imagine they are sitting next to a feisty nonna at mealtimes: whatever they eat should keep a smile on her face – not all of the time, but most of the time. She'll be happy if she sees us eating freshly made meals, made from good-quality ingredients – food that is delicious for us *and* our microbiome. Feed yourself and your family like this as much as possible, and everything else will sort itself out.

- **Mind and body** – Your mind is not separate from your body, and to assume otherwise is short sighted. The discovery of the microbiome has changed psychiatry irreversibly, and exploring the relationship between these bugs and our brain health is being dubbed 'psychobiome'. More research in this area is still needed, but what we do understand is that by feeding our bugs what they like (plenty of varied plants), we can alter their production of serotonin and dopamine which, in turn, dramatically alter mood. Exercise can also be not just as effective, but more effective than antidepressants, and should be actively prescribed by all doctors. This does not mean that I will stop prescribing antidepressants when necessary – they still have an important place – but it is thrilling to unearth proof of what we can each do to help ourselves.

    Exciting new discoveries are also shining a spotlight on our immune systems of all things. Amazingly, more and more evidence now suggests that chronic inflammation in the body is mirrored in the brain which, in turn, directly correlates with mental-health symptoms. When you improve this inflammation, believe it or not, the symptoms lift. A whole book* is needed to explore this fully but luckily, in a way, I have already told you everything you need

---

* I highly recommend *The Inflamed Mind* by Edward Bullmore to learn more.

to know to prevent the underlying mechanisms. Eating to boost your microbiome and minimise insulin resistance will protect your brain from inflammation and, thus, reduce your risk of mental-health conditions; secondly, learning to prevent chronically raised cortisol by managing stress and optimising sleep is equally important. As it turns out, what is good for your happiness is good for your physical health and vice versa.

- **Stress** – This is an inevitable part of life but sometimes our response to it is the real problem. Without meaning to, as a young doctor I was spending barely any time outside and did little to no exercise (other than running to crash calls). My sleep quality took a hit, and hurried by career pressures and ongoing exams, I invested less and less time in the cortisol-lowering activities which could have mitigated my stress. The consequences of doing this are not insignificant. Remember, chronically raised cortisol will conspire with insulin to drive disease, while also directly impacting mitochondria to shorten your life. I find it odd now to realise that I seemed to specifically avoid all the lifestyle interventions which could have helped. I was in a sickness behaviour cycle: I withdrew from friends, became lethargic, put minimal effort into my appearance (just like animals stop grooming) and lost motivation to do anything other than slump. Had I understood what was happening to me at the time, I could have corrected it. If you recognise this sickness behaviour in yourself the key is to have insight and consciously employ the pillars of happiness discussed in the last chapter.

Why was I so unwell?

I can now look back at my junior-doctor years and understand what happened to me. Other than a change in diet, my microbiome received other insults; firstly, I took a year-long course of antibiotics to treat my acne. Having had relatively few antibiotics in my life, this was likely a huge shock to my bugs! Ironically, feeding a healthy microbiome and optimising my blood sugar control could have improved my skin. But instead, I persisted with medication, even though I could see it wasn't working. Next, I was unlucky enough to have several episodes of gastroenteritis – this may not have been avoidable, but we know it can massively disrupt the microbiome and is a well-recognised trigger for IBS. The debilitating bloating and pain which followed now make perfect sense. (Hindsight is a wonderful thing!)

As I mentioned at the start of the book, the moment I became a doctor my attitude to food changed: it was no longer a priority. I reasoned I was 'too busy' to cook and so opted for convenient UPFs instead. On top of that, my shifts completely disrupted my circadian rhythm creating a perfect storm to worsen my metabolic health. But my mistakes are easy ones to make, and you don't have to be working shifts to make them. Many of us disrupt our circadian rhythms by going to bed late at night and eating at random times throughout the day. In hindsight, the next insult to my health was loneliness but I was not alone in this: many of us also spend a huge amount of time alone – and even in the company of others, we choose to look at our screens instead of interacting. Parts of my medical training proved to be an exceptionally isolating experience (doctors often have to move around the country, far away from friends and family) and I found I was spending almost no time with people who knew me as I knew myself. But again, anyone can have this experience and, increasingly, many of us do; we have never been lonelier than we are now. We never evolved to be alone so it is no surprise that social isolation is a well-recognised risk factor for all-cause mortality. If I could go back in time, I now recognise how a change in how I was living my life could have prevented so many of my health problems. Hopefully, my experience and series of epiphanies will save you from the same fate.

How to feel well and be well

With time, I have realised that the secret to feeling truly well is not a secret at all. Really, the answers are simple and humbling. No one really knows how long their life will be, nor is it really up to them. And so I would argue chasing immortality is both arrogant and foolish. To quote J.R.R. Tolkien's Gandalf: 'all we have to decide is what to do with the time that is given to us'.

My advice is twofold: firstly, eat *good* food – it should be a pleasure. My goal is to eat food that is delicious for both me and my microbiome. Unpalatable diet-culture concoctions are not my idea of good food. Instead, I only eat things I genuinely enjoy – I don't understand the logic of eating anything else. But on that point, my second bit of advice is to consider your body and mind as things that are under your guardianship: it is simply your job to look after them. And you now have a manual on how to do just that.

Ultimately, I encourage you to think carefully about living a *good* life. When it one day ends, many of the ego-led stresses of modern life won't be on your mind. We know the best predictor of a long and happy life is the people you invite into it. Essentially, I suggest we all try to copy Blue Zone centenarians: eat delicious whole foods in the company of many, help each other out, spend time outside and keep moving at every age. Let yourself live a *good* life. Everything else will work itself out when you do.

SUMMARY OF APPETITE GUT HORMONES IN APPETITE REGULATION

Group	Hormones	Effect	Released from
PP-Fold Protein	Neuropeptide Y (NPY) Peptide YY (PYY) Pancreatic polypeptide (PP)	Stimulate fullness.	NPY: central nervous system PYY: intestines (max distal small intestine) PP: pancreas
	Cholecystokinin (CCK)	Stimulates fullness.	Small intestine
Proglucagon-Derived Peptides	GLP-1 GLP-2 Oxyntomodulin (OXM) Glucagon Proglucagon-derived peptides	GLP-1: reduces food intake, suppresses glucagon secretion, and delays gastric emptying; stimulates insulin secretion in response to carbohydrates. Promotes nerve growth and prevents nerve death. GLP-2: no effect on food intake. Promotes intestine cell growth; reduction in gastric emptying. OXM: reduces food intake and increases energy expenditure. Glucagon: stimulates liver to produce glucose when blood levels are low. Proglucagon-derived peptides: influence GLPs and glucagon.	Proglucagon: pancreas/ small intestine/ brainstem Glucagon: pancreas OXM, GLP-1, GLP-2: intestines, brain
Hunger hormone	Ghrelin	Stimulates appetite, gastric-acid secretion, gastric motility, pancreatic protein output. Also affects heart function, bone/nerve/muscle formation.	Mostly the stomach; some from intestine, brain, lung, adrenal cortex, kidney, bone, testis, placenta, pancreas
Peripheral adiposity signals	Insulin Leptin	Insulin: moves glucose out of the bloodstream into cells in the form of glycogen and fat. Leptin: creates a general background effect of reduced appetite.	Insulin: pancreas Leptin: fat cells

MY TOP SLEEPING TIPS*

1) Use your bedroom for sleep and sex – nothing else. Your subconscious mind needs to associate bed with sleep, so don't use it to watch TV or scroll through your phone.

2) Don't allow yourself to feel stressed in bed – this creates an anxious association with bedtime, which makes falling asleep much harder. That means you should only attempt to go to bed if you genuinely feel tired enough to fall asleep. If you are lying awake for more than 30 minutes, get up and go read in another room. Only attempt to sleep again when you feel truly tired.

3) Honour your circadian rhythm! Timing matters and you need to set your internal clock to release melatonin at the correct time every day. Initially, if you are struggling with sleep this just means setting an alarm and waking up at the same time EVERY DAY (including weekends). Try to go outside promptly or get to a window so you can get 20 minutes of sunlight into your eyes. Conversely, evenings should be cosy and dimly lit with at least an hour of screen-free time before bed.

4) Eventually, once you have set this circadian rhythm and find it easier to fall asleep, you should aim to also go to bed at the same time every day.

---

* Based on NIH Medline Plus (Internet). Bethesda, MD: National Library of Medicine (US); summer 2012. Tips for getting a good night's sleep. Available from: https://magazine.medlineplus.gov/pdf/MLP_Summer2012web.pdf

5) Caffeine can take as long as 8 hours to wear off fully so if you are struggling to sleep, make sure you get all of your coffee, tea and chocolate in before noon. I would include energy drinks/soft drinks but, after reading this book, I hope you won't be drinking those! If you are still struggling to sleep, you may need to reduce your caffeine further (e.g. only have it first thing in the morning or not at all).

6) If you are going through a period of poor sleep my advice is to cut alcohol out completely for a few weeks until it has improved. When your sleep is better, be very mindful about how you reintroduce alcohol and aim to have several alcohol-free days a week.

7) If you are struggling to sleep, this is the time to increase your exercise! Firstly, because it is one of the most effective ways to reduce stress. Secondly, because it directly helps you build 'sleep pressure'. Ideally, avoid high intensity exercise 2–3 hours before bed.

8) If you are waking frequently in the night to pass urine, speak to your doctor! At the same time, be mindful of how much fluid you drink in the evening and try to frontload this earlier in the day instead.

9) Try to finish all eating 2–4 hours before going to bed to avoid indigestion, which contributes to poor sleep. (This will also be better for your metabolic health as insulin works more efficiently earlier in the day).

10) Body temperature matters when trying to fall asleep. Make sure the room isn't too hot (18°C is ideal) and have a warm bath/shower before bed – this counterintuitively helps you drop your core body temperature.

11) Avoid napping, if possible, especially if you are struggling with long-term insomnia. Ideally, you want to create enough sleep pressure as possible so that you can actually fall asleep at night. If you absolutely need a nap, avoid doing this after 3pm.

12) Finally, ask yourself why you are struggling to sleep. Typically, this is because your sympathetic nervous system or the 'fight or flight' mode is overstimulated. What in your life is causing this? Take a look at Chapter 10 and work hard on reducing your life stress. If you allow this to bubble away long term, a bad night's sleep will be the least of your worries!

ACKNOWLEDGEMENTS

Strange as it may sound, I need to start by thanking three men I have never met: Dan Buettner, Simon Bainbridge and Professor Tim Spector. You see, it is only with the benefit of hindsight that you can appreciate the peculiar butterfly effect of your own life. In the space of two months I went from having a thousand Instagram followers to a book deal because of strangers I've still never met! The point of my account was simply to teach my own patients about food – showing them what I actually ate seemed the most obvious way to do that. I only ever meant for it to be a teaching tool and hobby but, one day, an unassuming bean soup tickled the algorithm just enough to go viral. The ripple effect had begun. To my amazement, Dan Buettner (whose work on Blue Zones I had long admired) reposted my recipe on his own Instagram account! Overnight my following exploded exponentially with tens of thousands of new followers in no time. Two months later, a man named Simon Bainbridge stumbled across my recipe and decided to show his partner. I'm very grateful he did because she happened to be Sam Jackson, one of Penguin's editorial directors. I will be *eternally* indebted to her for the best birthday present of my life: I woke up to a message asking if I might want to write a book.

But, of course, having something to write about at all is where the real ripple began. It is not an exaggeration to say reading one book by Professor Tim Spector was the catalyst for my interest in lifestyle medicine. I don't think it's humanly possible to convey how grateful I am to him for writing it! But really the person I should thank most of all is my wonderful mother for 'lending' the book to me (I have yet to give it back). In truth, most of what I understand about being healthy I learned from her. To have braved offending me about my weight with a practical solution is something most mothers wouldn't have dared. Handing me a book, in a way, was the greatest act of maternal love and I will always be grateful for it. I absolutely could not have written this book without my other half (a term often misused by people who don't have a twin) who broke down in floods of happy tears when I got a book deal. To have someone who genuinely lives your happiness as if it were happening to them is a rarity which I don't take for granted. I can't count her hours of consoling phone calls; if you ever suffer from imposter syndrome, a twin sister is the best remedy! Rewind a few decades and perhaps the first ripple happened, aged 11, when my father convinced me I could become doctor. As a child I was crippled by a deep belief that I was the stupidest person I knew. He spent a lifetime insisting I was wrong, encouraging me to attempt everything I assumed I was incapable of, including writing this book. No one achieves anything alone. This book belongs to my family as much as it does to me.

I have been enormously lucky to have many professional mentors over the years. My GP trainer, Dr Richard Harper, deserves special mention. He too handed me a couple of lifestyle medicine books – this stamp of approval hugely motivated me to learn more. But mostly, he simply gave me an example of the type of doctor I wanted to be and I still ask myself 'what would Richard do?' I am now obscenely lucky to work in the same building as Sir Denis Pereira Gray whose kind words of wisdom on medicine, life and book-writing I will always cherish. But to have the flexibility to write a book and be a GP was only possible because of my wonderful GP colleagues (and bosses) Professor Alex Harding, Dr Al Buick, Dr.Anna Bullock, Dr.Briony Tebbutt, Dr David Bossano, Dr Dave Higgie and Dr Simon Ogilvie: thank you for adjusting my shifts and cheering me on. Writing would have been painfully lonely without you and all of your corridor pep talks are *genuinely* what got me through!

Other than Sam Jackson (who deserves a double mention for giving me an opportunity of a lifetime), I owe so much to everyone at Ebury involved in the mystical, military operation that is publishing a book. I could never have imagined the enormous teamwork behind the scenes! To Anne Newman, Marta Catalano, Jessica Anderson, Aisling O'Toole, Jasleen Dhindsa and Kaitlin Beranek thank you for all your hard work. But, finally, I save a special and heartfelt thanks to my main point of contact, Leah Feltham. I warned her I would be writing several paragraphs on the depths of my enormous gratitude to her but, having blindly ignored our original word-count, I suspect this wouldn't go down well! In short, I've realised writing a book is like herding sheep: my thoughts were the sheep but Leah was the wise shepherd gently and calmly organising them. Her patience, reassurance and (much needed) handholding were instrumental in the whole process. Many of the ideas shared are hers and, really, we came up with this book together. Thank you, Leah.

FURTHER RESOURCES

As mentioned in my introduction, I treat each appointment as a tutorial and tend to send my patients 'homework'. Here is a general list of the further learning I 'prescribe' them.

BOOKS

Every Body Should Know This by Dr Federica Amati (Penguin Random House, 2024)

Exercised by Prof. Daniel Lieberman (Knopf Doubleday, 2021)

Fast. Feast. Repeat. by Gin Stephens (Macmillan, 2020)

Fibre Fuelled by Dr Will Bulsiewicz (Penguin Random House, 2022)

Gene Eating by Dr Giles Yeo (Pegasus Books, 2019)

Glucose Revolution by Jessie Inchauspé (Hachette, 2022)

Spoon-Fed by Prof. Tim Spector (Penguin Random House, 2020)

The Circadian Code by Prof. Satchin Panda (Penguin Random House, 2018)

The Clever Guts Diet by Dr Michael Mosley (Hachette, 2017)

The Diet Myth by Prof. Tim Spector (Hachette, 2015)

The Feel Good Fix by Lavina Mehta (Penguin Random House, 2024)

The Food for Life Cookbook by Prof. Tim Spector (Penguin Random House, 2024)

The Full Diet by Dr Saira Hameed (Penguin Random House, 2022)

The Inflamed Mind by Prof. Edward Bullmore (Hachette, 2018)

The Obesity Code by Dr Jason Fung (Scribe, 2016)

The Pioppi Diet by Dr Aseem Malhotra and Donal O'Neill (Penguin Random House, 2017)

This Book May Save Your Life by Dr Karan Rajan (Penguin Random House, 2023)

Ultra-Processed People by Dr Chris van Tulleken (Cornerstone, 2023)

Why We Sleep by Prof. Matthew Walker (Penguin Random House, 2018)

DOCUMENTARIES

Hack your Health: The Secrets of Your Gut (Netflix, 2024)

Live to 100: Secrets of the Blue Zones (Netflix, 2023)

PODCASTS

Dr. Rangan Chatterjee's *Feel Better, Live More*

Microbiome Medics

The Doctor's Kitchen

ZOE Science & Nutrition

YOUTUBE

@feelgoodwithlavina – I send her workouts to my elderly patients

@joanmacdonald6346 (Instagram: @trainwithjoan) – further inspiration to move at any age

REFERENCES

CHAPTER 1: YOUR MICROBIOME – THE ORGAN YOU DIDN'T KNOW YOU HAD

When the Hungarian obstetrician Ignaz Semmelweis ... Tyagi, U. & Barwal, K. C. (2020). 'Ignac Semmelweis – Father of hand hygiene.' *Indian Journal of Surgery*, 82(3), 276–7. https://doi.org/10.1007/s12262-020-02386-6

We have known about placebos since the 1700s ... Jütte, R. (2013). 'The early history of the placebo.' *Complementary Therapies in Medicine*, 21(2), 94–7. https://doi.org/10.1016/j.ctim.2012.06.002

... in 2015 when Parkinson's patients received ... Espay, A. J. et al. (2015). 'Placebo effect of medication cost in Parkinson disease.' *Neurology*, 84(8), 794–802. https://doi.org/10.1212/wnl.0000000000001282

We also know placebos release ... Benedetti, F., Carlino, E. & Pollo, A. (2010). 'How placebos change the patient's brain.' *Neuropsychopharmacology*, 36(1), 339–54. https://doi.org/10.1038/npp.2010.81

... these isolated chemicals never produce the same health benefits as the actual food itself! Jacobs, D. R. & Tapsell, L. C. (2008). 'Food, not nutrients, is the fundamental unit in nutrition.' *Nutrition Reviews*, 65(10), 439–50. https://doi.org/10.1111/j.1753-4887.2007.tb00269.x

Pollan M. (2007). 'Unhappy Meals'. *New York Times*. Available at: https://www.nytimes.com/2007/01/28/magazine/28nutritionism.t.html

... it turns out that taking vitamin C ... Hemilä, H. & Chalker, E. (2013). 'Vitamin C for preventing and treating the common cold.' *Cochrane Library*, 5. https://doi.org/10.1002/14651858.cd000980.pub4

In fact, some vitamins are even dangerous ... Singal, M., Banh, H. L., Allan, G.M. (2013). 'Daily multivitamin to reduce mortality, cardiovascular disease, and cancer.' *Canadian Family Physician*, 59: 847

Bjelakovic, G., Nikolova, D., Gludd, L. L., Simonetti, R. G. & Gluud, C. (2012), 'Antioxidant supplements for prevention of mortality in healthy participants and patients with various diseases.' *Cochrane Database of Systematic Reviews*, 3

Just one piece of broccoli has several of these ... Liu, M., Zhang, L., Ser, L., Cumming, J. R., Ku, K. M. (2018). 'Comparative Phytonutrient Analysis of Broccoli By-Products: The Potentials for Broccoli By-Products Utilization.' *Molecules*, 23(4): 900.

In fact, of the 8,000 polyphenols we know of ... Liu, R. H. (2003). 'Health Benefits of Fruit and Vegetables Are from Additive and Synergistic Combinations of Phytochemicals.' *American Journal of Clinical Nutrition* 78(3): 517S–20S. https://doi.org/10.1093/ajcn/78.3.517S

Just under half the chemicals in our blood ... Visconti, A. et al. (2019). 'Interplay between the human gut microbiome and host metabolism.' *Nature Communications*, 10(1). https://doi.org/10.1038/s41467-019-12476-z

... discovered one particularly nasty strain of a bug called *Enterobacter.* Fei, N., Zhao, L. (2013). 'An opportunistic pathogen isolated from the gut of an obese human causes obesity in germfree mice.' *ISME J* 7, 880–884. https://doi.org/10.1038/ismej.2012.153

... when we truly value something, compliance isn't a problem. Spector, T. (2015). *The Diet Myth: The Real Science Behind What We Eat.* Hachette UK

... a 32-year-old lady developed a devastating gut infection ... Alang, N. & Kelly, C. R. (2015). 'Weight Gain after Fecal Microbiota Transplantation.' *Open Forum Infectious Diseases* 2(1). https://doi.org/10.1093/ofid/ofv004

... thousands are now getting it without setting foot in hospital ... Freeman et al. (2010). 'The Changing Epidemiology of *Clostridium Difficile* Infections' *Clinical Microbiology Reviews* 23(3), 529–549, https://doi.org/10.1128/cmr.00082-09; Lessa, F. C. et al. (2015). 'Burden of *Clostridium Difficile* Infection in the United States.' *New England Journal of Medicine* 372(9): 825–34, https://doi.org/10.1056/NEJMoa1408913

... this is something the ancient Chinese were doing 1,500 years ago. Rossen, N. G. et al. (2015). 'Fecal microbiota transplantation as novel therapy in gastroenterology: a systematic review.' *World Journal of Gastroenterology*, 21, 5359–71. https://doi.org/10.3748/wjg.v21.i17.5359

It is remarkably effective, curing 90 per cent of infections ... D'Haens, G. R. & Jobin, C. (2019b). 'Fecal microbial transplantation for diseases beyond recurrent *Clostridium difficile* infection.' *Gastroenterology*, 157(3), 624–36. https://doi.org/10.1053/j.gastro.2019.04.053

... the mouse with the obese twin's transplant grows obese ... Clarke, G. et al. (2014). 'Minireview: Gut Microbiota: The Neglected Endocrine Organ.' *Molecular Endocrinology* 28(8): 1221–38, https://doi.org/10.1210/me.2014-1108

Ridaura V. K. et al. (2013). 'Gut microbiota from twins discordant for obesity modulate metabolism in mice.' *Science* 341(6150), https://doi.org/10.1126/science.1241214

It's called *Christensenella* ... Goodrich, J. K., et al. (2014). 'Human genetics shape the gut microbiome.' *Cell*, 159(4), 789–99. https://doi.org/10.1016/j.cell.2014.09.053

One in 10 lucky humans is infected by this helpful critter ... Zierer, J. et al. (2018). 'The fecal metabolome as a functional readout of the gut microbiome.' *Nature Genetics*, 50(6), 790–5. https://doi.org/10.1038/s41588-018-0135-7

WHAT YOUR DOCTOR EATS

... it is a parasite called *Blastocystis* ... Spector, T. (2022). *Food for Life: Your Guide to the New Science of Eating Well*. Random House

... another study in Boston also found bacteria called *Lactobacillus* and *Bifidus* ... Wang, J. et al. (2014). 'Modulation of gut microbiota during probiotic-mediated attenuation of metabolic syndrome in high fat diet-fed mice.' *The ISME Journal*, 9(1), 1–15. https://doi.org/10.1038/ismej.2014.99

Some bacteria are just showing off ... Ley, R. E., Bäckhed, F., Turnbaugh, P., Lozupone, C. A., Knight, R. D. & Gordon, J. I. (2005). 'Obesity alters gut microbial ecology.' *Proceedings of the National Academy of Sciences of the United States of America*, 102(31), 11070–5. https://doi.org/10.1073/pnas.0504978102

Turnbaugh, P. J. et al. (2006). 'An obesity-associated gut microbiome with increased capacity for energy harvest.' *Nature*, 444(7122), 1027–31. https://doi.org/10.1038/nature05414

... when scientists try to guess who is more likely to gain weight ... Spector, T. (2015b). *The Diet Myth: The Real Science Behind What We Eat*. Hachette UK

... we also know a 'diverse' microbiome seems to help ... Cotillard, A. et al. (2013). 'Dietary intervention impact on gut microbial gene richness.' *Nature*, 500(7464), 585–8. https://doi.org/10.1038/nature12480

Asnicar, F. et al. (2021). 'Microbiome connections with host metabolism and habitual diet from 1,098 deeply phenotyped individuals.' *Nature Medicine*, 27(2), 321–32. https://doi.org/10.1038/s41591-020-01183-8

The main thing that seems to predict this diversity ... McDonald, D. et al. (2018). 'American Gut: an Open Platform for Citizen Science Microbiome Research.' *MSystems*, 3(3). https://doi.org/10.1128/msystems.00031-18

Twin studies show that those who had more fibre ... Menni, C., Jackson, M. A., Pallister, T., Steves, C. J., Spector, T. D. & Valdes, A. M. (2017). 'Gut microbiome diversity and high-fibre intake are related to lower long-term weight gain.' *International Journal of Obesity*, 41(7), 1099–1105. https://doi.org/10.1038/ijo.2017.66

... polyphenols show an independent benefit ... Mompeo, O. et al. (2020). 'Consumption of Stilbenes and Flavonoids is Linked to Reduced Risk of Obesity Independently of Fiber Intake.' *Nutrients*, 12(6), 1871. https://doi.org/10.3390/nu12061871

... in 2019, the PREDICT 1 study ... Asnicar, F. et al. (2021). 'Microbiome connections with host metabolism and habitual diet from 1,098 deeply phenotyped individuals.' *Nature Medicine*, 27(2), 321–32. https://doi.org/10.1038/s41591-020-01183-8

Amazingly, the microbiome can influence the release of GLP-1 ... Cani, P. D. et al. 'Gut microbiota fermentation of prebiotics increases satietogenic and incretin gut peptide production with consequences for appetite sensation and glucose response after a meal.' *American Journal of Clinical Nutrition*, 90(5), 1236–43 (2009). https://doi.org/10.3945/ajcn.2009.28095

... our bugs can even affect the very way we taste and crave food. Alcock, J., Maley, C. C. & Aktipis, C. A. (2014). 'Is eating behavior manipulated by the gastrointestinal microbiota? Evolutionary pressures and potential mechanisms.' *BioEssays*, 36(10), 940–9. https://doi.org/10.1002/bies.201400071

... people who admit to chocolate cravings ... Rezzi, S. et al. (2007). 'Human metabolic phenotypes link directly to specific dietary preferences in healthy individuals.' *J Proteome Res*, 6:4469–77.

... germ-free mice ... have altered taste receptors ... Duca, F. A., Swartz, T. D., Sakar, Y. & Covasa, M. (2012). 'Increased oral detection, but decreased intestinal signaling for fats in mice lacking gut microbiota.' *PLoS ONE*, 7

Swartz, T. et al (2012). 'Up-regulation of intestinal type 1 taste receptor 3 and sodium glucose luminal transporter-1 expression and increased sucrose intake in mice lacking gut microbiota.' *British Journal of Nutrition*, 107:621

Changes in taste-receptor expression ... Miras, A. D. & le Roux, C.W. (2013). 'Mechanisms underlying weight loss after bariatric surgery.' *Nat Rev Gastroenterol Hepatol*, 10:575–84

... this way of eating seems to trigger chronic inflammation ... Christ, A. et al. (2018). 'Western diet triggers NLRP3-Dependent innate immune reprogramming.' *Cell*, 172(1–2), 162–75. https://doi.org/10.1016/j.cell.2017.12.013

.... one French study found a junk-food diet ... Kong, L. C. et al. (2014). 'Dietary Patterns Differently Associate with Inflammation and Gut Microbiota in Overweight and Obese Subjects.' *PloS One*, 9(10). https://doi.org/10.1371/journal.pone.0109434

... your fat tissue is sort of like an 'endocrine' organ ... Huh, J. Y., Park, Y. J., Ham, M. & Kim, J. B. (2014). 'Crosstalk between Adipocytes and Immune Cells in Adipose Tissue Inflammation and Metabolic Dysregulation in Obesity.' *Molecules and Cells/Molecules and Cells*, 37(5), 365–71. https://doi.org/10.14348/molcells.2014.0074

Just over a hundred years ago a food allergy had never been seen ... Schloss, O. M. (1912). 'A case of food allergy to common foods.' *American Journal of Diseases of Children*, 3, 342–362.

Golbert, T. M. (August 1969). 'Systemic allergic reactions to ingested antigens.' *Journal of Allergy*, 44(2): 96–107.

As C-sections have increased, so have food allergies ... Cho, C. E. & Norman, M. (2013). 'Cesarean section and development of the immune system in the offspring.' *American Journal of Obstetrics and Gynecology*, 208(4), 249–54. https://doi.org/10.1016/j.ajog.2012.08.009

One meta-analysis even saw a 20 per cent increase in asthma ... Thavagnanam, S., Fleming, J., Bromley, A., Shields, M. D. & Cardwell, C. R. (2007). 'A meta-analysis of the association between Caesarean section and childhood asthma.' *Clinical & Experimental Allergy/Clinical and Experimental Allergy*, 38(4), 629–33. https://doi.org/10.1111/j.1365-2222.2007.02780.x

... in America, 35 per cent of people have the coeliac gene ... Bulsiewicz, W. (2022). *Fibre fuelled: The Plant-Based Gut Health Plan to Lose Weight, Restore Health and Optimise Your Microbiome*. Random House

... people with IBS appear to have very low microbiome diversity. Chong, P. P., Chin, V. K., Looi, C. Y., Wong, W. F., Madhavan, P. & Yong, V. C. (2019). 'The Microbiome and Irritable Bowel Syndrome – a review on the pathophysiology, current research and future therapy.' *Frontiers in Microbiology*, 10. https://doi.org/10.3389/fmicb.2019.01136

... trialling faecal transplants as a treatment for IBS ... Halkjær, S. I., Boolsen, A. W., Günther, S., Christensen, A. H. & Petersen, A. M. (2017). 'Can fecal microbiota transplantation cure irritable bowel syndrome?' *World J. Gastroenterol*, 23 4112–20. https://doi.org/10.3748/wjg.v23.i22.4112

... SIBO (or small intestinal bacterial overgrowth) ... Takakura, W. & Pimentel, M. (2020). 'Small intestinal bacterial overgrowth and irritable bowel syndrome – an update.' *Frontiers in Psychiatry*, 11. https://doi.org/10.3389/fpsyt.2020.00664

... anywhere between 4 and 78 per cent of IBS patients have SIBO. Ghoshal, U. C., Shukla, R. & Ghoshal, U. (2017). 'Small Intestinal Bacterial Overgrowth and Irritable Bowel Syndrome: A Bridge between Functional Organic Dichotomy.' *Gut And Liver*, 11(2), 196–208. https://doi.org/10.5009/gnl16126

... our brain can actually create and respond to nerve hormones ... Lyte, M. (2014). 'Microbial Endocrinology.' *Gut Microbes* 5(3): 381–9. https://doi.org/10.4161/gmic.28682

... the gut microbiome produces 90 per cent of our serotonin and 50 per cent of our dopamine ... Yano, J. M. et al. (2015). 'Indigenous Bacteria from the Gut Microbiota Regulate Host Serotonin Biosynthesis.' *Cell* 161(2), 264–76. https://doi.org/10.1016/j.cell.2015.02.047

... 'dysbiosis' doesn't just cause IBS symptoms ... Mayer, E. A. (2008). 'Irritable Bowel Syndrome.' *New England Journal of Medicine* 358(16): 1692–99. https://doi.org/10.1056/NEJMcp0801447

They are vital for repairing the crumbling cement ... Braniste, V. et al. (2014). 'The Gut Microbiota Influences Blood-Brain Barrier Permeability in Mice.' *Science Translational Medicine* 6(263): 263ra158. https://doi.org/10.1126/scitranslmed.3009759

... the microbiome can affect everything from Parkinson's ... Bourassa, M. W. et al. (2016). 'Butyrate, Neuroepigenetics and the Gut Microbiome: Can a High Fiber Diet Improve Brain Health?' *Neuroscience Letters*, 625(20): 56–63. https://doi.org/10.1016/j.neulet.2016.02.009

Lap, H. et al. (2018). 'Protective Roles of Intestinal Microbiota-Derived Short Chain Fatty Acids in Alzheimer's Disease-Type Beta-Amyloid Neuropathological Mechanisms.' *Expert Review of Neurotherapeutics* 18(1): 83–90, https://doi.org/10.1080/14737175.2018.1400909

Sharma, S., Taliyan, R. & Singh, S. (2015). 'Beneficial Effects of Sodium Butyrate in 6-OHDA Induced Neurotoxicity and Behavioral Abnormalities:

Modulation of Histone Deacetylase Activity.' *Behavioural Brain Research*, 291: 306–14. https://doi.org/10.1016/j.bbr.2015.05.052

... helps keep your immune system tough enough to clean up the cancer cells ... Sepich-Poore, G. D., Zitvogel, L., Straussman, R., Hasty, J., Wargo, J. A. & Knight, R. (2021). 'The microbiome and human cancer.' *Science*, 371(653 6). https://doi.org/10.1126/science.abc4552

Ciernikova, S., Sevcikova, A., Stevurkova, V. & Mego, M. (2022). 'Tumor microbiome – an integral part of the tumor microenvironment.' *Frontiers in Oncology*, 12. https://doi.org/10.3389/fonc.2022.1063100

... tumours actually host a separate microbiome ... Swidsinski, A. et al. (1998). 'Association between intraepithelial *Escherichia coli* and colorectal cancer.' *Gas troenterology*, 115(2), 281–6. https://doi.org/10.1016/s0016-5085(98)70194-5

... we now know of 11 pathogens which cause cancer ... (2012). 'IARC Working Group on the Evaluation of Carcinogenic Risks to Humans, Biological agents. Volume 100 B. A review of human carcinogens.' *IARC Monogr. Eval. Carcinog. Risks Hum*, 100, 1–441

... dangerous secondary bile acids which seem to promote cancers ... Yang, R. & Qian, L. (2022). 'Research on Gut Microbiota-Derived Secondary Bile Acids In Cancer Progression.' *Integrative Cancer Therapies*, 21. https://doi.org/10.1177/15347354221114100

... why do African Americans have 65 times more colon cancer than rural Africans? O'Keefe, S. J. D. et al. (2015). 'Fat, Fibre and Cancer Risk in African Americans and Rural Africans.' *Nature Communications*: 6342. https://doi.org/10.1038/ncomms7342

Participants in America and Africa provided stool samples ... O'Keefe, S. J. D. et al. (2015). 'Fat, fibre and cancer risk in African Americans and rural Africans.' *Nature Communications*, 6(1). https://doi.org/10.1038/ncomms7342

... our estrobolome: a 'clique' of gut bacteria ... Plottel, C. S. & Blaser, M. J. (2011). 'Microbiome and malignancy.' *Cell Host & Microbe*, 10(4), 324–35. https://doi.org/10.1016/j.chom.2011.10.003

... it is also characterised by too many male sex hormones ... Guo, Y., Qi, Y., Yang, X., Zhao, L., Wen, S., Liu, Y., Tang, L. (2016). 'Association between Polycystic Ovary Syndrome and Gut Microbiota.' *PLoS One*, 11(4). doi: 10.1371/journal.pone.0153196

If a man has leaky-gut syndrome ... Tremellen, K. (2016). 'Gut Endotoxin Leading to a Decline IN Gonadal function (GELDING) – a novel theory for the development of late onset hypogonadism in obese men.' *Basic Clin Androl*, 26:7. https://doi.org/10.1186/s12610-016-0034-7

Even chemotherapy is influenced by our microbiome ... Viaud, S. et al. (2013b). 'The intestinal microbiota modulates the anticancer immune effects of cyclophosphamide.' *Science*, 342(6161), 971–6. https://doi.org/10.1126/science.1240537

CHAPTER 2: HOW DO WE ACTUALLY GAIN WEIGHT?

... **Wilbur Atwater spent 20 years** ... Bray, G. A. (2020). 'In the Footsteps of Wilbur Olin Atwater: The Atwater Lecture for 2019.' *Advances in Nutrition*, 11(3), 743–50. https://doi.org/10.1093/advances/nmz128

Take the humble almond ... 'Are nuts bad for you? Why the calorie counts for almonds don't add up.' (n.d.). https://zoe.com/learn/podcast-nuts

... **manufacturers are legally allowed an error rate of 20 per cent** ... Novotny, J. A., Gebauer, S. K. & Baer, D. J. (2012). 'Discrepancy between the Atwater factor predicted and empirically measured energy values of almonds in human diets.' *The American Journal of Clinical Nutrition*, 96(2), 296–301. https://doi.org/10.3945/ajcn.112.035782

Restaurants now also provide 'helpful' calorie counts ... Urban, L. E., Dallal, G. E., Robinson, L. M., Ausman, L. M., Saltzman, E. & Roberts, S. B. (2010). 'The Accuracy of Stated Energy Contents of Reduced-Energy, Commercially Prepared Foods.' *Journal of the American Dietetic Association*, 110(1), 116–23. https://doi.org/10.1016/j.jada.2009.10.003

... **in the presence of a high-fat meal** ... Moorthy, M., Sundralingam, U. & Palanisamy, U. D. (2021). 'Polyphenols as Prebiotics in the Management of High-Fat Diet-Induced Obesity: A Systematic Review of Animal Studies.' *Foods*, 10(2), 299. https://doi.org/10.3390/foods10020299

They even fund the research that supports claims ... Spector, T. (2020). *Spoon-Fed: Why Almost Everything We've Been Told About Food is Wrong*. Random House

... **a 20-year-old also rapidly gained just over 10kg in the space of a year.** Sapountzi, P., Charnogursky, G., Emanuele, M. A., Murphy, D., Nabhan, F. & Emanuele, N. V. (2005). 'Case study: Diagnosis of insulinoma using continuous glucose monitoring system in a patient with diabetes.' *Clinical Diabetes*, 23(3), 140–3. https://doi.org/10.2337/diaclin.23.3.140

Giving diabetics insulin obviously makes them gain weight ... White, N. H. et al. (2001). 'Influence of intensive diabetes treatment on body weight and composition of adults with type 1 diabetes in the Diabetes Control and Complications Trial.' *Diabetes Care*, 24(10):1711–21

UK Prospective Diabetes Study Group (1998). 'Intensive blood-glucose control with sulphonylureas or insulin compared with conventional treatment and risk of complications in patients with type 2 diabetes.' (UKPDS 33). *Lancet*, 352(9131), 837–53. https://doi.org/10.1016/s0140-6736(98)07019-6

Holman, R. R. et al. (2007). 'Addition of biphasic, prandial, or basal insulin to oral therapy in type 2 diabetes.' *The New England Journal of Medicine*, 357(17), 1716–30.

... **in one study, patients gained 8.7kg** ... Henry, R. R., Gumbiner, B., Ditzler, T., Wallace, P., Lyon, R. & Glauber, H. S. (1993). 'Intensive conventional insulin therapy for type II diabetes.' *Diabetes Care*, 16(1), 23–31.

Many other medications also cause weight gain by spiking insulin ... Smith, C. J., Fisher, M., McKay, G. A. (2010). 'Drugs for diabetes: part 2 sulphony-lureas.' *The British Journal of Cardiology*, 17(6): 279–82

Domecq, J. P. et al.(2015). 'Drugs commonly associated with weight change: A systematic review and meta-analysis.' *Journal of Clinical Endocrinology & Metabolism*, 100(2), 363–70. https://doi.org/10.1210/jc.2014-3421

Ebenbichler, C. F. et al. (2003). 'Olanzapine induces insulin resistance: results from a prospective study.' *The Journal of Clinical Psychiatry*, 64(12): 1436–9

Suzuki, Y. et al. (2012). 'Quetiapine-induced insulin resistance after switching from blonanserin despite a loss in both bodyweight and waist circumference.' *Psychiatry and Clinical Neurosciences*, 66(6):534–5

Penumalee, S., Kissner, P. & Midal, S. (2003). 'Gabapentin induced hypogly-caemia in a long-term peritoneal dialysis patient.' *American Journal of Kidney Diseases*, 42(6), E3–5.

... people who live with obesity simply have higher levels of insulin ... Polonsky, K. S., Given, B. D. & van Cauter, E. (1988). 'Twenty-four-hour profiles and pulsatile patterns of insulin secretion in normal and obese subjects.' *Journal of Clinical Investigation*, 81(2), 442–8. doi: 10.1172/JCI113339

... they are permanently in a fat-storing state. Duncan, R. E., Ahmadian, M., Jaworski, K., Sarkadi-Nagy, E. & Sul, H. S. (2007). 'Regulation of lipolysis in adipocytes.' *Annu Rev Nutr*, 27:79–101. doi: 10.1146/annurev.nutr.27.061406.093734

... people living with obesity have been found to have high levels of long-term cortisol ... Wester, V. L. et al. (2014). 'Long-term cortisol levels measured in scalp hair of obese patients.' *Obesity*, 22(9):1956–8. doi: 10.1002/oby.20795

... many studies showing increased cortisol levels are linked to insulin resistance ... Pagano, G. et al. (1983). 'An in vivo and in vitro study of the mechanisms of prednisolone-induced insulin resistance in healthy subjects.' *J Clin Invest*, 72(5):1814–20

Rizza, R. A., Mandarino, L. J. & Gerich, J. E. (1982). 'Cortisol-induced insulin resistance in man: impaired suppression of glucose production and stimula-tion of glucose utilization due to a postreceptor defect of insulin action.' *J Clin Endocrinol Metab*, 54(1):131–8

Dinneen, S., Alzaid, A., Miles, J. & Rizza, R. (1993). 'Metabolic effects of the nocturnal rise in cortisol on carbohydrate metabolism in normal humans.' *J Clin Invest*, 92(5):2283–90.

... our perceived level of stress correlated beautifully with raised cortisol ... Rosmond, R. et al. (1998). 'Stress-related cortisol secretion in men: relation-ships with abdominal obesity and endocrine, metabolic and hemodynamic abnormalities.' *J Clin Endocrinol Metab*, 83(6):1853–9.

CHAPTER 3: APPETITE – WHERE DOES IT COME FROM?

... a hormone called leptin spikes in altitude sickness ... Tschöp, M., Strasburger, C. J., Hartmann, G., Biollaz, J. & Bärtsch, P. (1998). 'Raised leptin concentrations at high altitude associated with loss of appetite.' *Lancet*, 352(9134), 1119–20. https://doi.org/10.1016/s0140-6736(05)79760-9

The more fat we lay down, the higher our leptin levels are ... Considine, R. V. et al. (1996). 'Serum Immunoreactive-Leptin Concentrations in Normal-Weight and Obese Humans.' *New England Journal of Medicine*, 334(5), 292–5. https://doi.org/10.1056/nejm199602013340503

... their brains simply don't register the high leptin ... Zelissen, P. M. J. et al. (2005). 'Effect of three treatment schedules of recombinant methionyl human leptin on body weight in obese adults: a randomized, placebo-controlled trial.' *Diabetes, Obesity and Metabolism*, 7(6), 755–61. https://doi.org/10.1111/j.1463-1326.2005.00468.x

... insulin and oestrogen also have a similar way of feeding back ... Air, E. L., Benoit, S. C., Smith, K. A. B., Clegg, D. J. & Woods, S. C. (2002). 'Acute third ventricular administration of insulin decreases food intake in two paradigms.' *Pharmacology, Biochemistry and Behavior*, 72(1–2), 423–9. https://doi.org/10.1016/s0091-3057(01)00780-8

Porte, D. & Woods, S. C. (1981). 'Regulation of food intake and body weight by insulin.' *Diabetologia*, 20(S1), 274–80. https://doi.org/10.1007/bf00254493

Hirschberg, A. L. (2012). 'Sex hormones, appetite and eating behaviour in women.' *Maturitas*, 71(3), 248–256. https://doi.org/10.1016/j.maturitas.2011.12.016

... set-point theory, which was first proposed in 1982. Ganipisetti, V. M. & Bollimunta, P. (2023). 'Obesity and Set-Point Theory.' In: StatPearls [Internet]. Treasure Island (FL): StatPearls Publishing

If you get people to swirl something sweet in their mouth ... Just, T., Pau, H. W., Engel, U. & Hummel, T. (2008). 'Cephalic phase insulin release in healthy humans after taste stimulation?' *Appetite*, 51(3):622–7. doi:10.1016/j.appet.2008.04.271

In rats, if you cut the nerve connecting the brain to the tongue ... Tonosaki, K., Hori, Y., Shimizu, Y. & Tonosaki, K. (2007). 'Relationships between insulin release and taste.' *Biomed Res*, 28(2):79–83. doi: 10.2220/biomedres.28.79. PMID: 17510492

... people who live with obesity see a much bigger spike in their cephalic-phase insulin response ... Teff, K. L., Mattes, R. D., Engelman, K. & Mattern, J. (1993). 'Cephalic-phase insulin in obese and normal-weight men: Relation to postprandial insulin.' *Metabolism*, 442(12), 1600-8. doi:10.1016/0026-0495(93)90157-J

... chewing triggers fullness hormones. Miquel-Kergoat, S., Azais-Braesco, V., Burton-Freeman, B. & Hetherington, M. M. (2015). 'Effects of chewing on appetite, food intake and gut hormones: A systematic review and meta-analysis.' *Physiology & Behavior*, 151, 88–96. https://doi.org/10.1016/j.physbeh.2015.07.017

But there's a catch: they will enjoy it less. Ferriday, D., Bosworth, M. L., Evans, N. R., Ciborowska, A., Godinot, N., Martin, N., Rogers, P. J. & Brunstrom, J. M. (2016). 'Are the effects of eating slowly on satiation and satiety anticipated in meal planning?' *Appetite*, 107:681. doi: 10.1016/j.appet.2016.08.037.

As your stomach becomes stretched ... Phillips, R. J. & Powley, T. L. (1996). 'Gastric volume rather than nutrient content inhibits food intake.' *American Journal of Physiology*, 271(3):R766–R79.

Schwartz, G. J. (2000). 'The role of gastrointestinal vagal afferents in the control of food intake: current prospects.' *Nutrition*, 16(10):866–73

This is called the ileal break ... Wen, J., Phillips, S. F., Sarr, M. G., Kost, L. J. & Holst, J. J. (1995). 'PYY and GLP-1 contribute to feedback inhibition from the canine ileum and colon.' *American Journal of Physiology*, 269(6):G945–52

I have already mentioned our friend GLP-1 ... Bodnaruc, A. M., Prud'homme, D., Blanchet, R. & Giroux, I. (2016). 'Nutritional modulation of endogenous glucagon-like peptide-1 secretion: a review.' *Nutrition & Metabolism*, 13:92. doi: 10.1186/s12986-016-0153-3. PMID: 27990172; PMCID: PMC5148911

One study found 45 different bacterial strains capable of stimulating GLP-1 ... Tomaro-Duchesneau, C. et al. (2020). 'Discovery of a bacterial peptide as a modulator of GLP-1 and metabolic disease.' *Scientific Reports*, 10(1). https://doi.org/10.1038/s41598-020-61112-0

... people living with obesity get less of a GLP-1 spike from their food ... Holst, J. J. (2007). 'The physiology of glucagon-like peptide 1.' *Physiological Reviews*, 87(4):1409–39

... unlike CCK, it is mostly stimulated further down the gut. Suzuki, K., Jayasena, C. N. & Bloom, S. R. (2011). 'The gut hormones in appetite regulation.' *Journal of Obesity*, 1–10. https://doi.org/10.1155/2011/528401

... after a gastric bypass, patients trigger both more PYY and GLP-1 ... Cummings, D. E., Weigle, D. S., Scott Frayo, R. et al. (2002). 'Plasma ghrelin levels after diet-induced weight loss or gastric bypass surgery.' *New England Journal of Medicine*, 346(21):1623–30

Le Roux, C. W., Welbourn, R., Werling, M. et al. (2007). 'Gut hormones as mediators of appetite and weight loss after Roux-en-Y gastric bypass.' *Annals of Surgery*, 246(5):780–5.

One study evaluated the levels of gut hormones in healthy subjects ... Cani, P. D., Lecourt, E., Dewulf, E. M. et al. (2009). 'Gut microbiota fermentation of prebiotics increases satietogenic and incretin gut peptide production with consequences for appetite sensation and glucose response after a meal.' *American Journal of Clinical Nutrition*, 90(5):1236–43

Figure 1. Natalucci, G., Riedl, S., Gleiss, A., Zidek, T. & Frisch, H. (2005). 'Spontaneous 24-h ghrelin secretion pattern in fasting subjects: maintenance of a meal-related pattern.' *European Journal of Endocrinology*, 152(6), 845–50. https://doi.org/10.1530/eje.1.01919

A biology textbook will tell you ghrelin ... Panda, S. (2018). *The Circadian Code: Lose Weight, Supercharge Your Energy and Sleep Well Every Night.* Random House

Long story short, a combination ... Ubaldo-Reyes, L., Buijs, R., Escobar, C. & Ángeles-Castellanos, M. (2017). 'Scheduled meal accelerates entrainment to a 6-h phase advance by shifting central and peripheral oscillations in rats.' *European Journal of Neuroscience/EJN*, 46(3), 1875–86. https://doi.org/10.1111/ejn.13633

... 'eat little and often' has ingrained itself into wellness culture ... Ma, Y. et al. (2003). 'Association between eating patterns and obesity in a free-living US adult population.' *Am J Epidemiol* 1;158(1):85–92. doi: 10.1093/aje/kwg117

In 1970, snacks made up one tenth of our calories ... Kant, A. K. & Graubard, B. I. (2015). '40 year trends in meal and snack eating behaviours of American adults.' *Journal of the Academy of Nutrition and Dietetics*, 115(1): 50–63

American adults eat between 4.2 and 10.5 times a day ... Gill, S. & Panda, S. (2015). 'A smartphone app reveals erratic diurnal eating patterns in humans that can be modulated for health benefits.' *Cell Metabolism*, 22(5), 789–98. https://doi.org/10.1016/j.cmet.2015.09.005

In the 1970s, the vast majority of people only had three eating episodes ... Popkin, B. M. & Duffey, K. J. (2010). 'Does hunger and satiety drive eating anymore?' *Am J Clin Nutr*, 91(5):1342–7

... only half of Japanese people report regularly eating snacks ... Murakami, K., Livingstone, M. B. E., Masayasu, S. & Sasaki, S. (2022). 'Eating patterns in a nationwide sample of Japanese aged 1–79 years from MINNADE study: eating frequency, clock time for eating, time spent on eating and variability of eating patterns.' *Public Health Nutr*, 25(6):1515–27. doi: 10.1017/S1368980021000975

... just over 3 per cent of Japanese people are obese ... Yoshiike, N. & Miyoshi, M. (2013). '[Epidemiological aspects of overweight and obesity in Japan--international comparisons].' *Nihon Rinsho*, 71(2):207–16.

... if you take a stool sample from someone who is jet lagged ... Thaiss, C. A. (2014). 'Transkingdom control of microbiota diurnal oscillations promotes metabolic homeostasis.' *Cell*, 159(3):514–29. doi: 10.1016/j.cell.2014.09.048

... one night of sleep disruption can also reduce leptin and spike ghrelin ... van Egmond, L. T., Meth, E. M. S., Engström, J., Ilemosoglou, M., Keller, J. A., Vogel, H. & Benedict, C. (2023). 'Effects of acute sleep loss on leptin, ghrelin, and adiponectin in adults with healthy weight and obesity: A laboratory study.' *Obesity*, 31(3):635–41. doi: 10.1002/oby.23616

... if it shoots up briefly, like nature intended, you will lose your appetite ... Charmandari, E., Tsigos, C. & Chrousos, G. (2005). 'Endocrinology of the stress response.' *Annu Rev Physiol*, 67:259–84. doi: 10.1146/annurev.physiol.67.040403.120816

However, if you have low-level chronic stress ... Adam, T. C. & Epel, E. S. (2007). 'Stress, eating and the reward system.' *Physiol Behav*, 91(4):449–58. doi: 10.1016/j.physbeh.2007.04.011

... ghrelin has a powerful effect on several areas in the brain ... Malik, S., McGlone, F., Bedrossian, D. & Dagher, A. (2008). 'Ghrelin modulates brain activity in areas that control appetitive behavior.' *Cell Metabolism*, 7(5):400–9

... when people are given an injection of ghrelin, their thoughts of food become more vivid ... Schmid, D. A., Held, K., Ising, M., Uhr, M., Weikel, J. C. & Steiger, A. (2005). 'Ghrelin stimulates appetite, imagination of food, GH, ACTH, and cortisol, but does not affect leptin in normal controls.' *Neuropsychopharmacology*, 30(6):1187–92

... rats lose their appetite as their cortisol rises ... Adam, T. C. & Epel, E. S. (2007). 'Stress, eating and the reward system.' *Physiol Behav*, 91(4):449–58. doi: 10.1016/j.physbeh.2007.04.011

Humans aren't quite the same – about 30 per cent will lose their appetites ... Adam, T. C. & Epel, E. S. (24 July 2007). 'Stress, eating and the reward system.' *Physiol Behav*, 91(4):449–58. doi: 10.1016/j.physbeh.2007.04.011

... Dr Chris van Tulleken, offered himself up as tribute ... Van Tulleken, C. (2023). *Ultra-Processed People: Why Do We All Eat Stuff That Isn't Food ... and Why Can't We Stop?* Random House

... our blood sugar can influence appetite and eating habits. Mayer, J. (1996). 'Glucostatic mechanism of regulation of food intake.' *Obesity Research*, 4(5), 493–6. https://doi.org/10.1002/j.1550-8528.1996.tb00260.x

... in the 2019 PREDICT 1 study ... Wyatt, P. et al. (2021). 'Postprandial glycaemic dips predict appetite and energy intake in healthy individuals.' *Nature Metabolism*, 3(4), 523–9. https://doi.org/10.1038/s42255-021-00383-x

... blood-sugar control seems to influence our cravings ... Page, K. A. et al. (2011). 'Circulating glucose levels modulate neural control of desire for high-calorie foods in humans.' *Journal of Clinical Investigation* 121(10), 4161–9. https://doi.org/10.1172/jci57873

Endocrinologist Dr Saira Hameed describes this as eating 'packaged hunger' ... Hameed, S. (2022). *The Full Diet: The Revolutionary Guide to Ditching Ultra-Processed Foods and Achieving Lasting Health*. Penguin UK

We see this with artificial sweeteners ... Blundell, J. E. (2019). 'Low-calorie sweeteners: more complicated than sweetness without calories.' *Am J Clin Nutr* 1;109(5):1237–8. doi: 10.1093/ajcn/nqz015. PMID: 30997491

Hill, S. E., Prokosch, M. L., Morin, A. & Rodeheffer, C. D. (2014). 'The effect of non-caloric sweeteners on cognition, choice, and post-consumption satisfaction.' *Appetite*, 83:82–8. doi: 10.1016/j.appet.2014.08.003

Toews, I., Lohner, S., Küllenberg de Gaudry, D., Sommer, H. & Meerpohl, J. J. (2019). 'Association between intake of non-sugar sweeteners and health outcomes: systematic review and meta-analyses of randomised and non-randomised controlled trials and observational studies.' *BMJ*, 364. doi: 10.1136/bmj.k4718. Erratum in: *BMJ* (January 2019), 364. doi: 10.1136/bmj.l156

... artificial sweeteners probably increase your risk of diabetes ... Nettleton, J. A. et al. (2009). 'Diet soda intake and risk of incident metabolic syndrome and type 2 diabetes in the Multi-Ethnic Study of Atherosclerosis (MESA).' *Diabetes Care*, 32(4):688–94. doi: 10.2337/dc08-1799

Anderson, J. J. et al. (2020). 'The associations of sugar-sweetened, artificially sweetened and naturally sweet juices with all-cause mortality in 198,285 UK Biobank participants: a prospective cohort study.' *BMC Med*, 18(1):97. doi: 10.1186/s12916-020-01554-5

CHAPTER 4: CAN WE CHANGE OUR BIOLOGY?

... 45 per cent of people around the world are on a diet ... Purcell, S. & O'Brien, C. (2021). 'More than half of the global population would rather exercise more and/or eat more healthily' [press release]. Ipsos. https://www.ipsos.com/sites/default/files/ct/news/documents/2021-01/pr-global-weight-and-actions.pdf

In 2012, a Finnish study looked at 4,129 individual twins ... Pietiläinen, K. H., Saarni, S. E., Kaprio, J. & Rissanen, A. (2012). 'Does dieting make you fat? A twin study.' *International Journal of Obesity*, 36(3):456–64. doi: 10.1038/ijo.2011.160

... other studies have demonstrated the same results ... Lowe, M. R., Doshi, S. D., Katterman, S. N. & Feig, E. H. (2013). 'Dieting and restrained eating as prospective predictors of weight gain.' *Front Psychol*, 4:577. doi:10.3389/fpsyg.2013.00577

The first thing it will do is ramp up your appetite ... Melby, C. L., Paris, H. L., Foright, R. M. & Peth, J. (2017). 'Attenuating the biologic drive for weight regain following weight loss: Must what goes down always go back up?' *Nutrients*, 9(5). doi:10.3390/nu9050468

Both a drop in leptin and a rise in ghrelin will produce changes in MRI brain scans ... Rosenbaum, M., Sy, M., Pavlovich, K., Leibel, R. L. & Hirsch, J. (2008). 'Leptin reverses weight loss-induced changes in regional neural activity responses to visual food stimuli.' *J Clin Invest*, 118(7):2583–91. doi: 10.1172/JCI35055

Malik. S., McGlone, F., Bedrossian, D. & Dagher, A. (2008). 'Ghrelin modulates brain activity in areas that control appetitive behavior.' *Cell Metab*, 7(5):400–9. doi: 10.1016/j.cmet.2008.03.007

The most famous study to demonstrate this ... Fothergill, E. et al. (2016). 'Persistent metabolic adaptation 6 years after "The Biggest Loser" competition.' *Obesity*, 24(8):1612–19. doi:10.1002/oby.21538

Rosenbaum, M., Hirsch, J., Gallagher, D. A. & Leibel, R. L. (2008). 'Long-term persistence of adaptive thermogenesis in subjects who have maintained a reduced body weight.' *Am J Clin Nutr*, 88(4):906–12. doi:10.1093/ajcn/88.4.906

REFERENCES

Tremblay, A., Royer, M-M., Chaput, J-P. & Doucet, É. (2013). 'Adaptive thermogenesis can make a difference in the ability of obese individuals to lose body weight.' *Int J Obes*, 37:759–64. doi:10.1038/ijo.2012.124

... in 2011, researchers put 50 overweight or obese participants ... Sumithran, P., Prendergast, L. A., Delbridge, E., Purcell, K., Shulkes, A., Kriketos, A. & Proietto, J. (2011). 'Long-term persistence of hormonal adaptations to weight loss.' *N Engl J Med*, 365(17):1597–604. doi: 10.1056/NEJMoa1105816

... it doesn't take long for cortisol levels to rise and thyroid levels to fall ... Ebbeling, C. B. (2012). 'Effects of dietary composition on energy expenditure during weight-loss maintenance.' *JAMA*, 307(24):2627–34. doi: 10.1001/jama.2012.6607

If the body has too much insulin around, the fat-storing switch is turned on ... Duncan, R. E., Ahmadian, M., Jaworski, K., Sarkadi-Nagy, E. & Sul, H. S. (2007). 'Regulation of lipolysis in adipocytes.' *Annu Rev Nutr*, 27:79–101. doi:10.1146/

... even when they aren't eating and are in a 'fasted state' ... Polonsky, K. S., Given, B. D., Van Cauter, E. (1988). 'Twenty-four-hour profiles and pulsatile patterns of insulin secretion in normal and obese subjects.' *J Clin Invest*. 81(2):442–8. doi: 10.1172/JCI113339

... coined by Anton, et al. in their knockout paper ... Anton, S. D. et al. (2018). 'Flipping the metabolic switch: Understanding and applying the health benefits of fasting.' *Obesity*, 26(2):254–68. doi: 10.1002/oby.22065

When people first start IF, they might not enter fat burning ... Ruderman, N., Meyers, M., Chipkin, S. & Tornheim, K. 'Hormone-Fuel Interrelation-ships: Fed State, Starvation, and Diabetes Mellitus' | Oncohema Key. https:// oncohemakey. com/hormone-fuel-interrelationships-fed-state-starvation-and-diabetes-mellitus/

... one of the first was in 2012 and it completely baffled scientists ... Hatori, M. et al. (2012). 'Time-Restricted Feeding without Reducing Caloric Intake Prevents Metabolic Diseases in Mice Fed a High-Fat Diet.' *Cell Metabolism*, 15(6), 848–60. https://doi.org/10.1016/j.cmet.2012.04.019

... insulin works best earlier in the day ... Sturis, J., Scheen, A. J., Leproult, R., Polonsky, K. S. & Van Cauter, E. (1995). '24-hour glucose profiles during continuous or oscillatory insulin infusion. Demonstration of the functional significance of ultradian insulin oscillations.' *The Journal of Clinical Investigation* 95(4), 1464–71. https://doi.org/10.1172/jci117817

This burden of work and its downstream consequences ... Picard, M., Juster, R. P. & McEwen, B. S. (2014). 'Mitochondrial allostatic load puts the "gluc" back in glucocorticoids.' *Nat Rev Endocrinol*, 10(5):303–10. doi: 10.1038/nrendo.2014.22

Giri, B., Dey, S., Das, T., Sarkar, M., Banerjee, J. & Dash, S. K. (2018). 'Chronic hyperglycemia mediated physiological alteration and metabolic distortion leads to organ dysfunction, infection, cancer progression and other pathophysiological consequences: An update on glucose toxicity.' *Biomed Pharmacother*, 107:306–28. doi: 10.1016/j.biopha.2018.07.157

... mitochondrial dysfunction is something I see every day ... Hyman, M. (2023). *Young Forever*. Hachette UK

... mitochondrial dysfunction appears to be implicated in poorly understood conditions ... Molnar, T. et al. (2024). 'Mitochondrial dysfunction in long COVID: mechanisms, consequences, and potential therapeutic approaches.' *Geroscience*. doi: 10.1007/s11357-024-01165-5.

Meeus, M., Nijs, J., Hermans, L., Goubert, D. & Calders, P. (2013). 'The role of mitochondrial dysfunctions due to oxidative and nitrosative stress in the chronic pain or chronic fatigue syndromes and fibromyalgia patients: peripheral and central mechanisms as therapeutic targets?' *Expert Opin Ther Targets*, 17(9):1081–9. doi: 10.1517/14728222.2013.818657

In Spain, France and Italy over a third of the population skip breakfast ... Spector, T. (2015c). *The Diet Myth: The Real Science Behind What We Eat*. Hachette UK

... poor-quality, small-scale studies of people living with obesity ... Casazza, K. et al. (2013). 'Myths, presumptions, and facts about obesity.' *N Engl J Med*, 368(5):446–54. doi: 10.1056/NEJMsa1208051

... many studies show no effect on total calories consumed if skipping breakfast ... Sievert, K. et al (2019). 'Effect of breakfast on weight and energy intake: systematic review and meta-analysis of randomised controlled trials.' *BMJ*, 364:l42. doi: 10.1136/bmj.l42

Studies suggest hunter-gatherers regularly had long periods without food ... Crittenden, A. N. & Schnorr, S. L. (2017). 'Current views on hunter-gatherer nutrition and the evolution of the human diet.' *Am J Phys Anthropol*, 16263(Suppl):84–109

... studies show they still boost their microbiome ... Spector, T. (2015d). *The Diet Myth: The Real Science Behind What We Eat*. Hachette UK

It takes about 12 weeks for this to happen ... Panda, S. (2018). *The Circadian Code: Lose Weight, Supercharge Your Energy and Sleep Well Every Night*. Random House

In fact, it can take as little as four days ... Ravussin, E., Beyl, R. A., Poggiogalle, E., Hsia, D. S. & Peterson, C. M. (2019). 'Early Time-Restricted Feeding Reduces Appetite and Increases Fat Oxidation But Does Not Affect Energy Expenditure in Humans.' *Obesity*, 27(8), 1244–54. https://doi.org/10.1002/oby.22518

These ketones also reduce brain inflammation ... Panda, S. (2018). *The Circadian Code: Lose Weight, Supercharge Your Energy and Sleep Well Every Night*. Random House

... fasting results in less depression, better memory and reduces your risk of neurodegenerative diseases ... Lee, J., Seroogy, K. B. & Mattson, M. P. (2002). 'Dietary restriction enhances neurotrophin expression and neurogenesis in the hippocampus of adult mice.' *Journal of Neurochemistry*, 80(3), 539–47. https://doi.org/10.1046/j.0022-3042.2001.00747.x

Mattson, M. P. (2005). 'Energy intake, meal frequency, and health: a neurobiological perspective.' *Annual Review of Nutrition*, 25(1), 237–60. https://doi.org/10.1146/annurev.nutr.25.050304.092526

Mattson, M. P., Longo, V. D. & Harvie, M. (2017). 'Impact of intermittent fasting on health and disease processes.' *Ageing Research Reviews*, 39, 46–58. https://doi.org/10.1016/j.arr.2016.10.005

In fact, low BDNF is linked to depression ... Mattson, M. P. (2005). 'Energy intake, meal frequency, and health: a neurobiological perspective.' *Annu Rev Nutr*; 25:237–60. doi: 10.1146/annurev.nutr.25.050304.092526

Time-restricted eating helps by containing CCK ... Panda, S. (2018). *The Circadian Code: Lose Weight, Supercharge Your Energy and Sleep Well Every Night.* Random House

If mice are left to eat all day, they develop features of IBS ... Ibid

Speaking of your microbiome, it needs rest too ... Remely, M. et al. (2015). 'Increased gut microbiota diversity and abundance of Faecalibacterium prausnitzii and Akkermansia after fasting: a pilot study.' *Wien Klin Wochenschr*, 127(9-10):394–8. doi: 10.1007/s00508-015-0755-1

McDonald, D. (2018). 'American Gut: an Open Platform for Citizen Science Microbiome Research.' *mSystems*, 3(3):e00031–18. doi: 10.1128/mSystems.00031-18

The main bug that loves fasting is called *Akkermansia* ... Hyman, M. (2021). *The Pegan Diet: 21 Practical Principles for Reclaiming Your Health in a Nutritionally Confusing World.* Hachette UK

... people notice an improvement in rheumatoid-arthritis pain during Ramadan ... Said, M. S. M. et al. (2013). 'The effects of the Ramadan month of fasting on disease activity in patients with rheumatoid arthritis.' *Turkish I Rheumatol*, 28(3):189–94. doi:10.5606/tjr.2013.3147

Faris, M. A. et al. (2012). 'Intermittent fasting during Ramadan attenuates proinflammatory cytokines and immune cells in healthy subjects.' *Nutr Res*, 32(12):947–55. doi:10.1016/J.NUTRES.2012.06.021

... chemicals are involved in promoting asthma, allergies, autoimmune disease and inflammatory bowel disease ... Liu, Y., Yu, Y., Matarese, G. & La Cava, A. (2012). 'Fasting-induced hypoleptinemia expands functional regulatory T cells in systemic lupus erythematosus.' *Immunol*, 188(5):2070–3. doi:10.4049/jimmunol.1102835

This too has a circadian rhythm. Ibid.

... instead, protein can be used to build muscle. McPherron, A. C., Guo, T., Bond, N. D. & Gavrilova, O. (2013). 'Increasing muscle mass to improve metabolism.' *Adipocyte*;2(2):92–8. doi: 10.4161/adip.22500

TRE even has another clever way of building muscle ... Salgin, B., Marcovecchio, M. L., Hill, N., Dunger, D. B. & Frystyk, J. (2012). 'The effect of prolonged fasting on levels of growth hormone-binding protein and free growth hormone.' *Growth Horm IGF Res*, 22(2):76–81. doi: 10.1016/j.ghir.2012.02.003

... this is your body's own perfectly legal steroid ... Monson, J. P., Drake, W. M., Carroll, P. V., Weaver, J. U., Rodriguez-Arnao, J. & Savage, M. O. (2002). 'Influence of growth hormone on accretion of bone mass.' *Horm Res Paediatr*, 58(1):52–6. doi:10.1159/000064765

Bex, M. & Bouillon, R. (2003). 'Growth hormone and bone health.' *Horm Res Paediatr*, 60(3):80–6. doi:10.1159/000074507

Dioufa, N. et al. (2010). 'Acceleration of wound healing by growth hormone-releasing hormone and its agonists.' *Proc Natl Acad Sci USA*, 107(43):18611, doi:10.1073/PNAS.1013942107

... within an 11-hour window were significantly protected from breast cancer ... Marinac, C. R. et al. (2015). 'Prolonged Nightly Fasting and Breast Cancer Risk: Findings from NHANES (2009-2010).' *Cancer Epidemiol Biomarkers Prev*, 24(5):783–9. doi: 10.1158/1055-9965.EPI-14-1292

... fasting appears to reduce the speed of tumour growth and improves response to chemotherapy ... Lee, C. et al. (2012). 'Fasting cycles retard growth of tumors and sensitize a range of cancer cell types to chemotherapy.' *Sci Transl Med*, 4(124):124ra27. doi:10.1126/scitranslmed.3003293

... controlling insulin resistance between the ages of 20 and 30 reduced men's risk of a heart attack ... Eddy, D., Schlessinger, L., Kahn, R., Peskin, B. & Schiebinger, R. (2009). 'Relationship of insulin resistance and related metabolic variables to coronary artery disease: a mathematical analysis.' *Diabetes Care*, 32(2), 361–6. https://doi.org/10.2337/dc08-0854

TRE, believe it or not, is an excellent trick for optimising it. Panda, S., PhD. (2020). *The Circadian Code: Lose Weight, Supercharge Your Energy, and Transform Your Health from Morning to Midnight: Longevity Book*. Rodale Books

... bile acid ... is partly made of cholesterol ... Watanabe, M. et al. (2006). 'Bile acids induce energy expenditure by promoting intracellular thyroid hormone activation.' *Nature*, 439(7075):484–9. doi: 10.1038/nature04330

... an eating window of six hours was just as effective as blood-pressure medication. Sutton, E. F., Beyl, R., Early, K. S., Cefalu, W. T., Ravussin, E. & Peterson, C. M. (2018). 'Early time-restricted feeding improves insulin sensitivity, blood pressure, and oxidative stress even without weight loss in men with prediabetes.' *Cell Metab*, 27(6):1212–21.e3. doi: 10.1016/j.cmet.2018.04.010. Epub 10 May 2018

... a Japanese scientist called Dr Yoshinori Ohsumi ... The Nobel Prize in Physiology or Medicine 2016. (n.d.). NobelPrize.org. https://www.nobelprize.org/prizes/medicine/2016/press-release/

Rabinowitz, J. D. & White, E. (2010). 'Autophagy and metabolism.' *Science*, 330(6009): 1344–8. doi:10.1126/science.1193497

Kirkin, V. (2019). 'History of the selective autophagy research: How did it begin and where does it stand today?', *Journal of Molecular Biology*, 432(1):3-27. doi: 10.1016/j.jmb.2019.05.010

... **Dr Jason Fung has been reversing type 2 diabetes in his clinic** ... Furmli, S., Elmasry, R., Ramos, M. & Fung, J. (2018). 'Therapeutic use of intermittent fasting for people with type 2 diabetes as an alternative to insulin.' *BMJ Case Rep*;2018. doi:10.1136/bcr-2017-221854

Dr Unwin ... has also tired of only treating diabetes ... Unwin, D., Delon, C., Unwin, J., Tobin, S. & Taylor, R. (2023). 'What predicts drug-free type 2 diabetes remission? Insights from an 8-year general practice service evaluation of a lower carbohydrate diet with weight loss.' *BMJ Nutrition, Prevention & Health*, 6(1), 46–55. https://doi.org/10.1136/bmjnph-2022-000544

... **committing to long-term TRE will result in less fat and more muscle** ... de Cabo, R. & Mattson, M. P. (26 December 2019). 'Effects of Intermittent Fasting on Health, Aging, and Disease.' *N Engl J Med*, 381(26):2541–51. doi: 10.1056/NEJMra1905136.

Moro, T. et al. (2016). 'Effects of eight weeks of time-restricted feeding (16/8) on basal metabolism, maximal strength, body composition, inflammation, and cardiovascular risk factors in resistance-trained males.' *J Transl Med*, 14(1):290. doi: 10.1186/s12967-016-1044-0

CHAPTER 5: OUR HERITAGE – CAN WE INHERIT OBESITY?

... **National Food Surveys (NFS) at the time** ... Gwynn, M. & Coren, G. (2015). *Back in Time for Dinner: From Spam to Sushi: How We've Changed the Way We Eat.* https://openlibrary.org/books/OL27188208M/Back_in_time_for_dinner

My favourite study on genetic weight ... Stunkard, A. J., Sørensen, T. I., Hanis, C., Teasdale, T. W., Chakraborty, R., Schull, W. J. & Schulsinger, F. (23 January 1986). 'An adoption study of human obesity.' *N Engl J Med*, 314(4):193–8. doi: 10.1056/NEJM198601233140401

... **three out of four Americans still believe obesity is caused by a lack of will-power** ... Rosenthal, R. J., Morton, J., Brethauer, S., Mattar, S., de Maria, E., Benz, J. K., Titus, J. & Sterrett, D. (2017). 'Obesity in America.' *Surg Obes Relat Dis*, 13(10):1643–50. doi: 10.1016/j.soard.2017.08.002

... **in 2003, Chinese identical girls were accidentally separated at birth** ... https://www.pbs.org/independentlens/documentaries/twin-sisters. Accessed 2 July 2023.

... **children in the UK are, on average, 7cm shorter than other European children** ... NCD Risk Factor Collaboration (NCD-RisC). (7 November 2020). 'Height and body-mass index trajectories of school-aged children and adolescents from 1985 to 2019 in 200 countries and territories: a pooled analysis of 2181 population-based studies with 65 million participants.' *Lancet*, 396(10261):1511–24. doi: 10.1016/S0140-6736(20)31859-6

In fact, if you were to pluck any pair of identical twins off the street ... Referenced in: Spector, T. (2015). *The Diet Myth: The Real Science Behind What We Eat.* Hachette UK

... on average, 60–70 per cent of our weight is decided by genes ... Stunkard, A. J., Foch, T. T. & Hrubec, Z. (1986). 'A twin study of human obesity.' *JAMA*, 256(1):51–4

Llewellyn, C. H., van Jaarsveld, C. H., Boniface, D., Carnell, S. & Wardle, J. (December 2008). 'Eating rate is a heritable phenotype related to weight in children.' *Am J Clin Nutr*, 88(6):1560–6. doi: 10.3945/ajcn.2008.26175

Stubbe, J. H. et al (2006). 'Genetic influences on exercise participation in 37,051 twin pairs from seven countries.' *PLoS One*, 1(1), doi: 10.1371/journal.pone.0000022

If you have a sweet tooth, 50 per cent of this seems to come down to genes ... Keskitalo, K., Tuorila, H., Spector, T. D., Cherkas, L. F., Knaapila, A., Kaprio, J., Silventoinen, K. & Perola, M. (2008). 'The Three-Factor Eating Questionnaire, body mass index, and responses to sweet and salty fatty foods: a twin study of genetic and environmental associations.' *Am J Clin Nutr*, 88(2):263–71. doi: 10.1093/ajcn/88.2.263

... a propensity for obesity is strongly linked to sugar-loving genes ... Locke, A. E. et al. (2015). 'Genetic studies of body mass index yield new insights for obesity biology.' *Nature*, 518(7538), 197–206. https://doi.org/10.1038/nature14177

In 1990, researchers decided to purposely overfeed a group of identical twins ... Bouchard, C. et al. (1990). 'The response to long-term overfeeding in identical twins.' *N Engl J Med*, 322(21):1477–82. doi: 10.1056/NEJM199005243222101

... a rare genetic condition called Prader-Willi syndrome ... Butler, M. G., Manzardo, A. M., Heinemann, J., Loker, C. & Loker, J. (2017). 'Causes of death in Prader-Willi syndrome: Prader-Willi Syndrome Association (USA) 40-year mortality survey.' *Genetics in Medicine*, 19(6), 635–42. https://doi.org/10.1038/gim.2016.178

This genetic disease essentially interferes with hormones ... Rahman, Q. F. A., Jufri, N. F. & Hamid, A. (2023). 'Hyperphagia in Prader-Willi syndrome with obesity: From development to pharmacological treatment.' *IRDR*, 12(1), 5–12. https://doi.org/10.5582/irdr.2022.01127

In 1997, scientists discovered a rare leptin-deficiency gene ... Montague, C. T. et al. (1997). 'Congenital leptin deficiency is associated with severe early-onset obesity in humans.' *Nature*, 387(6636):903–8. doi: 10.1038/43185

Soon they started injecting it into everyone ... Heymsfield, S. B. et al. (1999). 'Recombinant leptin for weight loss in obese and lean adults: a randomized, controlled, dose-escalation trial.' *JAMA*, 282(16):1568–75. doi: 10.1001/jama.282.16.1568

Labradors technically have a genetic mutation which drives obesity ... Raffan, E. et al. (2016). 'A deletion in the canine POMC gene is associated with weight and appetite in obesity-prone Labrador retriever dogs.' *Cell Metab*, 23(5):893–900. doi: 10.1016/j.cmet.2016.04.012

REFERENCES

In 1998, researchers in Berlin discovered a similar POMC mutation ... Krude, H., Biebermann, H., Luck, W., Horn, R., Brabant, G. & Grüters, A. (1998). 'Severe early-onset obesity, adrenal insufficiency and red hair pigmentation caused by POMC mutations in humans.' *Nat Genet*, 19(2):155–7. doi: 10.1038/509

... a mutation of the MC$_4$R gene, which also blunts the brain's response to leptin ... Yeo, G. S., Farooqi, I. S., Aminian, S., Halsall, D. J., Stanhope, R. G. & O'Rahilly, S. (1998). 'A frameshift mutation in MC4R associated with dominantly inherited human obesity.' *Nat Genet*, 20(2):111–2. doi: 10.1038/2404

... up to 6 per cent of severely obese children ... Farooqi, I. S., Keogh, J. M., Yeo, G. S., Lank, E. J., Cheetham, T. & O'Rahilly, S. (2003). 'Clinical spectrum of obesity and mutations in the melanocortin 4 receptor gene.' *N Engl J Med*, 348(12):1085–95. doi: 10.1056/NEJMoa022050

... 1 per cent of people with a BMI greater than 30 ... Alharbi, K. K. et al. (2007). 'Prevalence and functionality of paucimorphic and private MC4R mutations in a large, unselected European British population, scanned by meltMADGE.' *Hum Mutat*, 28(3):294–302. doi: 10.1002/humu.20404

... there are around 100 genes that code for weight ... Locke, A. E. et al. (2015). 'Genetic studies of body mass index yield new insights for obesity biology.' *Nature*, 518(7538):197–206. doi: 10.1038/nature14177

And the more you have, the better you are at stripping out every last calorie ... Rukh, G., Ericson, U., Andersson-Assarsson, J., Orho-Melander, M. & Sonestedt, E. (2017). 'Dietary starch intake modifies the relation between copy number variation in the salivary amylase gene and BMI.' *Am J Clin Nutr*, 106(1):256–62. doi: 10.3945/ajcn.116.149831

... if a Chinese woman moves to America, she will double her risk of getting breast cancer ... Fung, J. (2020). *The Cancer Code: A New Paradigm for Understanding Cancer*. HarperThorsons

... a Ghanaian man is 11–15 times more likely to become obese after migrating to Europe ... Agyemang, C. et al. (2022). 'Cohort profile: Research on Obesity and Diabetes among African Migrants in Europe and Africa Prospective (RODAM-Pros) cohort study.' *BMJ Open*, 12(12), e067906. https://doi.org/10.1136/bmjopen-2022-067906

... how heritable obesity is seems to depend on which country you live in. Min, J., Chiu, D. T. & Wang, Y. (2013). 'Variation in the heritability of body mass index based on diverse twin studies: a systematic review.' *Obesity Reviews*, 14(11), 871–82. https://doi.org/10.1111/obr.12065

If we home in on a single country ... Rokholm, B., Silventoinen, K., Tynelius, P., Gamborg, M., Sorensen, T. I. & Rasmussen, F. (2011). 'Increasing genetic variance of body mass index during the Swedish obesity epidemic.' *PloS one*, 6(11):e27135

Rokholm, B., Silventoinen, K., Angquist, L., Skytthe, A., Kyvik, K. O. & Sorensen, T. I. (2011). 'Increased genetic variance of BMI with a higher prevalence of obesity.' *PloS One*, 6(6):e20816

... a child living in an obesogenic home has an 86 per cent heritability of obese genes ... Schrempft, S., van Jaarsveld, C. H. M., Fisher, A., Herle, M., Smith, A. D., Fildes, A. & Llewellyn, C. H. (2018). 'Variation in the heritability of child body mass index by obesogenic home environment.' *JAMA Pediatrics*, 172(12), 1153. https://doi.org/10.1001/jamapediatrics.2018.1508

... we seem to share a lot of microbiome similarities with anyone we live with ... Song, S. J. et al. (2013). 'Cohabiting family members share microbiota with one another and with their dogs.' *eLife*, 2. https://doi.org/10.7554/elife.00458

... growing up with pets reduces your risk of eczema ... Toyokuni, K. et al. (2024). 'Influence of household pet ownership and filaggrin loss-of-function mutations on eczema prevalence in children: A birth cohort study.' *Allergology International*. https://doi.org/10.1016/j.alit.2024.01.003

Prescott, S. L. et al. (2017). 'The skin microbiome: impact of modern environments on skin ecology, barrier integrity, and systemic immune programming.' *The World Allergy Organization Journal*, 10(29). https://doi.org/10.1186/s40413-017-0160-5

... some microbes are specifically influenced by your genes ... Pennisi, E. (2014). 'Genetics may foster bugs that keep you thin.' *Science*, 346(6210), 687. https://doi.org/10.1126/science.346.6210.687

One mouse study looked at how changing diets in each generation ... Sonnenburg, E. D. et al. (2016). 'Diet-induced extinctions in the gut microbiota compound over generations.' *Nature* 529, 7585: 212–5, https://doi.org/10.1038/nature16504

... if the mother was overweight, the baby was exposed to an environment in the womb ... Gaillard, R. (2015). 'Maternal obesity during pregnancy and cardiovascular development and disease in the offspring.' *European Journal of Epidemiology*, 30(11), 1141–52. https://doi.org/10.1007/s10654-015-0085-7

... if your mother had gestational diabetes, you are three times more likely to develop obesity. Meek, C. L. (2023). 'An unwelcome inheritance: childhood obesity after diabetes in pregnancy.' *Diabetologia*, 66(11), 1961–70. https://doi.org/10.1007/s00125-023-05965-w

... a study looking at child obesity between 1980 and 2001 ... Kim, J. et al. (2006). 'Trends in overweight from 1980 through 2001 among preschool-aged children enrolled in a health maintenance organization.' *Obesity*, 14(7):1107–12. doi: 10.1038/oby.2006.126

A study in Cambridge revealed ... Baker, P., Smith, J., Salmon, L., Friel, S., Kent, G., Iellamo, A., Dadhich, J. P. & Renfrew, M. J. (2016). 'Global trends and patterns of commercial milk-based formula sales: is an unprecedented infant and young child feeding transition underway?' *Public Health Nutr*, 19(14):2540–50. doi: 10.1017/S1368980016001117

... food industries have tweaked formulas to make them hyper-palatable ... Van Tulleken, C. (2023c). *Ultra-Processed People: Why Do We All Eat Stuff That Isn't Food . . . and Why Can't We Stop?* Random House

Obese children are 17 times more likely to be obese adults. Fung, J. (2016). *The Obesity Code: Unlocking the Secrets of Weight Loss.* Scribe Publications

... childhood obesity is directly linked to an increased risk of heart disease and overall mortality in adulthood ... Baker, J. L., Olsen, L. W. & Sørensen, T. I. (2007). 'Childhood body-mass index and the risk of coronary heart disease in adulthood.' *N Engl J Med*, 357(23):2329–37. doi: 10.1056/NEJMoa072515

Juonala, M. et al. (2011). 'Childhood adiposity, adult adiposity, and cardiovascular risk factors.' *N Engl J Med*, 365(20):1876–85. doi: 10.1056/NEJMoa1010112

If an overweight child develops a normal BMI by adulthood ... Ibid.

... the UK has the lowest rate of breastfeeding in the world ... 'International comparisons of health and wellbeing in early childhood.' (n.d.). Nuffield Trust. https://www.nuffieldtrust.org.uk/research/international-comparisons-of-health-and-wellbeing-in-early-childhood#:~:text=The%20UK%20has%20one%20of,compared%20with%2062.5%25%20in%20Sweden

Public-health campaigns have dramatically improved rates of breastfeeding ... World Health Organization, 'Exclusive breastfeeding under 6 months.' Data by country, 2022. Available at: https://www.who.int/data/gho/indicator-metadata-registry/imr-details/130. Accessed 27 October 2024

Figure 2. 'International comparisons of health and wellbeing in early childhood.' (n.d.). Nuffield Trust. https://www.nuffieldtrust.org.uk/research/international-comparisons-of-health-and-wellbeing-in-early-childhood#:~:text=The%20UK%20has%20one%20of,compared%20with%2062.5%25%20in%20Sweden

CHAPTER 6: A HISTORY LESSON – WHERE DID WE GO WRONG?

... some say its first depiction was 35,000 years ago ... Haslam, D. & Rigby, N. (2010). 'The art of medicine a long look at obesity.' *Lancet*, 376, 85– 6. https://www.thelancet.com/action/showPdf?pii=S0140-6736 per cent2810 per cent2961065-3

It seems as long as we have been worrying about obesity ... Foxcroft, L. (2013). *Calories & Corsets: A History of Dieting Over 2,000 Years.* Profile Books

Compare that to 8 per cent in the UK and 14 per cent in Europe today. Avison, Z. (2020). 'Why UK consumers spend 8 per cent of their money on food.' https://ahdb.org.uk/news/consumer-insight-why-uk-consumers-spend-8-of-their-money-on-food

Office of National Statistics (2017). 'Living Costs and Food Survey.' https://www.ons.gov.uk/peoplepopulationandcommunity/personalandhouseholdfinances/incomeandwealth/methodologies/livingcostsandfoodsurvey

Eurostat (2023). 'How much do households spend on food and alcohol?' *Eurostat.* https://ec.europa.eu/eurostat/web/products-eurostat-news/w/ddn-20230201-1#:~:text=In per cent202021 per cent2C per cent20households per cent20in per cent20the,14.3 per cent25 per cent20of per cent20total per cent20 household per cent20expenditure

In the 1950s, most men came home for lunch ... Gwynn, M. (2015). *Back in Time for Dinner: From Spam to Sushi: How We've Changed the Way We Eat.* Bantam Press

Many mothers were now employed ... Roantree, B. & Vira, K. (2017). 'The rise and rise of women's employment in the UK.' In Judith Payne (ed.), 'IFS Briefing Note BN234.' https://ifs.org.uk/sites/default/files/output_url_files/BN234.pdf

... these additives were 'generally regarded as safe' ... Van Tulleken, C. (2023d). *Ultra-Processed People: Why Do We All Eat Stuff That Isn't Food ... and Why Can't We Stop?* Random House

When US president Eisenhower had a heart attack in 1955 ... Spector, T. (2015e). *The Diet Myth: The Real Science Behind What We Eat.* Hachette UK

In 1900 the average male life expectancy ... Mills, J. (2012), *Mortality in England and Wales – Office for National Statistics.* https://www.ons.gov.uk/peoplepopulationandcommunity/birthsdeathsandmarriages/deaths/articles/mortalityinenglandandwales/2012-12-17

... a landmark paper named the 'Seven Countries Study' ... Keys, A. et al. (1984). 'The seven countries study: 2,289 deaths in 15 years.' *Preventive Medicine*, 13(2), 141–54. https://doi.org/10.1016/0091-7435(84)90047-1

Spector, T. (2015e). *The Diet Myth: The Real Science Behind What We Eat.* Hachette UK

Malhotra, A. & O'Neill, D. (2017). *The Pioppi Diet: A 21-Day Lifestyle Plan.* Penguin UK

Refined-grain consumption went up by almost 45 per cent ... USDA Factbook. 'Chapter 2: Profiling Food Consumption in America.' https://fliphtml5.com/nzsh/vvna/basic

In years to come, his sources would be re-analysed ... Harcome, Z., et al. 'Evidence from randomised controlled trials did not support the introduction of dietary fat guidelines in 1977 and 1983: A systematic review and meta-analysis'. *Open Heart* (2015), 2(I); doi: 10.1136/bmj.f6340

... he lived to regret the profound consequences of his research ... *Cholesterol: Debate Flares Over Wisdom In Widespread Reductions.* (1987). Retrieved 10 June 2024, from https://www.nytimes.com/1987/07/14/science/cholesterol-debate-flares-over-wisdom-in-widespread-reductions.html

However, I will let Ancel Keys redeem himself ... Kalm, L. M. & Semba, R. D. (2005). 'They starved so that others be better fed: Remembering Ancel Keys and the Minnesota Experiment.' *J Nutr*, 135(6):1347–52. doi: 10.1093/jn/135.6.1347

... the millions of European civilians who were dying from starvation. White, M. (2013). *Atrocities: The 100 Deadliest Episodes in Human History.* W. W. Norton

CHAPTER 7: HOW TO EAT FOOD WITHOUT WORRYING ABOUT IT

This is because we each have a unique subcutaneous fat capacity ... Lotta, L. A. et al. (2016). 'Integrative genomic analysis implicates limited peripheral adipose storage capacity in the pathogenesis of human insulin resistance.' *Nature Genetics*, 49(1), 17–26. https://doi.org/10.1038/ng.3714

... the catch with food that needs more chewing is that we enjoy it less ... Ferriday, D., Bosworth, M. L., Evans, N. R., Ciborowska, A., Godinot, N., Martin, N., Rogers, P. J. & Brunstrom, J. M. (2016). 'Are the effects of eating slowly on satiation and satiety anticipated in meal planning?' *Appetite*, 107:681. doi: 10.1016/j.appet.2016.08.037.

... Dr Chris van Tulleken describes these UPFs as 'pre-chewed' ... Van Tulleken, C. (2023). *Ultra-Processed People: Why Do We All Eat Stuff That Isn't Food . . . and Why Can't We Stop?* Random House

The effect you see in the brain is similar to that of addictive drugs ... Fletcher, P. C. & Kenny, P. J. (2018). 'Food addiction: a valid concept?' *Neuropsychopharmacology*, 43(13), 2506–13. https://doi.org/10.1038/s41386-018-0203-9

... because of the epigenetic expression of genes, it often takes about 12 weeks ... Panda, S. (2018b). *The Circadian Code: Lose Weight, Supercharge Your Energy and Sleep Well Every night*. Random House

... they create a gloopy 'net' between sugar molecules and your blood supply. Weickert, M. O. & Pfeiffer, A. F. (2008). 'Metabolic effects of dietary fiber consumption and prevention of diabetes.' *J Nutr*, 138(3):439–42. doi: 10.1093/jn/138.3.439. PMID: 18287346

... eat most of the fibre, fat and protein first ... Shukla, A. P., Iliescu, R. G., Thomas, C. E. & Aronne, L. J. (2015). 'Food order has a significant impact on postprandial glucose and insulin levels.' *Diabetes Care*, 38(7):e98–9. doi: 10.2337/dc15-0429

... the vinegar on the salad also helps in its own right ... Shishehbor, F., Mansoori, A. & Shirani, F. (2017). 'Vinegar consumption can attenuate postprandial glucose and insulin responses; a systematic review and meta-analysis of clinical trials.' *Diabetes Res Clin Pract*, 127:1–9. doi: 10.1016/j.diabres.2017.01.021

... my first meal will dramatically shape my blood sugar spikes ... Chandler-Laney, P. C., Morrison, S. A., Goree, L. L., Ellis, A. C., Casazza, K., Desmond, R. & Gower, B. A. (2018). 'Return of hunger following a relatively high carbohydrate breakfast is associated with earlier recorded glucose peak and nadir.' *Appetite*, 80:236–41. doi: 10.1016/j.appet.2014.04.031

... Keys had a fierce rivalry with a Professor John Yudkin ... Gwynn, M. (2015). *Back in Time for Dinner: From Spam to Sushi: How We've Changed the Way We Eat*. Random House

Even just in my lifetime average sugar consumption has gone up by 31.5 per cent ... Ibid.

... the average British child gets 12.3 per cent of their calories from added sugar. National Diet and Nutrition Survey Rolling Programme et al. 'National Diet and Nutrition Survey: Rolling Programme Years 9 to 11 (2016/2017 to 2018/2019).' In *National Diet and Nutrition Survey* [Report]. https://assets. publishing.service.gov.uk/government/uploads/system/uploads/attachment_ data/file/943114/NDNS_UK_Y9-11_report.pdf

Artificial sweeteners are no better and may be worse ... Sylvetsky, A. C., Figueroa, J., Zimmerman, T., Swithers, S. E. & Welsh, J. A. (2019). 'Consumption of low-calorie sweetened beverages is associated with higher total energy and sugar intake among children, NHANES 2011–2016.' *Pediatr Obes*, 14(10). doi: 10.1111/ijpo.12535

... part of the way they also achieve this is by disrupting your valuable microbiome. Suez, J. et al. (2014). 'Artificial sweeteners induce glucose intolerance by altering the gut microbiota.' *Nature*, 514(7521):181–6. doi: 10.1038/ nature13793

... our palates have become desensitised to it. May, C. E. & Dus, M. (2021). 'Confection confusion: interplay between diet, taste, and nutrition.' *Trends in Endocrinology and Metabolism*, 32(2): 95–105. https://doi.org/10.1016/j. tem.2020.11.011

CHAPTER 8: FOOD – WHAT SHOULD YOU EAT?

A similar phenomenon is seen in animals ... Holliday, R. J. (n.d.) 'Nutrition and Holistic Animal Health.' https://www.abcplus.biz/Doc_Holliday_Nutritional_ Holistic_Animal_Health

... Dr Chris van Tulleken proposes we are doing the exact same thing ... Van Tulleken, C. (2023b). *Ultra-Processed People: Why Do We All Eat Stuff That Isn't Food . . . and Why Can't We Stop?* Random House

... Dr Clara Davis, an American paediatrician ... Ibid.

Specially designed diets became the 'in' thing in the 1920s ... Fomon, S. J. (2001). 'Infant feeding in the 20th century: Formula and Beikost.' *Journal of Nutrition*, 131(2), 409S-420S. https://doi.org/10.1093/jn/131.2.409s

... in his book *The Dorito Effect* ... Schatzker, M. (2015) ... *The Dorito Effect: The Surprising New Truth About Food and Flavor.* Simon and Schuster

... the study comparing bowel cancer in rural Africans to African Americans ... O'Keefe, S. J. D. et al. (2015). 'Fat, fibre and cancer risk in African Americans and rural Africans.' *Nature Communications*, 6(1). https://doi.org/10.1038/ ncomms7342

... five pockets in the world, called the Blue Zones. Buettner, D. (2012). *The Blue Zones, Second Edition: 9 Lessons for Living Longer: From the People Who've Lived the Longest.* Simon and Schuster

The term 'prebiotic' wasn't even a recognised word ... Bulsiewicz, W. (2022). *Fibre Fuelled: The Plant-Based Gut Health Plan to Lose Weight, Restore Health and Optimise Your Microbiome.* Random House

Spector, T. (2022). *Food for Life: Your Guide to the New Science of Eating Well.* Random House

… breast milk contains hundreds of microbiome species … Lyons, K.E., Ryan, C. A., Dempsey, E. M., Ross, R. P., Stanton, C. (2020). 'Breast Milk, a Source of Beneficial Microbes and Associated Benefits for Infant Health.' *Nutrients*, 9;12(4):1039. doi: 10.3390/nu12041039

… people who eat at least 30 different plants a week have much healthier microbiomes. McDonald, D. et al. (2018). 'American Gut: an Open Platform for Citizen Science Microbiome Research.' *MSystems*, 3(3). https://doi.org/10.1128/msystems.00031-18

Put very simply, polyphenols are … Spector, T. (2022). *Food for Life: Your Guide to the New Science of Eating Well.* Random House

… polyphenols positively remove them and they go absolutely wild … Sun, H., Chen, Y., Cheng, M., Zhang, X., Zheng, X. & Zhang, Z. (2017). 'The modulatory effect of polyphenols from green tea, oolong tea and black tea on human intestinal microbiota in vitro.' *Journal of Food Science and Technology*, 55(1), 399–407. https://doi.org/10.1007/s13197-017-2951-7

They significantly lower inflammation in the blood vessels … Quiñones, M., Miguel, M. & Aleixandre, A. (2013). 'Beneficial effects of polyphenols on cardiovascular disease.' *Pharmacological Research*, 68(1), 125–31. https://doi.org/10.1016/j.phrs.2012.10.018

A diet high in polyphenols can reduce cardiovascular disease risk … Tresserra-Rimbau, A. et al. (2014). 'Inverse association between habitual polyphenol intake and incidence of cardiovascular events in the PREDIMED study.' *Nutrition Metabolism and Cardiovascular Diseases*, 24(6), 639–47. https://doi.org/10.1016/j.numecd.2013.12.014

In truth, we are only now scratching the surface of what polyphenols can do for us … Dayem, A. A., Choi, H., Yang, G., Kim, K., Saha, S. & Cho, S. (2016). 'The anti-cancer effect of polyphenols against breast cancer and cancer stem cells: Molecular mechanisms.' *Nutrients*, 8(9), 581. https://doi.org/10.3390/nu8090581

Afaq, F. & Katiyar, S. K. (2011). 'Polyphenols: skin photoprotection and inhibition of photocarcinogenesis.' *Mini-Reviews in Medicinal Chemistry*, 11(14), 1200–15. https://doi.org/10.2174/13895575111091200

Socci, V., Tempesta, D., Desideri, G., de Gennaro, L. & Ferrara, M. (2017). 'Enhancing Human Cognition with Cocoa Flavonoids.' *Frontiers in Nutrition*, 4. https://doi.org/10.3389/fnut.2017.00019

Especially when there is enormous evidence behind fermented foods … Leeuwendaal, N. K., Stanton, C., O'Toole, P. W. & Beresford, T. P. (2022). 'Fermented foods, health and the gut microbiome.' *Nutrients*, 14(7), 1527. https://doi.org/10.3390/nu14071527

… the French each put away 24kg of cheese per year … Spector, T. (2015c). *The Diet Myth: The Real Science Behind What We Eat.* Hachette UK

... **when full-fat dairy products are fermented with bacteria** ... Martinez-Gonzalez, M. A., Sayon-Orea, C., Ruiz-Canela, M., de la Fuente, C., Gea, A., Bes-Rastrollo, M. (2014). 'Yogurt consumption, weight change and risk of overweight/obesity: the SUN cohort study.' *Nutr Metab Cardiovasc Dis*, 24(11):1189–96. doi: 10.1016/j.numecd.2014.05.015

... **fresh fruit and vegetables are often teeming with bugs** ... Lang, J. M., Eisen, J. A. & Zivkovic, A. M. (2014). 'The microbes we eat: abundance and taxonomy of microbes consumed in a day's worth of meals for three diet types.' *PeerJ*, https://doi.org/10.7717/peerj.659

... **healthy fat in the form of omega-3** ... Menni, C., Zierer, J., Pallister, T. et al. (2017). 'Omega-3 fatty acids correlate with gut microbiome diversity and production of N-carbamylglutamate in middle aged and elderly women.' *Sci Rep* 7, 11079. https://doi.org/10.1038/s41598-017-10382-2

We know artificial sweeteners and other added chemicals, like emulsifiers ... Chassaing, B., Koren, O., Goodrich, J. K., Poole, A. C., Srinivasan, S., Ley, R. E. & Gewirtz, A. T. (2015). 'Dietary emulsifiers impact the mouse gut microbiota promoting colitis and metabolic syndrome.' *Nature*, 519(7541), 92–6. https://doi.org/10.1038/nature14232

Suez, J. et al. (2014). 'Artificial sweeteners induce glucose intolerance by altering the gut microbiota.' *Nature*, 514(7521):181–6. doi: 10.1038/nature13793

Worryingly, for every 10 per cent of calories you get from UPFs in your diet ... Schnabel, L., Kesse-Guyot, E., Allès, B., Touvier, M., Srour, B., Hercberg, S., Buscail, C. & Julia, C. (2019). 'Association Between Ultraprocessed Food Consumption and Risk of Mortality Among Middle-aged Adults in France.' *JAMA Intern Med*, 179(4):490–8. doi: 10.1001/jamainternmed.2018.7289

Fiolet, T. et al. (2018). 'Consumption of ultra-processed foods and cancer risk: results from NutriNet-Santé prospective cohort.' *BMJ*, k322. https://doi.org/10.1136/bmj.k322

... **some 13 million kilograms of antibiotics are used today in agriculture** ... Spector, T. (2015d). *The Diet Myth: The Real Science Behind What We Eat*. Hachette UK

... **in the 1960s, farmers realised animals gained weight faster if they were given antibiotics.** Visek, W. J. (1978). 'The mode of growth promotion by antibiotics.' *Journal of Animal Science*, 46(5), 1447–69. https://doi.org/10.2527/jas1978.4651447x

... **up to 75 per cent of wild fish also contain them.** Burridge, L., Weis, J. S., Cabello, F., Pizarro, J., & Bostick, K. (2010). 'Chemical use in salmon aquaculture: A review of current practices and possible environmental effects.' *Aquaculture*, 306(1–4), 7–23. https://doi.org/10.1016/j.aquaculture.2010.05.020

Being vegan doesn't afford protection from unwanted antibiotics ... Karthikeyan, K. G. & Meyer, M. T. (2006). 'Occurrence of antibiotics in wastewater treatment facilities in Wisconsin, USA.' *Sci Total Environ*, 361(1–3):196–207. doi: 10.1016/j.scitotenv.2005.06.030

Examples of foods worth buying organic include ... Hyman, M. (2021c). *The Pegan Diet: 21 Practical Principles for Reclaiming Your Health in a Nutritionally Confusing World.* Hachette UK

In fact, not only is a faster transit time generally associated with better health outcomes ... Asnicar, F. et al. (2021). 'Blue poo: impact of gut transit time on the gut microbiome using a novel marker.' *Gut*, 70(9), 1665–74. https://doi.org/10.1136/gutjnl-2020-323877

Spector, T. (2022b). *Food for Life: Your Guide to the New Science of Eating Well.* Random House

The main difference he discovered was in their poo ... Hyman, M. (2023). *Young Forever: The Secrets to Living Your Longest, Healthiest Life.* Hachette UK

... a gluten-free diet in non-coeliacs has been found to worsen the microbiome. Spector, T. (2022b). *Food for Life: Your Guide to the New Science of Eating Well.* Random House

... you are 'what you eat eats'. Hyman, M. (2021b). *The Pegan Diet: 21 Practical Principles for Reclaiming Your Health in a Nutritionally Confusing World.* Hachette UK

Highly processed meats like bacon, hot dogs and ham are a recognised carcinogen ... 'Cancer: Carcinogenicity of the consumption of red meat and processed meat.' (n.d.). https://www.who.int/news-room/questions-and-answers/item/cancer-carcinogenicity-of-the-consumption-of-red-meat-and-processed-meat

I make an exception for good-quality Italian cured meats ... Spector, T. (2022b). *Food for Life: Your Guide to the New Science of Eating Well.* Random House

Interestingly, there seems to be a clear link in European studies ... Pan, A., Sun, Q., Bernstein, A. M., Schulze, M. B., Manson, J. E., Stampfer, M. J., Willett, W. C. & Hu, F. B. (2012). 'Red meat consumption and mortality: results from 2 prospective cohort studies.' *Arch Intern Med*, 172(7):555–63. doi: 10.1001/archinternmed.2011.2287

Lee, J. E. et al. (2013). 'Meat intake and cause-specific mortality: a pooled analysis of Asian prospective cohort studies.' *Am J Clin Nutr*, 98(4):1032–41. doi: 10.3945/ajcn.113.062638

... an unhelpful byproduct called 'TMAO', which increases heart disease. Tang, W. H., Wang, Z., Levison, B. S., Koeth, R. A., Britt, E. B., Fu, X., Wu, Y. & Hazen, S. L. (2013). 'Intestinal microbial metabolism of phosphatidylcholine and cardiovascular risk.' *N Engl J Med*, 25;368(17):1575–84. doi: 10.1056/NEJMoa1109400

Heianza, Y. et al. (2020). 'Long-term changes in gut microbial metabolite trimethylamine N-oxide and coronary heart disease risk.' *J Am Coll Cardiol*, 75(7):763–72. doi: 10.1016/j.jacc.2019.11.060

Our centenarian friends in the Blue Zones ... Buettner, D. (2012b). *The Blue Zones, Second Edition: 9 Lessons for Living Longer: From the People Who've Lived the Longest.* Simon and Schuster

As many as 90 per cent of us aren't getting enough fibre ... Gallagher, J. (2019). 'The lifesaving food 90 per cent aren't eating enough of.' BBC News. https://www.bbc.co.uk/news/health-46827426

Amazingly, even eating just an extra 7 grams of fibre per day ... Threapleton, D. E. (2013). 'Dietary fibre intake and risk of cardiovascular disease: systematic review and meta-analysis.' BMJ, 347:f6879. doi: 10.1136/bmj.f6879

... their gut microbiome plays a huge role in optimising blood cholesterol. Khare, A. & Gaur, S. (2020). 'Cholesterol-Lowering Effects of Lactobacillus Species.' Curr Microbiol, 77(4):638–44. doi: 10.1007/s00284-020-01903-w

Morrison, D. J. & Preston, T. (2016). 'Formation of short chain fatty acids by the gut microbiota and their impact on human metabolism.' Gut Microbes, 7(3), 189–200. https://doi.org/10.1080/19490976.2015.1134082

... TRE improves cholesterol ... Panda, S. (2018d). The Circadian Code: Lose Weight, Supercharge Your Energy and Sleep Well Every Night. Random House

It will give you an optimised cholesterol profile ... Falkenhain, K., Roach, L. A., McCreary, S., McArthur, E., Weiss, E. J., Francois, M. E. & Little, J. P. (2021). 'Effect of carbohydrate-restricted dietary interventions on LDL particle size and number in adults in the context of weight loss or weight maintenance: a systematic review and meta-analysis.' American Journal of Clinical Nutrition, 114(4), 1455–66. https://doi.org/10.1093/ajcn/nqab212

Ma, Y., Li, Y., Chiriboga, D. E., Olendzki, B. C., Hebert, J. R., Li, W., Leung, K., Hafner, A. R. & Ockene, I. S. (2006). 'Association between Carbohydrate Intake and Serum Lipids.' Journal of the American College of Nutrition, 25(2), 155–63. https://doi.org/10.1080/07315724.2006.10719527

Some people are especially good at clearing fat from their blood quickly after a meal ... Berry, S. E. et al. (2020). 'Human postprandial responses to food and potential for precision nutrition.' Nature Medicine, 26(6), 964–73. https://doi.org/10.1038/s41591-020-0934-0

My favourite heart health study is called PREDIMED ... Estruch, R. et al. (2013). 'Primary Prevention of Cardiovascular Disease with a Mediterranean Diet.' New England Journal of Medicine, 368(14), 1279–90. https://doi.org/10.1056/nejmoa1200303

One famous study, called the Lyon Diet Heart Study ... De Lorgeril, M., Salen, P., Martin, J., Monjaud, I., Delaye, J. & Mamelle, N. (1999). 'Mediterranean diet, traditional risk factors, and the rate of cardiovascular complications after myocardial infarction.' Circulation, 99(6), 779–85. https://doi.org/10.1161/01.cir.99.6.779

... as long as you are getting enough omega-3 in your diet ... 'Fats and fatty acids in human nutrition. Report of an expert consultation.' FAO Food Nutr Pap. 2010;91:1–166

Harris W. S. 'The omega-6/omega-3 ratio and cardiovascular disease risk: uses and abuses.' Curr Atheroscler Rep. 2006 Nov;8(6):453-9. doi: 10.1007/s11883-006-0019-7

Pischon T., Hankinson S. E., Hotamisligil G. S., Rifai N., Willett W. C., Rimm E. B. 'Habitual dietary intake of n-3 and n-6 fatty acids in relation to inflammatory markers among US men and women.' *Circulation.* 2003 Jul 15;108(2):155-60. doi: 10.1161/01.CIR.0000079224.46084.C2

Just 4g trans fats a day ... Merchant, A. T., Kelemen, L. E., de Koning, L., Lonn, E., Vuksan, V., Jacobs, R., Davis, B., Teo, K. K., Yusuf, S. & Anand, S. S. (2008). 'Interrelation of saturated fat, *trans* fat, alcohol intake, and subclinical atherosclerosis. *American Journal of Clinical Nutrition,* 87(1), 168–74. https://doi.org/10.1093/ajcn/87.1.168

CHAPTER 9: WHAT YOUR DOCTOR EATS

We now know alcohol consumption costs the NHS £3.5 billion a year ... Commission on Alcohol Harm, Finlay, B., Action for Children, The Children's Society, the National Association for Children of Alcoholics, Institute of Alcohol Studies, NHS Ayrshire and Arran Fetal Alcohol Advisory & Support Team & Daisy. (n.d.). '"It's everywhere" – alcohol's public face and private harm.' https://ahauk.org/wp-content/uploads/2020/09/Its-Everywhere-Commission-on-Alcohol-Harm-final-report.pdf

GOV.UK (21 March 2019). 'Health Matters: tobacco and alcohol CQUIN.' https://www.gov.uk/government/publications/health-matters-preventing-ill-health-from-alcohol-and-tobacco/health-matters-preventing-ill-health-from-alcohol-and-tobacco-use

... less than 2 units of alcohol a day is associated with an increase in breast, mouth, throat and oesophagus cancer? Committee on Carcinogenicity of Chemicals in Food, Consumer Products and the Environment (COC) & COC Secretariat (2015). 'Statement on consumption of alcoholic beverages and risk of cancer.' https://assets.publishing.service.gov.uk/government/uploads/system/uploads/attachment_data/file/490584/COC_2015_S2__Alcohol_and_Cancer_statement_Final_version.pdf

Alcohol can also cause detrimental brain changes ... Topiwala, A. et al. (2017). 'Moderate alcohol consumption as risk factor for adverse brain outcomes and cognitive decline: longitudinal cohort study.' *BMJ,* j2353. https://doi.org/10.1136/bmj.j2353

On top of that, it's linked to abnormal heart rhythms ... Commission on Alcohol Harm, Finlay, B., Action for Children, The Children's Society, the National Association for Children of Alcoholics, Institute of Alcohol Studies, NHS Ayrshire and Arran Fetal Alcohol Advisory & Support Team & Daisy. (n.d.-b). '"It's everywhere" – alcohol's public face and private harm.' https://ahauk.org/wp-content/uploads/2020/09/Its-Everywhere-Commission-on-Alcohol-Harm-final-report.pdf

UK Chief Medical Officers. (2016). 'UK Chief Medical Officers' Alcohol Guidelines Review Summary of the proposed new guidelines.' https://assets.publishing.service.gov.uk/government/uploads/system/uploads/attachment_data/file/489795/summary.pdf

CHAPTER 10: CONTROL STRESS –
THE BRIDGE BETWEEN MIND AND BODY

Take a look at the 'Life Change Index Scale' ... Holmes, T. H. & Rahe, T. H. (1967). 'Life Change Index Scale (The Stress Test).' *Journal of Psychosomatic Research*, 11, 213. https://www.dartmouth.edu/eap/library/lifechangestresstest.pdf

This scale is based on the Holmes and Rahe stress scale ... Noone, P. A. (2017). 'The Holmes–Rahe stress inventory.' *Occupational Medicine*, 67(7), 581–82. https://doi.org/10.1093/occmed/kqx099

It is the concept of 'flow state' ... Gold, J. & Ciorciari, J. (2020). 'A review on the role of the neuroscience of flow states in the modern world.' *Behavioral Sciences*, 10(9), 137. https://doi.org/10.3390/bs10090137

Krueger, J. (2015). 'Flow and happiness: Do you have to be an expert to be happy?' Retrieved from: https://www.psychologytoday.com/gb/blog/one-among-many/201502/flow-and-happiness

Alameda, C., Sanabria, D. & Ciria, L. F. (2022). 'The brain in flow: A systematic review on the neural basis of the flow state.' *Cortex*, 154, 348–64. https://doi.org/10.1016/j.cortex.2022.06.005

... flow state seems to inhibit your prefrontal cortex ... Fuster, J. M. (2015). 'Anatomy of the prefrontal cortex.' In *Elsevier eBooks* (pp. 9–62). https://doi.org/10.1016/b978-0-12-407815-4.00002-7

Friedman, N. P. & Robbins, T. W. (2021). 'The role of prefrontal cortex in cognitive control and executive function.' *Neuropsychopharmacology*, 47(1), 72–89. https://doi.org/10.1038/s41386-021-01132-0

The research coming out about nature's impact on health ... Van den Bosch, M. & Bird, W. (2018). *Oxford Textbook of Nature and Public Health: The Role of Nature in Improving the Health of a Population*. Oxford University Press

... putting patients in hospital beds with a view of nature speeds up their recovery. Ulrich, R. S. (1984). 'View through a window may influence recovery from surgery.' *Science*, 224(4647), 420–21. https://doi.org/10.1126/science.6143402

Crime rates plummeted where there was greenery. Kuo, F. & Sullivan, W. (2001). 'Environment and crime in the inner city: Does vegetation reduce crime?' *Environment and Behavior*, 33(3), 343–67. https://doi.org/10.1177/0013916501333002

... being in nature relaxes us, opens us up and promotes prosocial behaviour. Zhang, J. W., Piff, P. K., Iyer, R., Koleva, S. & Keltner, D. (2014). 'An occasion for unselfing: Beautiful nature leads to prosociality.' *Journal of Environmental Psychology*, 37, 61–72. https://doi.org/10.1016/j.jenvp.2013.11.008

... if their education is taken outside to a place of natural beauty ... Evans, N. M. (2023). 'Trauma-informed environmental education: Helping students feel safe and connected in nature.' *Journal of Environmental Education*, 54(2), 85–98. https://doi.org/10.1080/00958964.2022.2163220

... people are actively encouraged to engage in 'shinrin-yoku' or 'forest bathing'. Park, B. J., Tsunetsugu, Y., Kasetani, T., Kagawa, T. & Miyazaki, Y. (2009). 'The physiological effects of *Shinrin-yoku* (taking in the forest atmosphere or forest bathing): evidence from field experiments in 24 forests across Japan.' *Environmental Health and Preventive Medicine*, 15(1), 18–26. https://doi.org/10.1007/s12199-009-0086-9

Chatterjee, R. (2018). *The Stress Solution: The 4 Steps to a Calmer, Happier, Healthier You*. Penguin UK

We know mothers who spend a decent chunk of their pregnancy out in nature have healthier children. Van den Bosch, M. & Bird, W. (2018). *Oxford Textbook of Nature and Public Health: The Role of Nature in Improving the Health of a Population*. Oxford University Press

If those children then grow up playing outside, they will develop a larger hippocampus ... Kühn, S. et al. (2020). 'Brain structure and habitat: Do the brains of our children tell us where they have been brought up?' *Neuroimage*, 222:117225. doi: 10.1016/j.neuroimage.2020.117225

When our homes are cluttered and messy ... Chatterjee, R. (2018). *The Stress Solution: The 4 Steps to a Calmer, Happier, Healthier You*. Penguin UK

It is therefore completely logical that to feel content ... Van den Bosch, M. & Bird, W. (2018). *Oxford Textbook of Nature and Public Health: The Role of Nature in Improving the Health of a Population*. Oxford University Press

Waldinger, R. & Schulz, M. (2023). *The Good Life: Lessons from the World's Longest Scientific Study of Happiness*. Simon and Schuster

... those who had the most meaningful social connections ... Harvard Second Generation Grant and Glueck Study. 'Study of Adult Development.' (n.d.). https://www.adultdevelopmentstudy.org/grantandglueckstudy

Shetty, M. (2024). 'How social connection supports longevity.' Stanford Lifestyle Medicine. https://longevity.stanford.edu/lifestyle/2023/12/18/how-social-connection-supports-longevity/

We know that people who are lonely are 30 per cent more likely to die from a heart attack or stroke ... Chatterjee, R. (2018). *The Stress Solution: The 4 Steps to Reset Your Body, Mind, Relationships and Purpose*. Penguin UK

... over time you become resistant ... Montag, C., Zhao, Z., Sindermann, C., Xu, L., Fu, M., Li, J., Zheng, X., Li, K., Kendrick, K. M., Dai, J. & Becker, B. (2018). 'Internet Communication Disorder and the structure of the human brain: initial insights on WeChat addiction.' *Scientific Reports*, 8(1). https://doi.org/10.1038/s41598-018-19904-y

Westbrook, A., Ghosh, A., van den Bosch, R., Määttä, J. I., Hofmans, L. & Cools, R. (2021). 'Striatal dopamine synthesis capacity reflects smartphone social activity.' *iScience*, 24(5), 102497. https://doi.org/10.1016/j.isci.2021.102497

This is explored in one of my favourite books, *The Top Five Regrets of the Dying*. Ware, B. (2019). *The Top Five Regrets of the Dying: A Life Transformed by the Dearly Departing*. Hay House, Inc

We all know that not getting enough sleep ... Walker, M. (2017). *Why We Sleep: The New Science of Sleep and Dreams*. Penguin UK

Panda, S. (2018c). *The Circadian Code: Lose Weight, Supercharge Your Energy and Sleep Well Every Night*. Random House

Foster, R. (2022). *Life Time: The New Science of the Body Clock, and How It Can Revolutionize Your Sleep and Health*. Penguin UK

These pills don't simulate true sleep ... Arbon, E. L., Knurowska, M. & Dijk, D. J. (2015). 'Randomised clinical trial of the effects of prolonged-release melatonin, temazepam and zolpidem on slow-wave activity during sleep in healthy people.' *J Psychopharmacol*, 29(7):764–6. doi: 10.1177/026988 1115581963

... giving yourself 'fake sleep' in a pill ... Kripke, D. F., Langer, R. D. & Kline, L. E. (2012). 'Hypnotics' association with mortality or cancer: a matched cohort study.' *BMJ Open*, 2(1):e000850. doi: 10.1136/bmjopen-2012-000850

... if an average person usually sleeps fewer than seven hours a night ... Hyman, M. (2023a). *Young Forever*. Hachette UK

Figure 4. The National Sleep Foundation. (2024). 'How much sleep do you really need?' National Sleep Foundation. https://www.thensf.org/how-many-hours-of-sleep-do-you-really-need/

... shift workers can be more vulnerable to infections. Mohren, D. C. et al. (2002). 'Prevalence of common infections among employees in different work schedules.' *J Occup Environ Med*, 44(11):1003–11. doi: 10.1097/00043764-200211000-00005 Erratum in: *J Occup Environ Med*. January 2003;45(1):105.

... women who simply sleep at their preferred bedtime actually have better breast-cancer survival rates. Hahm,B. J. et al. (2014). 'Bedtime misalignment and progression of breast cancer.' *Chronobiol Int*, 31(2):214–21. doi: 10.3109/07420528.2013.842575 Epub 24 October 2013.

In fact, we know suicide rates increase in winter ... Davis, G. E. & Lowell, W. E. (2002). 'Evidence that latitude is directly related to variation in suicide rates.' *Can J Psychiatry*, 47(6):572–4. doi: 10.1177/070674370204700611

... if you transplant a stool sample from a shift worker ... Thaiss, C. A. et al. (2014). 'Transkingdom control of microbiota diurnal oscillations promotes metabolic homeostasis.' *Cell*, 159(3):514–29. doi: 10.1016/j.cell.2014.09.048

... one of them is called IL-15, which also directly supports sleep. Kubota, T., Brown, R. A., Fang, J. & Krueger, J. M. (2001). 'Interleukin-15 and interleukin-2 enhance non-REM sleep in rabbits.' *Am J Physiol Regul Integr Comp Physiol*, 281(3):R1004–12. doi: 10.1152/ajpregu.2001.281.3.R1004

... an exercise programme called PD Warrior. PD Warrior. (23 January 2024). Dr. Melissa McConaghy – PD Warrior. https://pdwarrior.com/speaker/melissa-mcconaghy/

... Daniel Lieberman explores this eloquently in his book *Exercised* ... Lieberman, D. (2020). *Exercised: The Science of Physical Activity, Rest and Health*. Penguin UK

... exercise is not just as effective, but often *more* effective than most antidepressants. Cooney, G. M., Dwan, K., Greig, C. A., Lawlor, D. A., Rimer, J., Waugh, F. R., McMurdo, M. & Mead, G. E. (2013). 'Exercise for depression.' *Cochrane Database Syst Rev*, 2013(9): CD004366. doi: 10.1002/14651858. CD004366.pub6

... only 20 per cent of psychiatrists recommend exercise ... Melville, N. A. (2018). 'Few psychiatrists recommend exercise for anxiety disorders.' *Medscape*. https://www.medscape.com/viewarticle/894987?form=fpf

Well, our muscles serve more functions than we ever realised ... Lin, T. W. & Kuo, Y. M. (2013). 'Exercise benefits brain function: the monoamine connection.' *Brain Sci*, 3(1):39–53. doi: 10.3390/brainsci3010039 PMID: 24961306

Maddock, R. J., Casazza, G. A., Fernandez, D. H., Maddock, M. I. (2016). 'Acute modulation of cortical glutamate and GABA content by physical activity.' *J Neurosci*, 36(8):2449–57. doi: 10.1523/JNEUROSCI.3455-15.2016

Meyer, J. D., Crombie, K. M., Cook, D. B., Hillard, C. J. & Koltyn, K. F. (2019). 'Serum endocannabinoid and mood changes after exercise in major depressive disorder.' *Med Sci Sports Exerc*, 51(9):1909–17. doi: 10.1249/MSS.0000000000002006

Duclos, M. & Tabarin, A. (2016). 'Exercise and the hypothalamo-pituitary-adrenal axis.' *Front Horm Res*, 47:12–26. doi: 10.1159/000445149

... they protect us from things like cancer and diabetes ... Hood, D. A., Uguccioni, G., Vainshtein, A. & D'souza, D. (2011). 'Mechanisms of exercise-induced mitochondrial biogenesis in skeletal muscle: implications for health and disease.' *Compr Physiol*, 1(3):1119–34. doi: 10.1002/cphy. c100074

Gianni, P., Jan, K. J., Douglas, M. J., Stuart, P. M. & Tarnopolsky, M. A. (2004). 'Oxidative stress and the mitochondrial theory of aging in human skeletal muscle.' *Exp Gerontol*, 39(9):1391–400. doi: 10.1016/j.exger.2004.06.002

It's also why building muscle mass is a genius way ... Sylow, L., Kleinert, M., Richter, E. A. & Jensen, T. E. (2017). 'Exercise-stimulated glucose uptake – regulation and implications for glycaemic control.' *Nat Rev Endocrinol*, 13(3):133–48. doi: 10.1038/nrendo.2016.162

... moderate exercise reduces the risk of breast cancer by 30–40 per cent and colon cancer by 40–50 per cent ... Friedenreich, C. M. & Orenstein, M. R. (2002). 'Physical activity and cancer prevention: etiologic evidence and biological mechanisms.' *J Nutr*, 132(11 Suppl):3456S–64S. doi: 10.1093/jn/132.11.3456S

It is the best-known protection from dementia ... Hamer, M. & Chida, Y. (2009). 'Physical activity and risk of neurodegenerative disease: a systematic review of prospective evidence.' *Psychol Med*, 39(1):3–11. doi: 10.1017/S0033291708003681

Interestingly, exercise can be a surprisingly inefficient weight-loss tool ... Turner, J. E., Markovitch, D., Betts, J. A. and Thompson, D. (2010).

'Nonprescribed physical activity energy expenditure is maintained with structured exercise and implicates a compensatory increase in energy intake.' *Am J Clin Nutr*, 92(5):1009–16. doi: 10.3945/ajcn.2010.29471

Williams, P. T. & Wood, P. D. (2005). 'The effects of changing exercise levels on weight and age-related weight gain.' *International Journal of Obesity*, 30(3), 543–51. https://doi.org/10.1038/sj.ijo.0803172

If you look at foraging populations from Australia to South America ... Hawkes, K., O'Connell, J. F. & Jones, N. G. B. (1997). 'Hadza women's time allocation, offspring provisioning, and the evolution of long post-menopausal life spans.' *Current Anthropology*, 38(4), 551–77. https://doi.org/10.1086/204646

Centenarians in the Blue Zones are the same ... Buettner, D. (2012c). *The Blue Zones, Second Edition: 9 Lessons for Living Longer: From the People Who've Lived the Longest.* Simon and Schuster

Put bluntly, people who engage in charitable acts live longer. Brown, S. L., Nesse, R. M., Vinokur, A. D. & Smith, D. M. (2003). 'Providing social support may be more beneficial than receiving it.' *Psychological Science*, 14(4), 320–7. https://doi.org/10.1111/1467-9280.14461

Dossey, L. (2018). 'The helper's high.' *EXPLORE*, 14(6), 393–9. https://doi.org/10.1016/j.explore.2018.10.003

Unnecessary acts of kindness flood our brains ... Fehr, E. & Fischbacher, U. (2003). 'The nature of human altruism.' *Nature*, 425(6960), 785–91. https://doi.org/10.1038/nature02043

Warneken, F., Hare, B., Melis, A. P., Hanus, D. & Tomasello, M. (2007). 'Spontaneous altruism by chimpanzees and young children.' *PLoS Biol*, 5(7):e184. doi: 10.1371/journal.pbio.0050184

Interestingly, we see similar evolutionary reactions ... Bullmore, E. (2019). *The Inflamed Mind: A Radical New Approach to Depression.* Hachette UK

Van den Bosch, M. & Bird, W. (2018). *Oxford Textbook of Nature and Public Health: The Role of Nature in Improving the Health of a Population.* Oxford University Press

APPENDIX 1: SUMMARY OF APPETITE GUT HORMONES IN APPETITE REGULATION

Suzuki, K., Jayasena, C. N. & Bloom, S. R. (2011). 'The gut hormones in appetite regulation.' *Journal of Obesity*, 1–10. https://doi.org/10.1155/2011/528401

Abdalla, M. M. I. (2015). 'Ghrelin – Physiological functions and regulation.' *European Endocrinology*, 11(2), 90. https://doi.org/10.17925/ee.2015.11.02.90

INDEX

Note: page numbers in **bold** refer to images.

INDEX

microwaves 139
migratory motor complex (MMC)
98–9, 156, 201–2, 296
Minnesota Starvation experiment
141–3, 145, 217, 283
mirror cells 266–7
mitochondria 87–91, 94–6, 101,
105, 170, 252, 282–3, 299
modern diet 65, 88, 96–7, 100,
138
mood 28, 142, 151, 271, 275,
281–2
'moon face' 54
mouse studies 18, 23, 86–7, 93,
96–7, 117, 276
'germ-free' mice 18, 22, 27, 72
mouth 63–4, 154
movement 258, 278–85, 292, 304
MRI scans 75, 77, 82, 259, 263
muesli, Bircher 228–9
muhammara-ganoush dip 234–5
muscle mass 285
gain 99–100, 104, 153–4, 283–4
loss 99–100, 142, 275

'nachos', sweet potato 245–6
napping 305
nature 258, 262–4, 277, 292
near-death experiences 253–4
nervous system 36–7, 273
neuropeptide Y (NPY) 303
neuroplasticity 96
neurotransmitters 36
nicotine 158, 304
nomophobia 267
non-alcoholic fatty-liver disease
(NAFLD) 172–3
'nonna test' 185, 203–4, 211–12,
298
nonsteroidal anti-inflammatories
(NSAIDs) 195
nutrition, personalised 3, 115, 209
nutritional deficiencies 15–16, 180,
182
nutritional supplements 15–17
nuts 169, 188, 201, 209–11, 216,
219–20, 224, 226–8, 234, 236–7,
247, 296

obesity 3–4, 72, 99–100, 124, 155,
276
and appetite 66
and breakfast skipping 92
and calories 48
central/abdominal 54, 118
childhood 3, 110–13, 118–21,
125–6, 162
complexity 20, 42, 136
and cortisol 56
and Covid-19 complications 31
and dieting 83–4
and the French Paradox 192
and genetics 75, 106–27
and GLP-1 66
and the gut microbiome 18–19,
20, 21, 23, 30
history of 128–45
and the in utero environment
118–19
as infection 18–19, 20–3
and insulin levels 64, 85
and intermittent fasting 87
and lack of exercise 48
and leptin 61–2
morbid 18, 20, 110–13, 130
one-way street to 136–9
and Ozempic 26
prevalence 126, 140
and sleep 72, 273
stigma 111, 118, 121, 128–30,
133, 135, 145
and time-restricted eating 164
and ultra-processed foods 75,
124
oestrogen 30, 40, 62, 197
olive oil 209–10
omega-3 fatty acids 193, 210–11
omega-6 fatty acids 210
omeprazole 195
onion, 'quickled' red 238–9
online-disinhibition effect 269
opiates 15
opioids 282
organelles 88, 103
organic produce 196, 205–6
orthorexia 124, 195
ovaries 30, 40, 123

satiety (fullness) hormones 26,
60–2, 65–8, 78, 83, 150, 157,
170, 303
see also GLP-1; leptin; peptide YY
sauce, romesco-ish 233–4
sauerkraut 27
science 5, 7–9, 31, 80–2, 86, 129
seasonal affective disorder (SAD)
274
seasonal eating 189, 222–3
seeds 45, 185, 188, 193, 201,
210–11, 213, 219–20, 224, 226,
228–32, 234, 240–2, 247, 248,
296
self-soothing 267–8
serotonin 36, 298
set-point theory 62
sex hormones, metabolism 40
shift work 72, 100, 273–4, 276
short-chain fatty acids (SCFAs) 37,
39, 207
sickness behaviour 289–90, 293,
299
skin 28–9, 40–2, 116–17, 191, 254,
296, 300
microbiome 17, 32, 117
see also acne
sleep 4, 258, 263, 271–8, 274,
291–2, 296, 299, 304–6
poor 71–3, 100, 254, 271–8,
281, 304–6
sleep hormones 87, 156, 159, 276,
277, 296
sleep pressure 276
sleeping pills 271–3, 276
slow food 138
small intestinal bacterial overgrowth
(SIBO) 34–5
smartphones 267–70
smoking 158, 218, 304
smoothies 158, 195
snacks 71–2, 98, 155–6, 177
social jetlag 73, 274
social media 267–70, 291
socioeconomic status 116
soda bread, microbiome-boosting
240–1
soup 169

Spector, Tim 3, 18–19, 153, 190,
205
sperm count 40, 142, 276
standard American diet (SAD) 22–3,
28, 39
staples 221–2, 239–43
starch 114, 169, 173, 208
resistant 186
starvation 82–4, 100, 132, 141–3,
145, 154, 217
statins 190–1
steroids 55, 100, 251
stomach 63–6, 70–1
stretch receptors 65, 77, 158,
265
stomach acid 63, 77, 87, 97
stress 89–90, 301
and appetite 73–4
chronic 73–4, 90–1, 266, 273,
278, 286, 291
impact on health 33, 57
management 251–93, 299
physical 90
psychological 90, 91
triggers 255–8
and weight gain 55–6, 57
stress hormones 55–6, 291
see also cortisol
stroke 25, 47, 52–3, 151, 154, 191,
208, 252, 265
sugar 30, 47, 63, 88, 89, 91, 96,
114, 125, 140, 169, 171–5, 177,
208
added 171–2
desensitisation of the palate to
173–4
refined 76, 165, 172
sugar hangovers 167
sugar-free drinks 64, 70, 78, 164
suicide 256, 272, 274, 289
sumac 219–20
suprachiasmatic nucleus (SCN) 70,
72, 87
survival 68, 82–3, 105, 265, 285
sweet drinks 170–2, 174, 177,
304
sweet foods 171–7, 216, 224–5
sweet potato 'nachos' 245–6

INDEX

symbiosis 17
sympathetic nervous system 273

T cells (TREGS) 30–1
tahini dressing 237–8
taste, sense of 27–8, 64
telomeres 90
testicles 30
testosterone 40, 74, 276
texture of food 247
thinness 20, 43, 57, 107, 135–6,
151, 155, 281, 283
thyroid 30, 84, 112
time-restricted eating (TRE)
92–104, 105, 155–64, 177, 195,
202, 206–7
TMAO 205
toast, avocado 231–2
TOFIs (Thin on the Outside but Fat
on the Inside) 283
trans fats 209, 210–11
treatment prices 15–16
triglycerides (blood fats) 25, 118,
185
tumours 38–9, 40–1, 51–2, 101
see also insulinoma

twin studies 24–5, 81, 136
identical 22, 81, 95
non-identical 27, 81

ultra-processed foods (UPFs) 7, 48,
158–9, 182, 185, 192, 194–5,
197, 201, 203, 206, 213–14, 216,
300
baby milk 119–20, 122
and children 125, 161, 194
and the gut microbiome 19, 30
and hedonic hunger 74–5, 79
lack of nutrients 180
meats 205
and obesity 116, 124
percentage of calories gained
from 194
and satiety bypass 65, 183, 247
swaps 224–5
urinary tract infections (UTIs) 197

vaginal delivery 23, 32, 116–17
vaginal microbiome 23, 32, 116–17,
197
Van Tulleken, Chris 74–5, 158,
180–1, 183, 195, 224
vegan diet 196, 205, 206
vegetarian diet 205, 206
vinaigrette, basil 238, 245
vinegar 168–70
vitamin C 16, 20
vitamin D 182, 207
vitamin E 15–16

waist circumference 100
water retention 154–5
weighing yourself 100, 153
weight
determinants of 20
healthy 126
inherited 106–27
and long-term dieting 81
set-point theory of 62
stable 83
stopping thinking about 152–4
see also obesity; overweight
weight gain 1, 2, 4, 58, 92, 154–5,
155
and appetite 26, 58
and artificial sweeteners 78
and cortisol 54–6
and dieting 136
and the gut microbiome 20–1,
23–5
mechanisms of 43–57
pregnancy 124
rapid 6–7
and steroids 251
and stress 251–2, 291
unique nature of 43
weight loss 155
and breastfeeding 123
and calorie reduction 44–5
and cortisol levels 55
and fasting 104, 164
and the gut microbiome 18–19,
22, 24, 45–6
and leptin 112–13
and low-carb diets 133